Illustrated Atlas of Esthetic Mesotherapy

Active Substances | Dosage | Administration

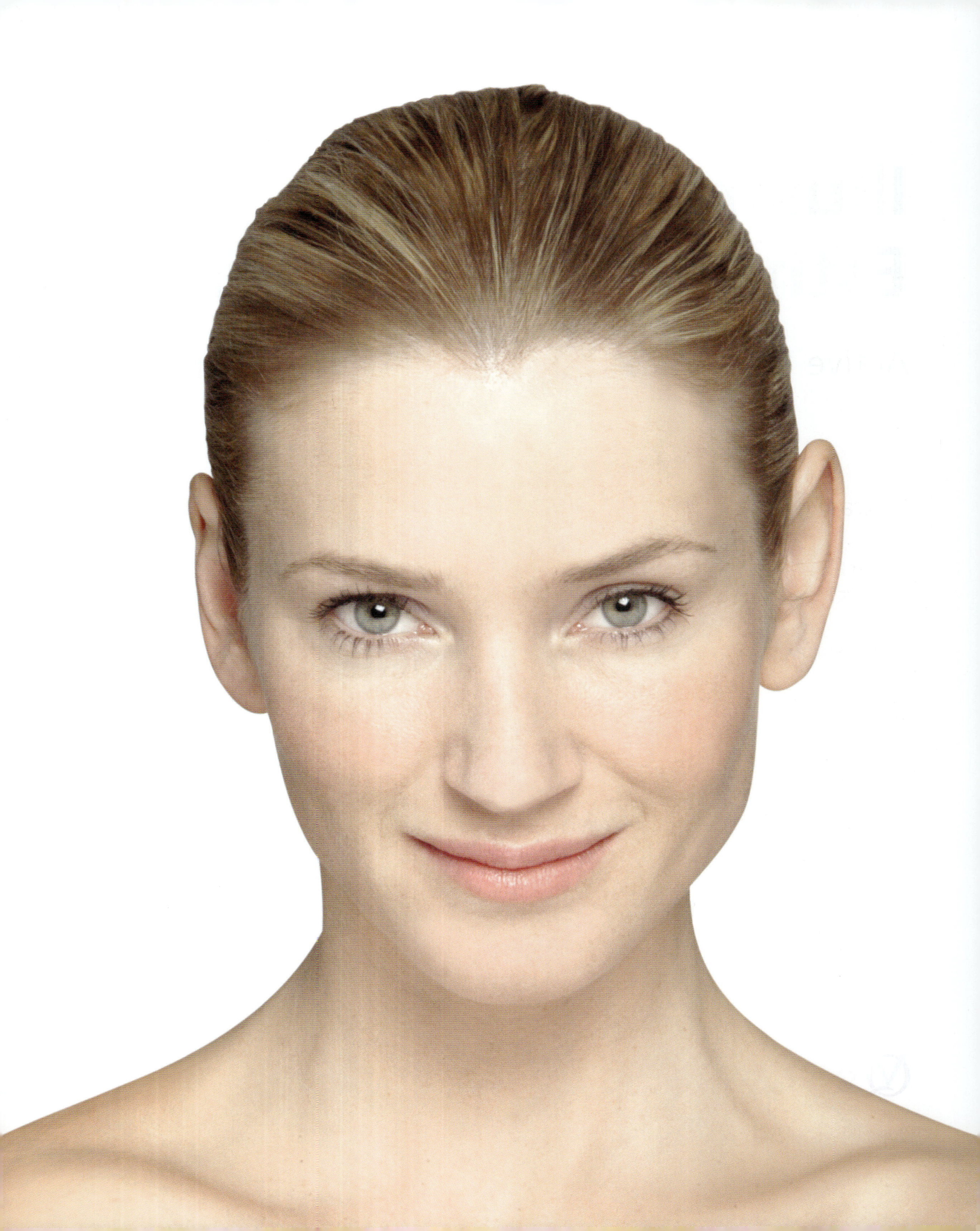

Illustrated Atlas of Esthetic Mesotherapy

Active Substances | Dosage | Administration

Britta Knoll

Edited by
Gerhard Sattler

With 165 figures

QUINTESSENCE PUBLISHING

London, Berlin, Chicago, Tokyo, Barcelona, Beijing, Istanbul, Milan,
Moscow, New Delhi, Paris, Prague, São Paulo, Seoul, Singapore and Warsaw

Abbreviations and symbols

The following abbreviations and symbols are used in this book:

ACH	Acetylcholine
AOC	Arterial occlusive disease
Botox	Botulinum toxin
BMI	Body Mass Index
CE	Conformité Européenne (in accordance with EU Guidelines)
cm	Centimeter
DC	Deoxycholate
DHE	Dihydroergotamine
DHT	Dihydrotestosterone
F	France
HA	Hyaluronic acid
IU	International Unit
LA	Local anesthetic
ml	Milliliter
meso	μέσος = central, middle
mm	Millimeter
PPC	Phosphatidylcholine
POM	Prescription-only medicine
ROS	Reactive oxygen species
™	Trademark
®	Registered brand name
↑	Increase
↓	Decrease
→	Direction of movement
.....	Epidermal injection technique, linear nappage (pulse/salvo mode)
***	One-by-one injections
o	Infiltration

Important note

Like every other science, medicine is subject to constant development. Research and clinical experience widen our knowledge base, particularly with regard to medicines and other forms of treatment. If any active substances, dosages or specific methods of administration are mentioned in this book, the reader may have confidence that the authors, editors and publisher have taken great care to ensure that this information is in line with the latest knowledge available at the time of publication. However, the publisher cannot give guarantees for any information regarding dosages, mixtures and methods of administration. *The use of any dose or method of administration takes place at the user's own risk.* All users must ensure that they attend a training course in the practical application of mesotherapy, and take great care to check the manufacturer's information of the products used, including the doses and contraindications given therein. The author and publisher appeal to all users to inform the publisher if they spot any obvious inaccuracies. This sort of check is particularly important with rarely used products or those which have been recently launched and have not yet been granted a CE certificate or a marketing authorization.

Editor's Foreword

Mesotherapy is a highly versatile, user-friendly method. This Atlas describes the techniques of mesotherapy in esthetic medicine. While many of our colleagues have heard of mesotherapy, they are not always quite clear as to what exactly mesotherapy is. Is it *minimally invasive lipolysis,* often referred to as the *fat-away injection* by the yellow press? Or does it have something to do with homeopathy or acupuncture? All the possible (mis)interpretations are explained here. Furthermore, this Atlas is the first German publication that I know of in this area. I am very happy to have been able to bring on board my colleague Dr. Britta Knoll as its highly qualified author. She has been involved in mesotherapy for more than 25 years, having acquired her knowledge at first hand from the method's founder, Michel Pistor, in France. And if anyone has been linked with introducing mesotherapy to Germany, it must be Dr. Knoll. For many years, she has been giving lectures and courses to promote mesotherapy in Germany. She is also President of the German Mesotherapy Association and Vice-President of the International Mesotherapy Society. Taken together, there were all excellent reasons for offering her the authorship within this series.
Sadly, these are as yet few scientific studies of the effect of mesotherapy. However, very positive patient reactions have vastly heightened its popularity, leading to a progressive rise in demand for this type of treatment. It is my view, therefore, that physicians can confidently include mesotherapy in their individual treatment portfolios and offer it when required. Mesotherapy is minimally invasive and the training input involved in learning it is highly justifiable. Therefore, I hope that this work, with its practical focus, will help the reader to learn the basics of the method and to use it when required.
I wish all my colleagues great treatment successes and many happy patients.

Darmstadt, May 2010
Gerhard Sattler

Table of contents

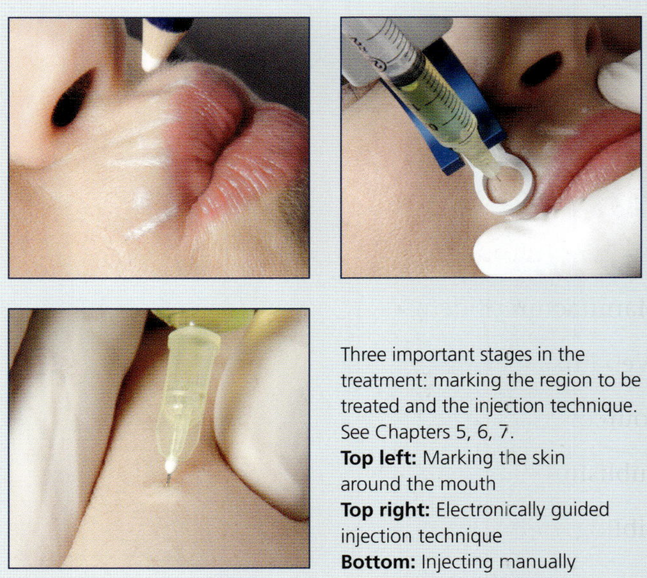

Three important stages in the treatment: marking the region to be treated and the injection technique. See Chapters 5, 6, 7.
Top left: Marking the skin around the mouth
Top right: Electronically guided injection technique
Bottom: Injecting manually

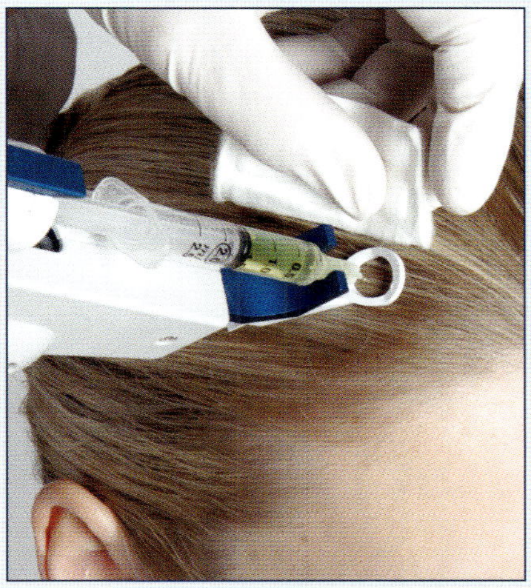

The revitalization cocktail injected into the scalp in MesoHair leads to stimulation and regeneration of the hair roots. See Chapter 9.2.

Introduction

As a young doctor, when I was introduced to Michel Pistor and his mesotherapy in Paris, I never suspected that this would result in my lifelong involvement in this novel treatment. At the time, I probably had an intuitive realization of the potential of this simple but ingenious method, which involves the targeted administration of known medical active substances into the skin of the affected area in the form of microinjections, according to the motto of "little – infrequently – in the right place". Now, twenty-five years on, both my experiences in everyday practice, and my involvement in research, training and exchanges with colleagues have confirmed this potential.

Fifty years ago, the country doctor Michel Pistor had already identified a variety of mesotherapy indications – and designed the appropriate treatment protocols – not only in general medicine and the treatment of pain, but also cross-disciplinary indications in dermatology, dentistry and geriatric medicine, i.e. what would be known as anti-aging treatment today. In his early books, he already gives indications of the method's potential uses in esthetic medicine, calls the skin rejuvenation method "Mesolift", and describes the treatment of hair loss and cellulite. Since then, esthetic mesotherapy has carved out a permanent niche for itself in the beauty market in many countries, alongside plastic surgery and established dermatological methods. For more than ten years, the German Mesotherapy Association has offered a structured mesotherapy training program, which is open to all interested medical practitioners.

Any therapist who takes the trouble (and there is not a lot of trouble involved) to learn the theory and practice of mesotherapy correctly, will be able to chalk up successes quickly and without a lot of costly investment, in an area which can assure our survival and quality of life in today's tough times: private-payer medicine. Our achievement-oriented society has created a frantic need for everlasting health and attractiveness. Thus, as the population's life expectancy continues to increase, so does its need to support and maintain the body's physical functions and an appearance appropriate to a youthful attitude to life. In only 20 years' time, every third citizen will be more than 60 years old, and many will attempt to meet their increased needs and demands through the second healthcare market of private medicine. While the demand for natural and environmentally friendly treatment methods generally takes first place on this wish list, requirements that follow closely include effectiveness, a long-term result and safety. Mesotherapy can offer all of these. Last but not least, there is a brisk demand for it among the general public, as it is not only versatile and effective, but also relatively reasonably priced. These "beauty-shots" enhance attractiveness, usually without any down-time, and can be tailored perfectly to individual circumstances.

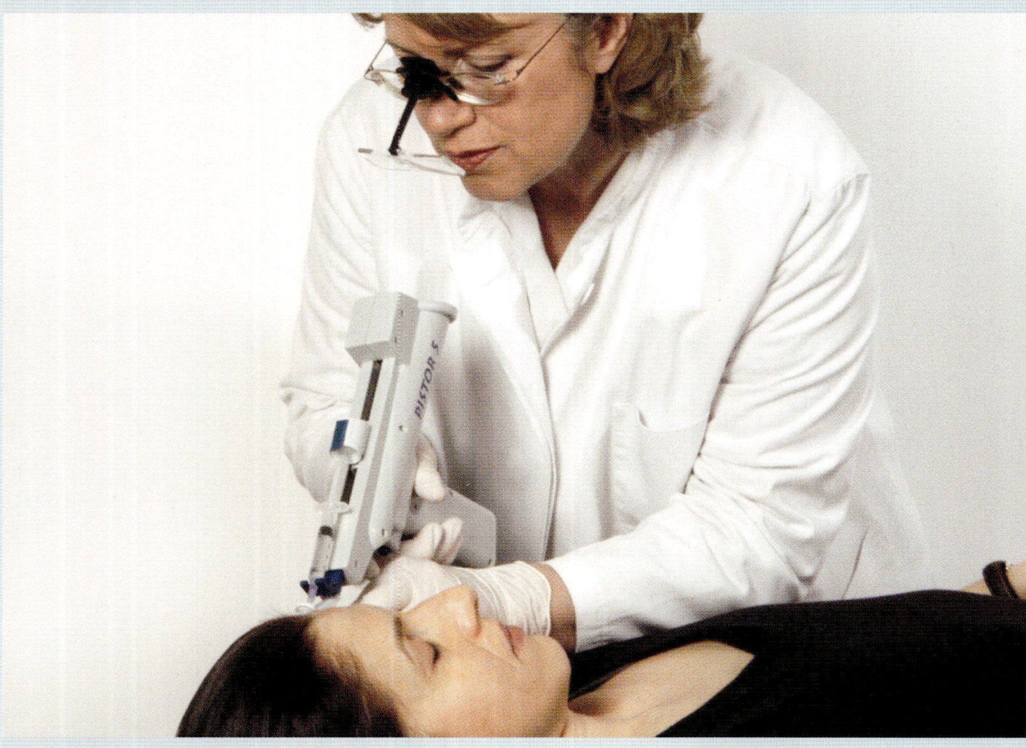

A calm and relaxed atmosphere is as important for the patient as a pleasant environment. The therapist will often need loupe glasses.

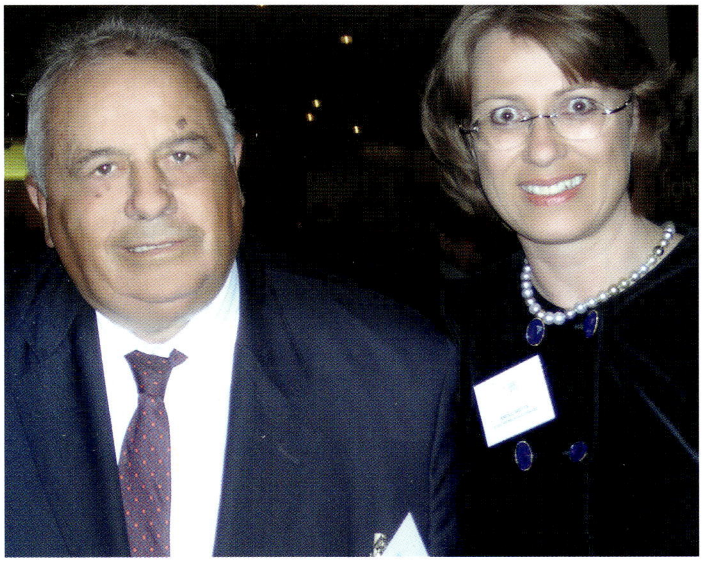

Michel Pistor and Britta Knoll at the International Mesotherapy Conference in 2003

I would like to thank all those who have helped this book come into being: my husband Wilfried, who takes on so many of my organizational burdens, my big daughter Isabelle, whose independence gave me the time I needed for this project, my assistant Yvonne, who has been my ever-reliable support at the practice for 20 years, as well as Mr. Sattler, Mr. Kolster and the many other colleagues who support mesotherapy and have carried out true pioneering work in this area.

The future of esthetic medicine

Key guidelines for future success and survival on a global market involve the following points:

- Relevance of the services on offer
- Quality and efficacy of the service
- Plausibility of the service provider
- Evidence of lasting effect and safety

What is needed here are holistic solutions, tailored closely to the requirements of the target group in question. Aspects of cost-benefit and risk-benefit ratios are becoming increasingly prominent. In esthetic medicine and anti-aging treatment, the key factors are trustworthy concepts of holistic and long-lasting prevention and treatment of individually perceived defects in appearance and well-being. In times when the idea of wellness is on the upsurge, and there is a bewildering range of cosmetic methods and products on offer, it is natural that much greater demands are placed on the effectiveness of therapeutic interventions in medicine, when compared with the paramedical field. The American "pay for performance" principle applies.

Process optimization
In this context, this means doing what it necessary and leaving out what is not, i.e. developing and following an individual, long-term treatment strategy for the patient.

Cost optimization
This means reaching the best possible result at the lowest possible cost. Thus, for example, luxury cosmetics and care products, as well as many lifestyle medicines, can be replaced by a medical treatment from which patients derive a great deal more benefit.

Esthetic mesotherapy
As a stand-alone branch of treatment, this has in recent years seen many modifications of the classical, orthodox medical mesotherapy as developed by the French physician Dr. Michel Pistor. These modifications were necessary for this specialized area of treatment, and have since become more widespread and established worldwide. The boundaries of Pistor's original mesotherapy, according to the guiding principle of

Little – Infrequently – In the right place

have been extended, that is:

Little
Appreciable quantities of active substances may be administered in some cases. The volumes of the drug mixtures used range between a few tenths of a ml (Mesobotox) to 100 ml in lipolysis. However, the true increase has been slight, due to the use of extremely low-dose dilutions, extending the action spectrum at the molecular pharmacology level.

Infrequently
The treatment intervals vary from one to six weeks during the initial treatment, generally followed by a maintenance phase of monthly, quarterly or even annual booster doses. Depending on the baseline situation, repeated sessions are usually necessary to begin with, in order to achieve the desired effect (additive effects).

In the right place
If the skin is defined as the target organ of classical curative mesotherapy, in esthetics this also includes the subcutaneous adipose connective tissue.

Example

Lipolysis or the treatment of sagging skin

Large public surveys have shown that 80% of Germans want gentle medicine focusing on natural remedies, while 70% would consent to an esthetic treatment that *does not draw blood*. With the concurrent increase in the average age of our population, this means a huge potential for conservative esthetic treatment methods. Prerequisites for the therapist are not only to acquire thorough knowledge of the theory of mesotherapy, but also to learn how to implement it in practice, preferably in the form of hands-on training. The medical consultant must know the potential of his or her methods and their alternatives, and must be able to explain them. *Before-and-after images* provide helpful and necessary evidence. However, a medical practice is not permitted to use these in public advertising. It is essential for standardized information to be provided to the patient and for all consultations and treatments to be documented.
Most important of all is to clearly define the treatment goals and to end up with a happy and satisfied patient. New findings – particularly in physics, whether they involve the subtle energetic properties of water, the atoms, molecules and active substances, the resonance of the extracellular matrix or the cybernetic regulatory systems of the human body – will have a decisive effect in determining the future of applied medicine. Direct effects on basic regulation, the functional interplay between the terminal vessels, the matrix and the cells provide the scientific basis for the efficacy of minimally invasive injection methods like mesotherapy.

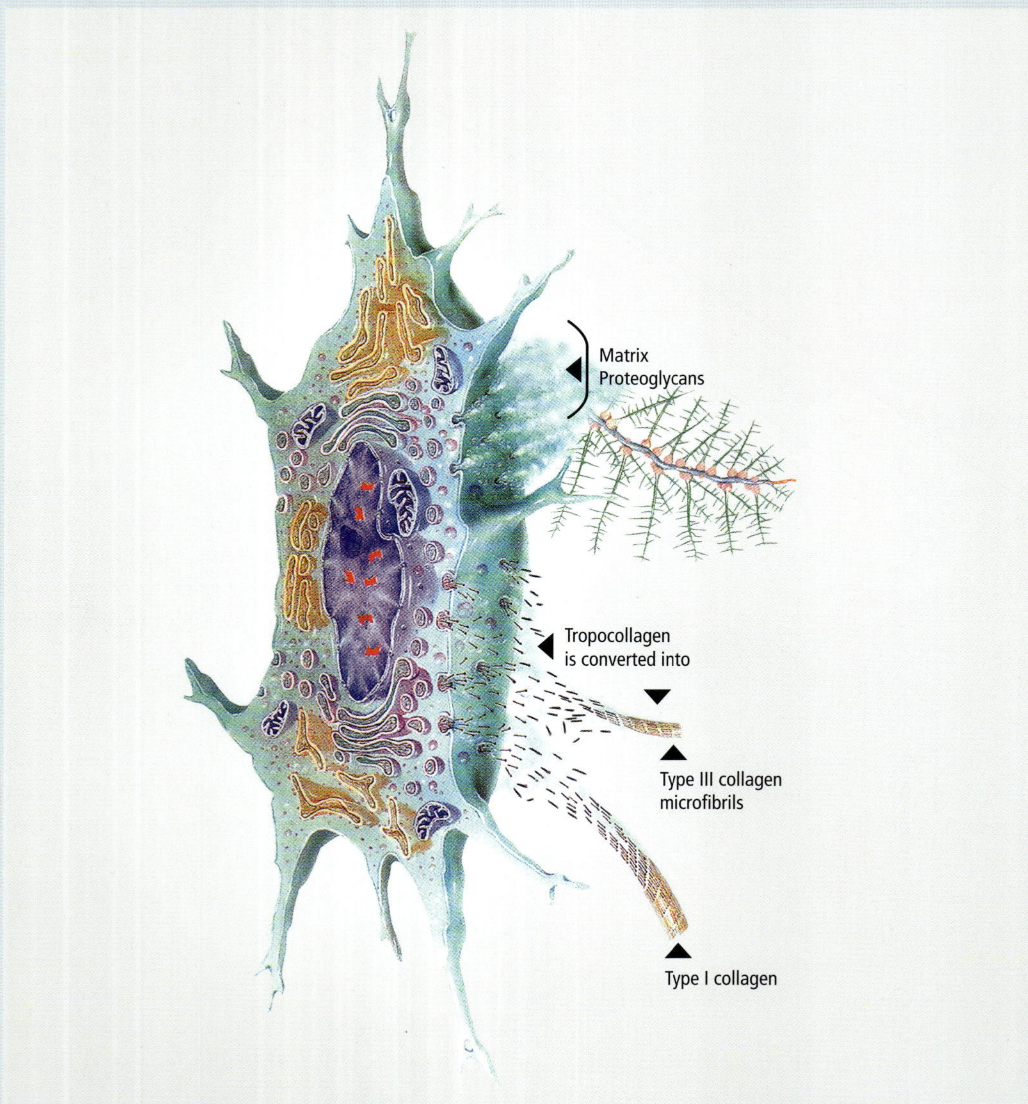

The fibroblasts of the connective tissue play an important role in the synthesis of the intercullular substance (extracellular matrix). They produce collagen and proteoglycans, which give the skin greater strength and stability. The microinjections given in mesotherapy stimulate the proliferation of the fibroblasts and increase the secretion of cytokines.

1 Definition of mesotherapy

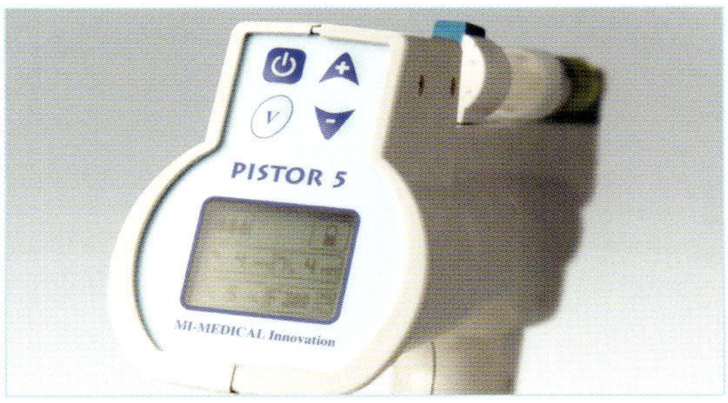

The use of a defined injection technique …

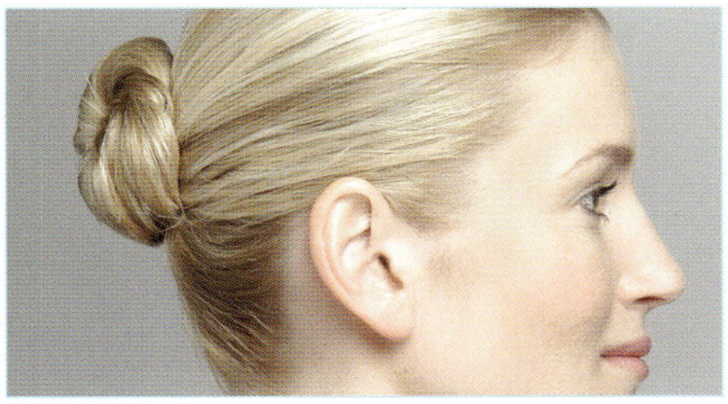

… means that mesotherapy can be used for the face and hair…

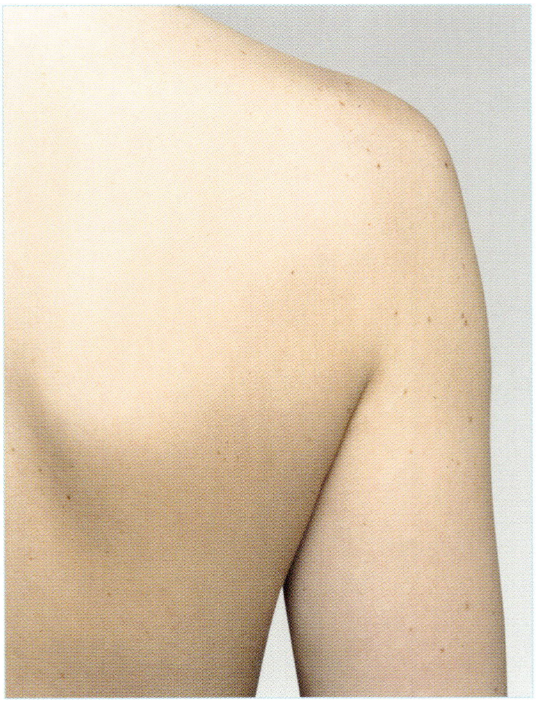

… and for local problem areas.

1

Definition of mesotherapy

meso = μέσος= central, middle

Mesotherapy is a minimally invasive injection technique, which is used to administer active substances directly into the area of skin on which they are intended to act, thus allowing a low dose to be given with no significant systemic side-effects. It is a method of conservative medicine. The Greek word meso means *between, middle* and refers to the embryonic mesodermal origin of the skin and connective tissue. When associated with mesotherapy, it stands for the skin and subcutaneous region, into which individually selected and adapted active substances are administered. Mesotherapy thus combines elements of orthodox medicine (pharmacology, medicinal products) with natural cures (physical stimuli, salutogenesis, orthomolecular, herbal and homeopathic active substances). Its target organ, the skin, enables targeted local treatment with a specific depot effect. The various injection techniques allow not only the rate of delivery of the active substances to be controlled, but also the length of time they remain in the tissue. While these active substances can also reach deeper regions by diffusion, they do not generally get into the systemic circulation, as the connective tissue and its matrix already ensure that these agents are metabolized. Since gastrointestinal absorption problems do not apply and there is no loss of the active substance as a result of enterohepatic passage, the active substances can and must be used at considerably reduced doses (low-dose treatment).

Medical and therapeutic acceptance

Mesotherapy was developed in 1952 by the French physician Dr. Michel Pistor, since when it has spread worldwide. Furthermore, since 2003, training in this discipline has become an established university subject in France, in the form of a one-year postgraduate course. In that country, mesotherapy has been approved by the statutory health insurance agencies as a treatment for pain, so that the therapy costs are covered.

In many other countries, however, mesotherapy has found a place mainly in the area of medical esthetics. In Germany, it may only be used by doctors and therapists who have a certificate to practice medicine. The German Association for Mesotherapy (*Deutsche Gesellschaft für Mesotherapie, DGM)* was founded in Germany as early as 1983, as an independent, non-profit organization. It provides qualified training and certification, protects the interests of its members and also provides up-do-date information to the public about this innovative treatment method.

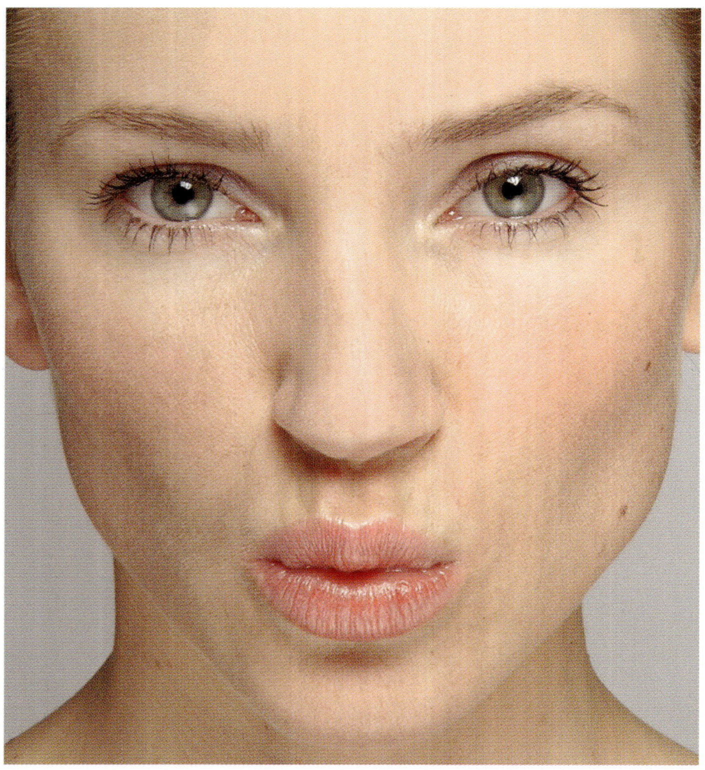

Mesotherapy is administered directly into the area to be treated by means of multiple microinjections.

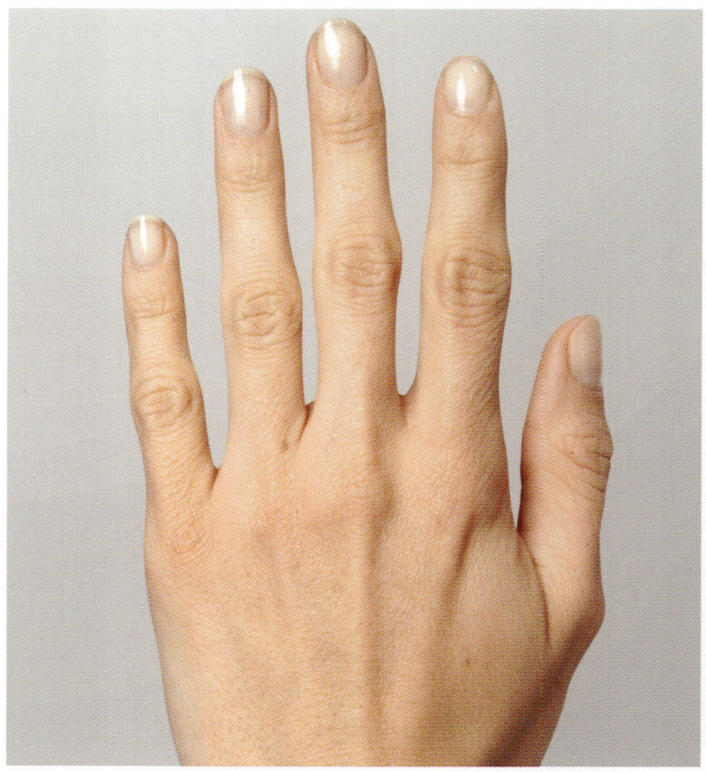

The gentle epidermal technique allows sensitive areas such as the hand or mouth region to be treated painlessly.

2 The active substances

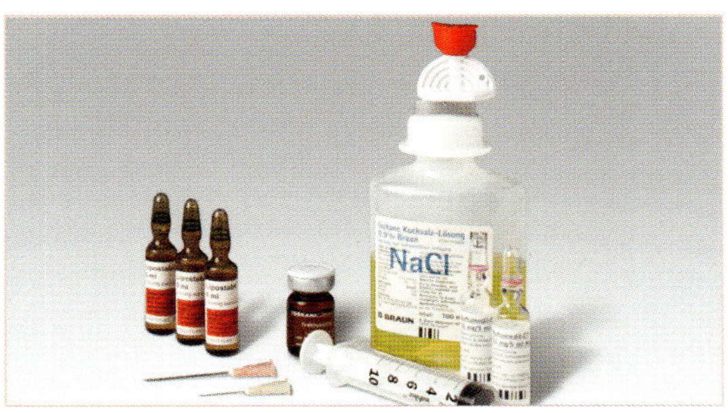

Active substances are mixed and diluted in mesotherapy and lipolysis.

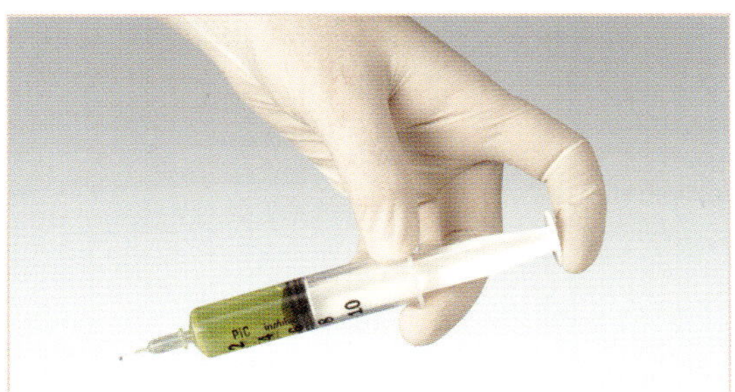

The cocktail is adjusted to individual requirements and accurately administered to the target area.

2

The active substances

These days, an individual's general appearance can be optimized without appearing artificial, by combining a variety of individually selected active substances and injecting them locally. European esthetic perception demands a relaxed, naturally youthful radiance. We like to receive compliments, but we do not want people to suspect us of having "work" done. Consequently, there is every reason for a gradual, long-term strategy, where it is preferable to start with a milder mixture, and then, if required, to follow it up with stronger active substances or concentrations later on in the treatment.

Note
Many years of positive experience and also some study results are available for many of the procedures, such as Mesolift, lipolysis or MesoHair. The choice of materials in this book, be it instruments or injectable agents, does not claim to be comprehensive. The treatment protocols are individually devised; ideally, they address not only the objective pathophysiology of each case, but also the wishes of the patients themselves.

2.1 Individual active substances in esthetic mesotherapy

2.1.1 Active substances in Mesolift

If the desired skin rejuvenation effect is to be achieved, we need the correct choice and combination of active substances matching the pathophysiology of each case. Knowledge of the pharmacological properties of many of the potential individual agents is therefore an essential prerequisite.

Description of selected active substances

Monomethyl trisilanol salicylate
(E.g. Conjonctyl® in F, Silicor Toskani)

Organic silicon is found here in a polymeric structure of silicic acid salts. Silicon is the most important natural semi-conductor; in the body's tissues, it acts as a nanospacer and catalyst in a variety of reactions. Uses include stimulation of collagen synthesis (not in salicylate allergy), tightening and regeneration of the skin, as a possible replacement for procaine and as a universal adjuvant for the improvement of connective tissue structures. It is also available linked to DMAE for skin tightening and firming (DM-silk), improving the latter's local tolerability.

Sodium pyruvate
(E.g. in Cocktail anti-aging Toskani)

This α-keto-derivative of lactic acid encourages amino acid and dermal collagen synthesis. It is an antioxidant (ROS destruction) and stimulates cell metabolism.
Uses: Particularly for sun-damaged skin, smoker's skin DMAE for skin tightening and firming (DM-silk), improving the latter's local tolerability.

Overview – active substances in Mesolift	
Carrier solutions	PROCAINE 1–2 % or lidocaine 1–2 %, NaCl 0.9% Conjonctyl® (monomethyl trisilanol salicylate)
Biostimulants	Non-cross-linked hyaluronic acid, Na-DNA Collagen, elastin, retinol, glycolic acid
Stem cell activators of plant origin	Proliferation of epidermal stem cells ↑, growth factors (IGF-1, bFGF, VEFG, TGF-β1)
Herbal remedies	Ginkgo biloba, Centella asiatica
Vitamins	A, B, C, E, dexpanthenol
Building blocks for protein synthesis	Amino acids for collagen and elastin production ↑, e.g. taurine Ubiquinone (coenzyme Q 10), glutathione, pyruvate
Regulation of muscle tone	Muscle tone ↓ (relaxation): botulinum toxin (POM), argireline Muscle tone ↑ (stretching): DMAE (anti-sagging)

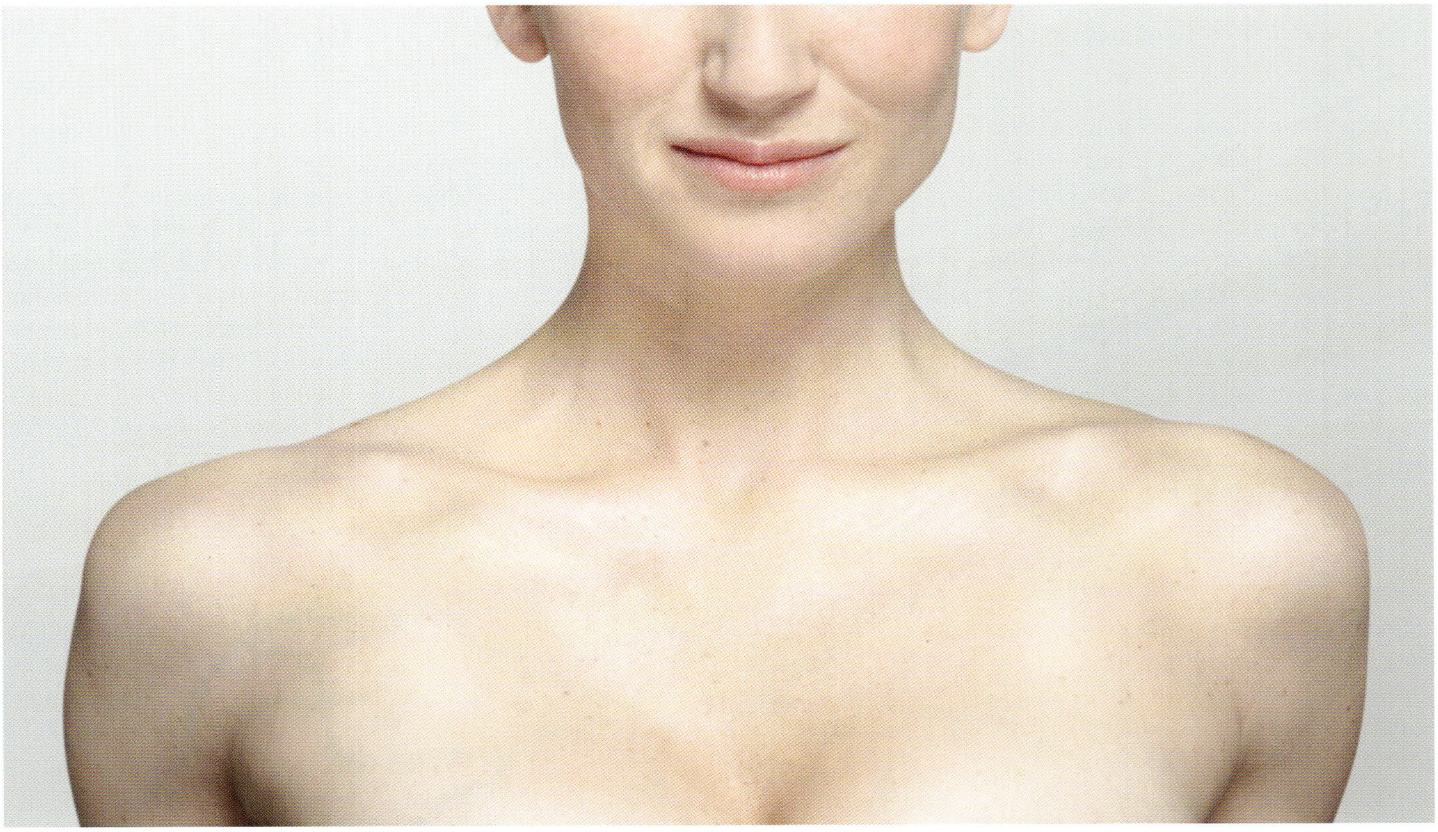

Mesolift is most frequently used on the face, neck and cleavage/neckline area.

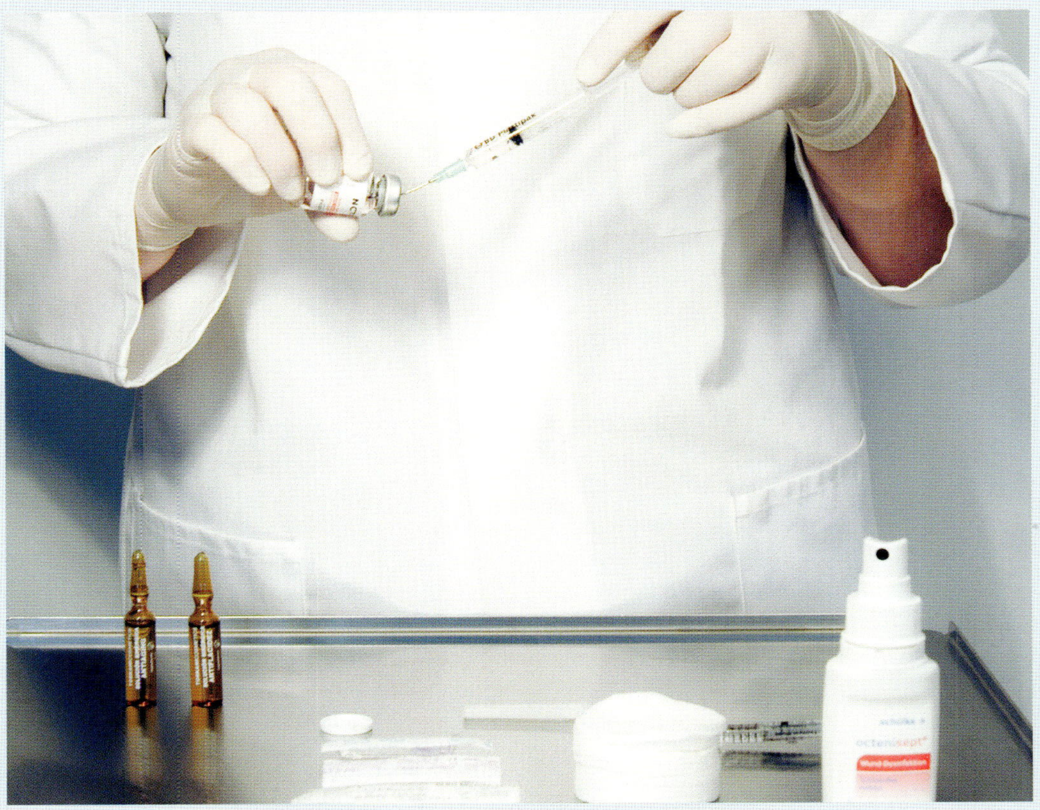

Once the individual components of the treatment have been selected, they are mixed in the correct way immediately before use on the patient.

2

Non-cross-linked hyaluronic acid
(E.g. Teosyal Meso, Redensity I, TKN HA MW 2%)

The glucosaminoglycan polysaccharide HA, also known simply as Hyaluron, is a universal and essential component of skin and connective tissue, possesses a high water-binding capacity and improves the viscoelastic properties of the dermis and epidermis. It counteracts skin thinning (by c. 6% every 10 years) and age-related skin atrophy. Produced in the fibroblasts, it has a significant role in the proliferation, migration and differentiation of the keratinocytes. Only HA produced by biotechnological methods, rather than the substance of animal origin, may be used in esthetics. There are many products on the market, but they differ with respect to quality, purity and HA concentration.
Uses: Universal. The nature-identical gel is an essential component of the Mesolift cocktail. It is water-soluble and can be homogenized. In non-cross-linked form, its long-term effect sets in only on epidermal or superficial intradermal administration; following deep injection, it is rapidly transported away from the skin and metabolized. Its half-life in perfused tissue is only 15 days.

Vitamin C
(Ascorbic acid 200 mg/ml)

Stimulates collagen synthesis, promotes wound healing and skin regeneration, protects from light, regulates melanogenesis.
Uses: Prevention of sun aging, Mesoglow, melasma.

Vitamin B5
(Pantothenic acid, dexpanthenol)

Involved in the acetylation of proteins and peptides, promotes glutathione synthesis, is essential for the hair roots and skin (nutrition, moisture binding), protects from oxidative stress and UV-radiation, has an antiviral and anti-inflammatory effect. Fibroblast proliferation ↑. Activates wound healing genes.
Uses: Stretch marks (striae), melasma.

L-glutathionen
(E.g. Glutamax Toskani)

Tripeptide, antioxidant, involved in the detoxification of free radicals and peroxides, causes depigmentation through tyrosinase block, reduces melanin formation.
Uses: Melasma, anti-aging, prevention and treatment of age spots.

Glycolic acid
(E.g. Glycomax 1% Toskani)

This alpha-hydroxy acid, obtained from sugar cane, is a well-known peeling agent, but can also be added to the Mesolift cocktail. It enables the effective treatment of acne or shallow acne scars, blemished and large-pored skin, age-related pigment spots and lines, as well as dull, lifeless and coarse skin. It causes superficial, fine reddening of the skin with subsequent peeling, dissolving and removing the layers of skin cells lying on the surface. After the treatment, the skin's sensitivity to light is heightened. Serious side-effects or risks have not been observed when the substance is used correctly.

Taurine
(E.g. Tauricol Toskani)

2-aminoethane-sulfonic acid is a semi-essential amino acid containing sulfur. It has an antioxidant, anti-inflammatory effect and vasoprotective effect. Stimulates keratinocytes, collagen synthesis and the storage of moisture in the skin.
Uses: Anti-aging, smoker's skin, skin regeneration, energy carrier.

DMAE
(E.g. in DM-Silk Toskani, Cocktail skin tightening Toskani)

Dimethylaminoethanol is a specific substance with a lifting effect on the face and body (anti-sagging). It increases skin muscle tone due to increased acetylcholine secretion and counteracts skin ptosis. Potential side-effects: toxic dermatitis and fibroblast damage at excessive concentrations. Its tolerability is considerably better when used in the form of DM-Silk (complex containing organic silicon).
Uses: Mesolift, skin tightening, stretch marks.

Polidocanol
(POM) (Aethoxysklerol®)

Its sclerosing effect may also be used for extravascular applications (*Note:* this is an off-label use), connective tissue firming, potent skin tightening, treatment of fresh stretch marks; concentration and dose depend on the depth of injection and the target structure. Potential side-effects: inflammation or even necrosis at excessive concentrations.
Uses: Tightening and firming of the skin, stretch marks, microsclerotherapy with DHE (dihydroergotamine, F), e.g. treatment of spider burst veins, couperose, small hemangiomas.

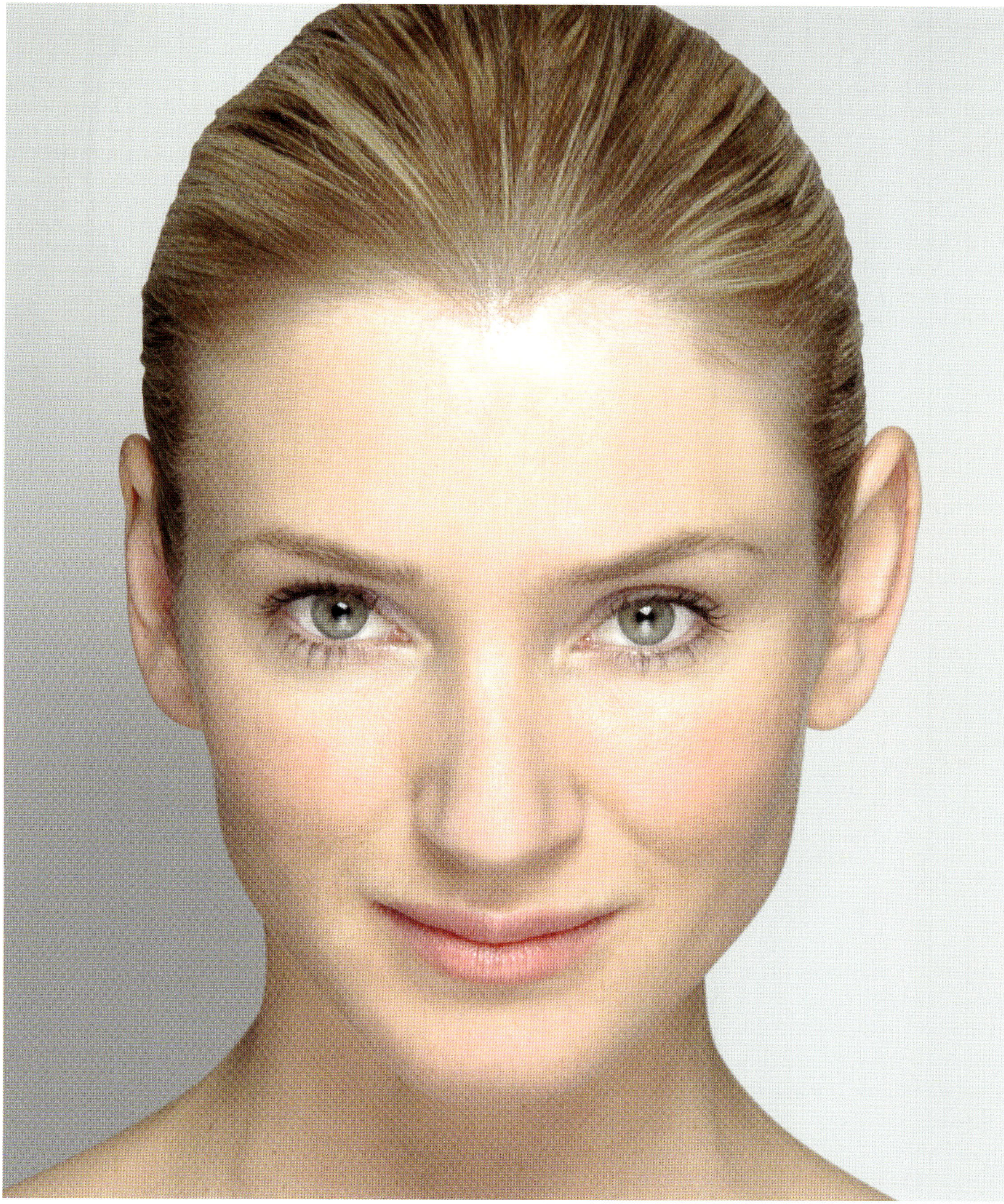

Inspection and assessment of the anatomy of the face and of the individual structure of the skin and connective tissue allow the therapist to select the correct active substance combination for mesotherapy, or a combination of methods for a more complex "face composition".

Argireline®
(E.g. in Cocktail antiaging Toskani)

A synthetic hexapeptide, its effect (though weaker) resembles that of Botulinum toxin, causes relaxation by reducing muscular acetylcholine secretion, skin muscle contraction is reduced, thus preventing the development of facial expression lines.

Centella asiatica
(E.g. in Cocktail antistriae Toskani)

A pentacyclic triterpene, anti-inflammatory, antioxidant, antisclerotic. Promotes skin elasticity and the formation of glucosaminoglycans (GAGs).
Uses: Skin regeneration, stretch marks, early keloids, acne, scars.

Vitamins and minerals
(Various)

Whereas the multivitamins, as antioxidants, primarily prevent and repair sun damage to skin, micro-dosed minerals act as co-factors of the cell enzymes to ensure a smoothly running cell metabolism. The body's own repair enzymes are supported by large-molecule antioxidants, e.g. superoxide dismutase, and by small-molecule antioxidants such as the lipophilic substances tocopherol or ubiquinone, and the hydrophilic agents ascorbate or glutathione. Antioxidants work together in networks, scavenging free radicals. Cell damage occurs when there is an imbalance between reactive oxygen species and repair enzymes or antioxidants. Micronutrients, particularly when applied locally, are effective in regenerating cell functions, and thus improving skin quality.
Uses: Universal, contained in most mesotherapy revitalization cocktails.

Amino acids, nucleic acids
(e.g. NCTF 135, Cocktail antiaging plus Mesolift Toskani)

NCTF contains, among other things, 24 water-soluble and stabilized amino acids. Building blocks for the structural proteins of the skin's matrix strengthen the specific synthesis function of skin cells. A reduction in the number of fibroblasts and keratinocytes, together with weakening of the interstitial links between skin layers, are the histological signs of aging skin. When combined with nucleic acids (DNA and RNA), a complex revitalization cocktail has been demonstrated to increase in-vitro fibroblast activity significantly and for a prolonged period

2.1.2 Active substances in MesoHair

Description of selected active substances

Procaine
(E.g. von Loges, Steigerwald, Lophacomp®)

Local anesthetic, universally used in mesotherapy. Also available specifically for intradermal use at a concentration of 0.5%, e.g. from Deltaselect. Should only be used with added adrenaline if vasoconstriction is desired, e.g. in special local anesthetic procedures. The only contraindications are severe cardiac arrhythmias, myasthenia gravis or the rare procaine allergy. Its local effects are many and varied:

- anesthetic
- analgesic
- membrane-stabilizing
- stimulates circulation
- neurovegetative stabilizer
- cell metabolism stabilizer
- anti-inflammatory
- anti-allergic.

Overview – active substances in Meso-Hair	
Carrier solutions	Procaine 0.5, 1, 2 % or lidocaine 0.5, 1, 2 %, NaCl 0.9 %
Vasoactive substances	Buflomedil (POM), pentoxifylline (POM), caffeine
Biostimulants, non-cross-linked	Non-cross-linked hyaluronic acid, Na-DNA
Stem cell activators of plant origin	Proliferation of local stem cells, growth factors (IGF-1, bFGF, VEFG, TGF-β1)
Vitamins	A, B, C, E, biotin, dexpanthenol
Herbal remedies	Ginkgo biloba, Centella asiatica, Silicea complex
Building blocks for protein synthesis	Amino acids for hair production↑, e.g. taurine, cystine Ubiquinone (coenzyme Q 10)

Caution: Larger containers (50 ml bottles) always contain a *preservative,* usually benzyl alcohol. For this reason, patients with severe allergies will either need to be treated with small ampoules (2 or 5 ml) or will require lidocaine. The latter is also available as *Lidocaine sine* (without preservatives). Local anesthetics are a popular choice as additives to mesotherapy mixtures, as this makes the injections considerably less painful.

Stem cell activators, growth factors
(E.g. in Cocktail FCE Toskani or from Toskani)

Stem cell activators of plant origin, human-identical growth factors and cytokines can now be manufactured using biotech methods. These "cosmeceuticals" are also available in lyophilized form for mesotherapy. However, there is as yet no consensus with respect to the products, the protocols or their effectiveness.
IGF-1 (insulin-like growth factor): Stimulation of the hair follicle, cell repair, HA biosynthesis
bFGF (basic fibroblast growth factor): For improvement of microcirculation and revitalization, increasing cell activity, biosynthesis of collagen and elastin
VEFG (vascular-endothelial growth factor): Neovascularization and improvement of micronutrition
TGF-β1 (transforming growth factor): Controls cell proliferation and cell differentiation.
Uses: Alopecia, Mesolift.

Biotin
(B-Hidroxin Toskani, in Cocktail Hair Toskani)

2

Vitamin H is a water-soluble vitamin of the B-complex. It plays a significant role in cell metabolism as a prosthetic group of enzymes, but is also of importance in the cell nucleus for the epigenetic regulation of gene functions. Has a trophic effect.
Uses: Hair loss, dry hair, seborrheic dermatitis.

Vitamin B5
(E.g. Dexanyl Toskani, in Cocktail Hair Toskani)

Pantothenic acid (or its analog dexpanthenol) is involved in the acetylation of proteins and peptides, promotes glutathione synthesis, is essential for the hair roots and skin (nutrition, moisture binding), protects from oxidative stress and UV radiation, has an antiviral and anti-inflammatory effect. Fibroblast proliferation . Activates wound healing genes.
Uses: Alopecia.

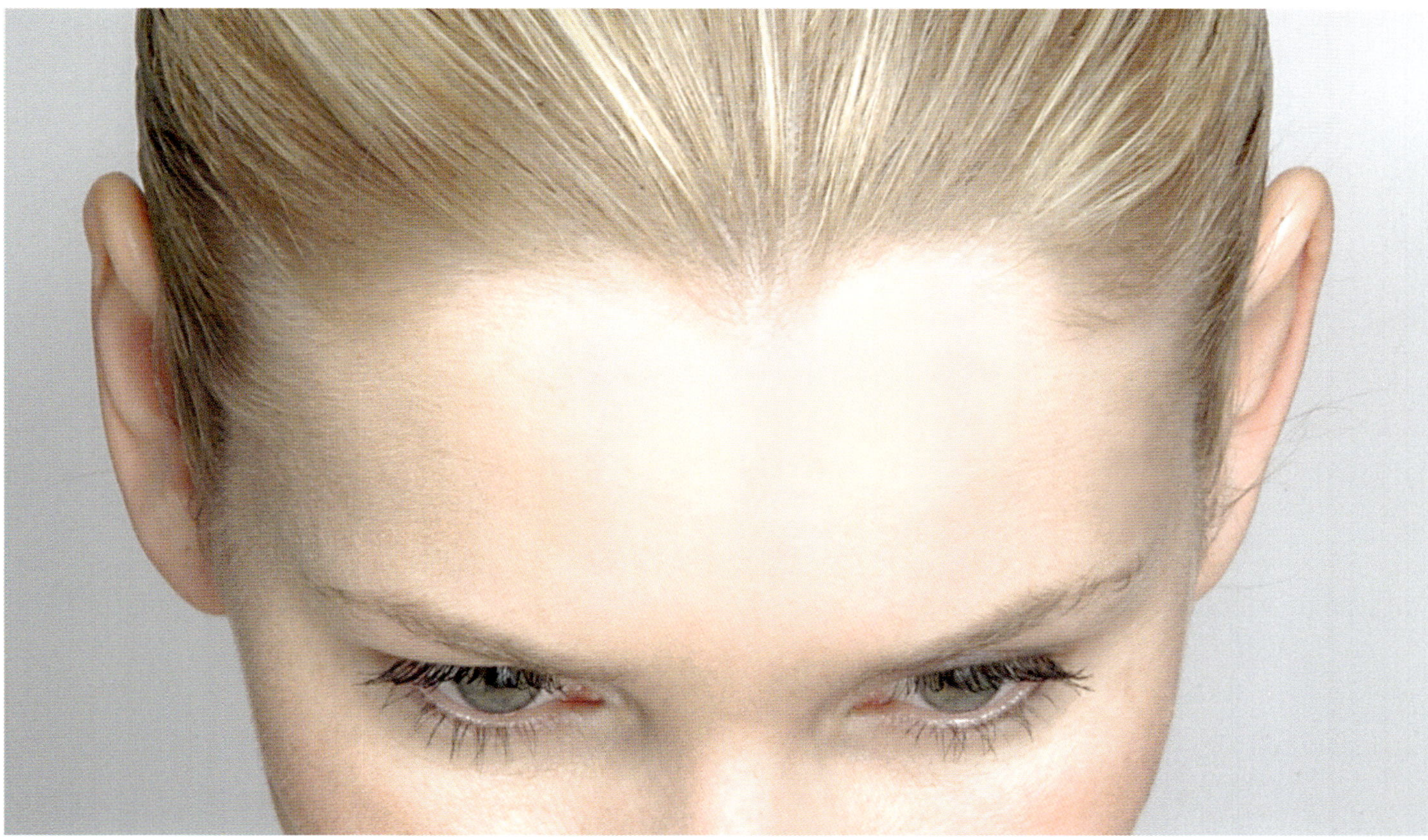

Hair loss in women usually affects the parietal region, but can also occur at the temples

Iron-gluconate
(E.g. in Cocktail Hair Toskani)

Iron-gluconate diminish the activity of 5α-reductase at the hair follicle and can thus counteract hair loss due to elevated local dihydrotestosterone (DHT) levels. They can be used not only in genetically predisposed men, but also in women. The effect is comparable to that of finasteride, but is free from side-effects.
Uses: Androgenic alopecia.

Taurine
(E.g. Tauricol Toskani)

2-aminoethane-sulfonic acid is a semi-essential amino acid containing sulfur. It has an antioxidant, anti-inflammatory and vasoprotective effect. Stimulates keratinocytes, collagen synthesis and the storage of moisture in the skin.
Uses: Anti-aging, alopecia, lipolysis.

Ubiquinone
(Coenzyme Q 10, e.g. in Ubichinon comp. Heel, Idebenyl Toskani, Cocktail FCE)

A natural protein, energy regenerator, universal mitochondrial enzyme catalyst and the most effective endogenous radical scavenger of the cell membranes. Since it is water-insoluble, it needs to be present in dispersed form.
Uses: Anti-aging, alopecia.

Argireline®
(E.g. in Cocktail antiaging Toskani, Myotec Toskani)

A synthetic hexapeptide, its effect (though weaker) resembles that of Botulinum toxin. Muscle contraction in the scalp is reduced, and the resultant relaxation promotes microcirculation and thus also hair growth.

2.1.3 Active substances used against cellulite

Description of selected active substances

Buflomedil
(POM)

A neurotropic vasodilator, it produces α-receptor blockade, thus opening the precapillary sphincters. It also has a papaverine-type (myotropic) effect and improves microcirculation.
Uses: In all cases where heating of the treated tissue is desired, e.g. cellulite, all hypotrophic tissues, all chronic disorders.

Dicynone®
(Ethamsylate, F)

A vasoactive, anti-edematous active substance, used particularly in Mesodrain treatment. The aim is to achieve decongestion and improved perfusion, particularly in the legs. Do not use in salicylate allergy.
Uses: Particularly in venolymphatic insufficiency, predisposition to edema, edematous cellulite.

Pentoxifylline
(POM)

A methylxanthine and peripheral vasodilator. Improves microcirculation. Has antioxidant and anti-inflammatory effects. Its main effect is to improve erythrocyte motility. Effects of interest when applied locally include its antifibrotic properties and induction of lipolysis through PDE3 inhibition. It also controls connective tissue water retention, which frequently occurs in localized estrogen overload.
Uses: Especially in the fibrous and edematous form of cellulite.

Overview – active substances in cellulite	
Carrier solutions	Procaine 1–2% or lidocaine 1–2%, NaCl 0.9% Conjonctyl® (monomethyl trisilanol salicylate) (F)
Vasoactive substances	Buflomedil (POM), Dicynone® (F) Xanthine derivatives: pentoxifylline (POM), theophylline (POM), aminophylline (POM), caffeine
Fat burn stimulation	Calcitonin (POM) in a hypo-osmolar solution = Mesodissolution® in France L-Carn® (L-carnitine) Lipostabil® (POM) phosphatidylcholine+deoxycholate
Vitamins	A, B, C, E, dexpanthenol
Herbal remedies	Ginkgo biloba Cynomax (artichoke extract) Asiacen (Centella asiatica, Fucus vesiculosus, Hedera helix) Rutinel (rutin, sweet clover extract)

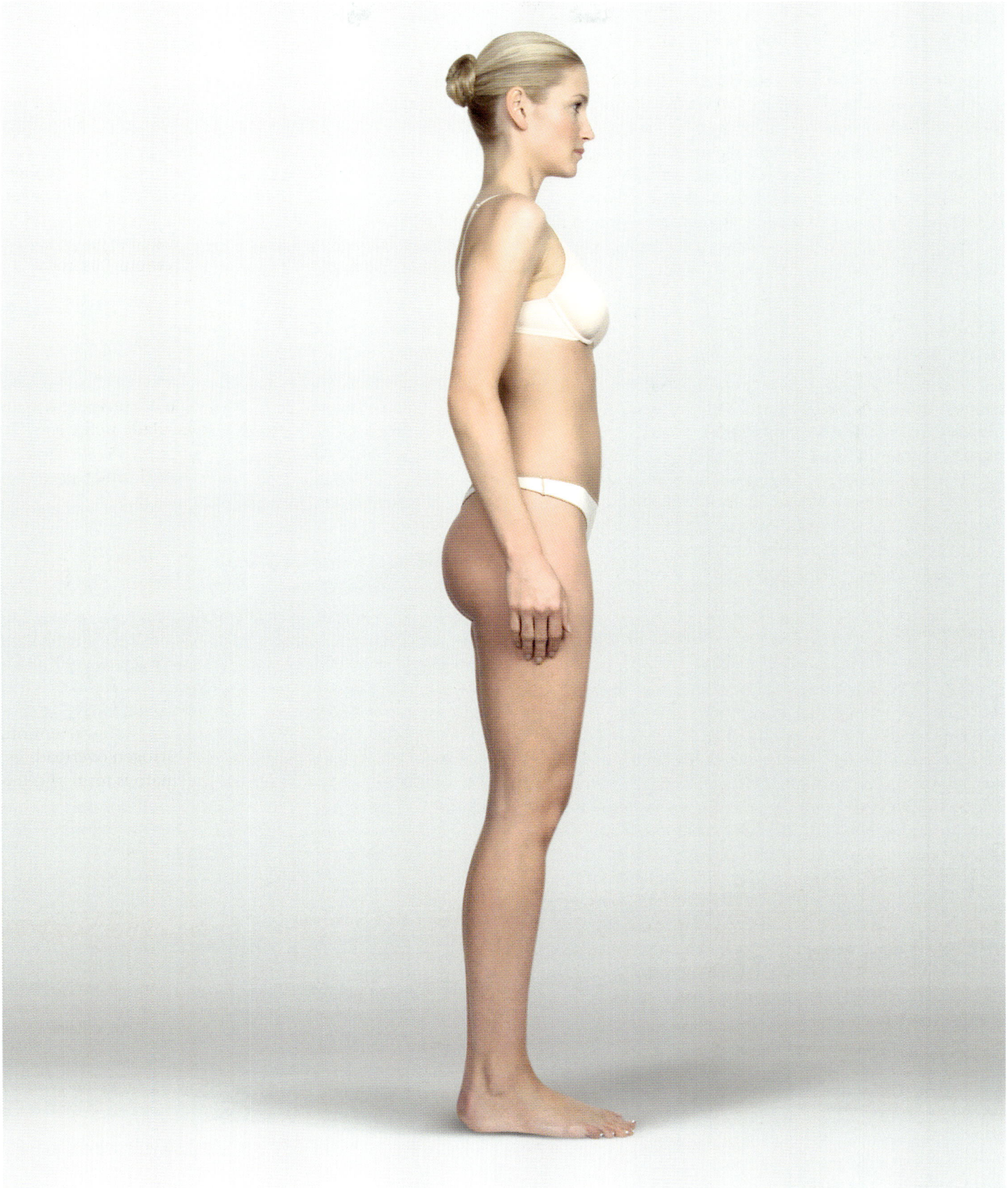

Inspection and assessment of the anatomy of the body and of the individual structure of the skin and connective tissue allow the therapist to select the correct active substance combination for mesotherapy, or a combination of methods for more complex "body-shaping".

Caffeine
(e.g. Cofinet Toskani, in Cocktail anticellulite Toskani)

A methylxanthine, its main effect is blockade of the adenosine receptors. It also inhibits specific phosphodiesterases which are responsible for the breakdown of cyclic to non-cyclic AMP. The inhibition of this breakdown results in an increased cAMP concentration in the cells. When applied topically, it increases fat breakdown in the adipocytes and stimulates the microcirculation, tissue drainage and diuresis. The surface of the skin becomes softer and smoother.
Uses: Cellulite, lipolysis, hair loss, Mesolift.

L-Carn®
(POM) (Carnitine)

L-Carnitine is a natural cell component and is a key contributor to energy generation in the mitochondria of the muscles. It specifically transports fatty acids through the mitochondrial membrane, where beta-oxidation, and thus fat burning, takes place. The more L-carnitine is present in the tissue, the more fat can be burned. When combined with physical activity and sports, this can contribute to weight loss and increased physical energy.
Uses: Cellulite, local fat deposits.

Lipostabil®
(POM) (PPC/DC)

Consists of phosphatidylcholine (PPC) and deoxycholate (DC). PPC is an essential phospholipid, a lecithin-like active substance which is obtained from the soy bean. It is ubiquitous in the cell membranes of higher forms of life. It has a lipotrophic effect and, by increasing the permeability of the adipocyte membrane, facilitates fat mobilization. Taurine is often added to the mixture as a solution stabilizer. As a bile acid, deoxycholate stabilizes the solution and contributes significantly to the fat-dissolving and skin-tightening effects of the preparation. Care is needed with the often severe local side-effects, which manifest in the form of reddening, swelling, pain and the formation of nodules. Unlike superficial mesotherapy, in lipolysis substances are injected directly into the subcutaneous adipose connective tissue. The two methods are generally combined. A down-time of at least 3 days needs to be factored in with PPC/DC. The results are often apparent only after 6–8 weeks. The intervals between injections should be of the same length.
Uses: Small localized fat deposits on the body, face and neck area, also when associated with sagging of the skin, in normal-weight or only slightly overweight patients. Small lipomas. Cellulite with a high fat content.

Gingko
(E.g. Gybilon Toskani)

Rich in terpenes, phytosterol and flavonoids. Has vasoregulatory activity (arterial vasodilator, venous vasoconstrictor, improves capillary microcirculation). Increases cell stability through improved utilization of glucose, oxygen and ATP. Is a neuroprotector and antioxidant. The half-life of intracellular nitric oxide (endothelial relaxation factor) is increased.
Uses: Cellulite, edema and venous-lymphatic insufficiency, accompanying inflammatory symptoms, varicose veins.

Artichoke extract
(Cynomax Toskani, in Cocktail anticellulite Toskani)

In addition to its choleretic effect (up to 30% increase in bile production and secretion), the artichoke has a local effect as a fat-mobilizing agent. It also possesses hepatoprotective and diuretic properties. In addition, cynarin lowers the levels of cholesterol and triglycerides in the blood.
Uses: Localized edematous cellulite.

Herbal anti-adipose cocktail
(Asiacen Toskani, Fuculacca Magnet Aktiv)

Asiacen is a combination of three purified plant extracts: Hedera helix (ivy), Fucus vesiculosus (bladder wrack) und Centella asiatica (gutu kola, the Indian pennywort). Centella has curative properties in the treatment of cellulite: it is venotonic, antifibrotic and improves the flexibility of connective tissue. Fucus is rich in iodine, which aids thyroid function. When used locally, it leads to increased lipolysis through the oxidation of fatty acids. The ivy extract is rich in rutin, thus acting as an arterial vasodilator and venous vasoconstrictor, with a pronounced draining and detoxifying effect. Consequently, this combination has a vasoactive, metabolic and tissue-regulating effect.
Fuculacca is a complex homeopathic preparation consisting of:

- 0.11 ml Rhamnus purshianus D3
- 0.11 ml Sulfur D12
- 0.11 ml Kalium carbonicum D8
- 0.11 ml Adonis vernalis D6
- 0.11 ml Graphites D15
- 0.11 ml Phytolacca americana D5
- 0.11 ml Calcium carbonicum Hahnemanni D15
- 0.11 ml Capsicum annuum D8
- 0.11 ml Fucus vesiculosus D6

It is injected locally or even intramuscularly (always mixed with a few drops of procaine to potentiate its effect); when used clinically, it markedly reduces the feeling of hunger,

thus facilitating weight loss, without being associated with side-effects or risks. According to homeopathic teaching, patients should tend to be adynamic and exhausted or show signs of hypothyroidism. When applied locally it is used for restructuring fatty connective tissue.
Uses: Cellulite, fat pads, connective tissue weakness, Mesodrain, weight loss.

Rutinel Toskani
(Sweet clover extract)

Rutins and coumarins are members of the flavonoids group. Both have antioxidant, anti-inflammatory, antithrombotic, cytoprotective and vasoprotective properties. They prevent the oxidation of vitamin C and block lipid peroxidation. Coumarin also has certain anticoagulant properties. Its effect extends not only to the arteries, but also the veins and lymph vessels.
Uses: Vascular cellulite, weak veins, venous edema, heavy legs, lymphedema, post-traumatic and postoperative edema, Mesodrain.

2.1.4 Special active substances

Polidocanol
(POM) (Aethoxysklerol® 0.25 – 0.5 – 1 – 2 – 4 %)

For potent skin tightening and firming through fibrosis. Extravascular administration leads to irritation and reddening of the skin. It can cause skin necroses at excessive doses. Established in the intravascular treatment of venous dilatation. In dilute form, it is an established agent for the microsclerotherapy of various skin structures.
Uses: Fresh stretch marks, couperose, spider burst veins, small skin hemangiomas, destruction of sweat glands.

Botulinum toxin (POM)
→ See also Sattler: Bildatlas der ästhetischen Botulinumtoxin-Therapie (Atlas of Esthetic Botulinum Toxin Therapy)

Highly potent bacterial toxin, which is turned into a medicinal product by extreme dilution. It is highly sensitive to handling, but can be mixed with isotonic orthomolecular

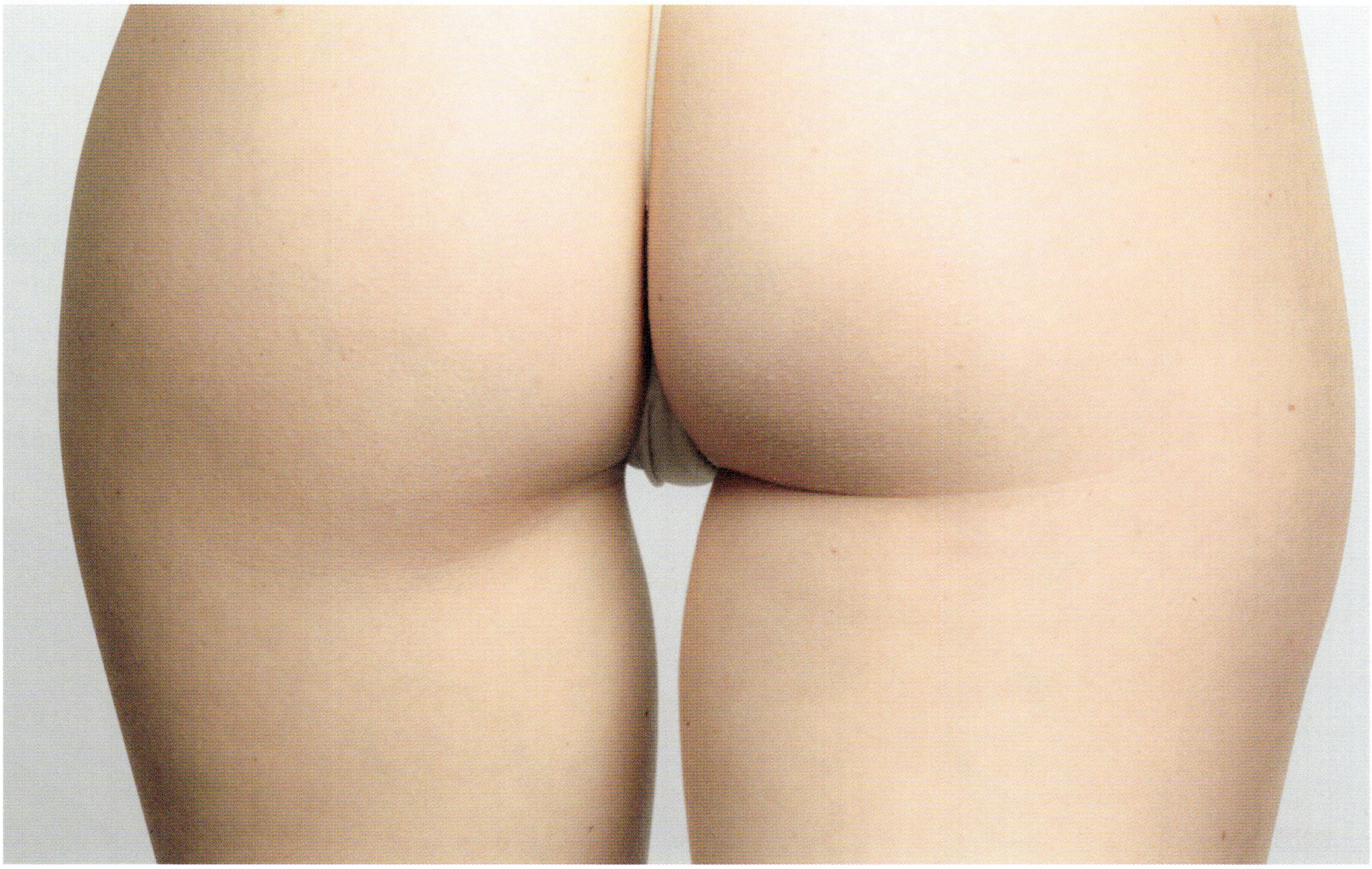

Typische Bereiche weiblicher Fettpölsterchen und Celluliteformationen: Hüften, Glutäalregion, Oberschenkelinnen-, -außen- und -rückseite.

solutions without any loss of effect. Supplements regenerative Mesolift if relaxation of large areas of the face (particularly the areas around the eyes and mouth), neck or cleavage are desired. The most recent observations indicate that this neurotoxin helps promote hair growth.
Uses: Mesobotox, epidermal and intradermal, rejuvenation and relaxation of the face, reducing the size of large skin pores. Hyperhydrosis of the axillae, scalp, palms and soles of the feet.

Salmon calcitonin (POM)
(50 or 100 IU) (must be kept refrigerated)

An oligopeptide, licensed as an osteoporosis agent of second choice, this hormone-like active substance has traditionally been used in mesotherapy for many years. Calcitonin is locally effective in all forms of chronic pain; in France, it is also widely used in the esthetic treatment of cellulite, fat pads and for Mesoglow. Its efficacy is explained by its regulation of calcium metabolism, together with its anti-inflammatory, vasodilatory and analgesic properties. It is regarded as a local repair and regeneration agent for universal use. In anti-aging medicine, it has become established in conditions including presbyobia, hearing loss, atrophy of the gums and loose teeth. Side-effects occur only in responders and at higher doses.

Collagenase
(USA, Mesomedica)

Dissolves fibrosclerotic structures in connective tissue.
Uses: Acne nodules, old scars, nodular cellulite, bull neck, encapsulated lipomas.

Dihydroergotamine (F)

Mild vasoconstriction through α-receptor stimulation. Increases venous tone. Microsclerotherapy, Mesodrain.
Uses: Venolymphatic insufficiency, cellulite, migraine.

Dutasteride (USA)

A 5α-reductase inhibitor which, like finasteride, acts on testosterone metabolism. In genetically predisposed individuals, the hair follicles react to DHT with a reduction in the anagen phase (growth phase). Finasteride and dutasteride also inhibit the local conversion of testosterone to DHT. The hair follicles react to this with a prolongation of the anagen phase and improved hair growth. Can be combined with a regeneration cocktail to improve the trophic situation and microcirculation.
Uses: Androgenic alopecia in men and women (not during pregnancy and exclusively for local use).

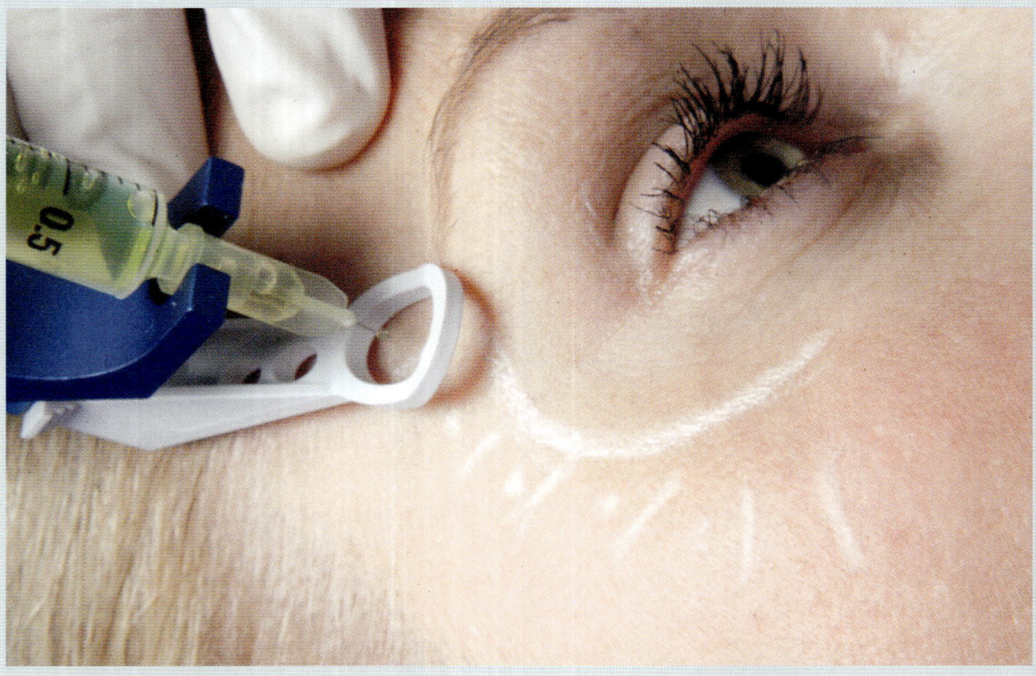

Mesobotox simultaneously provides optimum-dose muscle relaxation, skin regeneration and skin rehydration for fine lines around the eyes and mouth.

Wiedemann Homöokomplex BH
(Connective tissue/skin)

Complex homeopathic preparation consisting of:
- 0.5 ml Acidum hydrofluoricum D8
- 0.5 ml Hamamelis virginiana D4
- 0.5 ml Graphites D12
- 0.5 ml Kreosotum D10.

It is always added to mixtures used in patients with skin indurations, poor skin tolerability, wound healing problems and an increased predisposition to hematomas.
Uses: Fibrous cellulite, scars, stretch marks, skin damage.

2.2 Ready-made cocktails in esthetic mesotherapy

Examples of premixed cocktails which can also be used for skin rejuvenation include the following commercially available Mesolift cocktails of European origin:
- NCTF 135® (CE) with more or less HA (3-ml ampoule)
- Reparestim®HA (CE)
- Revitacare® (CE)
- TKN HA oligovit or TKN HA glowcomplex

Toskani offer a whole range of special Mesotherapy cocktails in 5-ml ampoules (source: www.mesotherapie-shop.de).

2.3 Mixing rules in mesotherapy

Local anesthetics (mostly procaine or lidocaine), physiological saline or monomethyl trisilanol salicylate (Conjonctyl®, Silicor) are used as carrier solutions. Allopathics licensed for intramuscular or intravenous use should be highly diluted in these carriers (generally by a factor of 10). The carriers and adjuvants are drawn into the syringe first, and the allopathic or viscous products (e.g. non-cross-linked hyaluronic acid) added afterwards. The mixture is then shaken briefly to homogenize it and the air evacuated. Care must be taken to ensure that no undiluted allopathics remain in the cone of the syringe. It is only then that the appropriate needle should be fitted onto the syringe. In contrast to systemic treatment, only fractions of the usual doses are needed for local administration. The first-pass effect of systemic administration does not apply, so that the active substances reach the target structure in their full extent. This often means that therapists need to switch to the microdose range and abandon any "more is more" mentality they may have. Adjuvants (special mesotherapy products, orthomolecular products or homeopathic preparations) can be mixed undiluted or used in their pure state. A maximum of three allopathic medicinal products may be mixed in one cocktail. Care must be taken to use only water-soluble substances, to ensure pH equivalence and to use only clear and isotonic solutions for injection. This is the only way to ensure that the procedure is tolerated by the skin. Ideally, the mixtures should be synergistic, with a mu-

Overview – Toskani ready-made cocktails

Skin and hair		
Cocktail FCE	*Composition:*	Composition: natural stemcell-activator (non-animal, wheat germ extract) 0,1% + Na-DNA 0,3% + Coenzym Q 10 0,01% + ferulic acid 0,05%
Cocktail antiaging	*Composition:*	DMAE bitartrate 3 % + carnitine 3 % + pyruvate 2 % + HA 0.5 % + sodium hydroxide 0.88 % + Argireline® 0.05 %
Cocktail antiaging plus Mesolift	*Composition:*	Na-DNA 3 % + HA 2 % + polyvitamin BCAE + organic Silicea 0.5 % + DMAE-Bitartrat 0.5 %
Skin tightening cocktail	*Composition:*	elastin 5 % + DMAE-bitartrate 3 % + sodium ascorbate 2 %
Cocktail antistriae	*Composition:*	Organic Silicea 2.5 % + dexpanthenol 2.5 % + Centella asiatica 2.5 % + elastin 2.5 % + collagen 2.5 % + Mimosa tenuiflora 1 %
Hair cocktail	*Composition:*	dexpanthenol 10 % + pyridoxine 2 % + Thiamin 1 % + biotin 0.05 % + iron gluconate 0.05 %
Cellulite and fat pad cocktails		
Cocktail anticellulite	*Composition:*	caffeine 5 % + Cynara scolymus 3 % + Equisetum arvense 1 % + PPC/DC 1 %
Cocktail anticellulite spot	*Composition:*	Hamamelis 2 % + Ruscus 2 % + PPC/DC 2 %
Natural stem cell activator	(Non-animal) for the skin: additives may include Q 10 und ferulic acid	

All the cocktails may be used in their pure state; where there is local sensitivity (e.g. Meso-Hair) add a local anesthetic: e.g. 0.5 ml procaine 1 % + 1.5 ml hair cocktail. The stem cell activator is mixed 1:1 (only for skin and hair).

tually potentiating effect. Cortisone is not used in mesotherapy, with a few exceptions (treatment of keloids, alopecia areata, inflammatory complications). Cortisone can lead to necrosis in the skin. An established option for the aforementioned exceptional indications consists of dexamethasone palmitate in the form of a microsphere emulsion (Lipotalon®), although care must be taken to check compatibility. For example, it cannot be mixed with lidocaine.

2.4 Individual preparation or ready-made cocktails

While it was previously the rule for the therapist to make up his or her mesotherapy mixtures individually for each patient, increasing numbers of ready-made products for esthetic indications are now appearing on the market. They are packaged according to indication and are user-friendly. While classical mesotherapy still requires a certain degree of special pharmacological know-how and a certain amount of time for the individual preparation of the cocktails, these ready-mades are more convenient, but generally also a bit more expensive. The decision about which way to go depends on the frequency of mesotherapy treatments at the practice and on the practitioner's knowledge and experience. Whichever product we use, we must always be able to rely on its sterility and impeccable manufacturing conditions, i.e. they should only be purchased from a trustworthy source. Not only the therapist, but also the manufacturer has to accept liability.

2.5 Contraindications

2.5.1 Absolute contraindications

As a matter of principle, for safety reasons, pregnant women should not have any esthetic treatments, particularly not to the abdomen. Other contraindications include: known intolerance or allergy to any of the active substances used, a predisposition to hypertrophic scars or pigmentation disorders, highly active autoimmune processes, severe cardiovascular or metabolic disorders, acute viral or bacterial infections, acute inflammatory skin conditions, epilepsy.

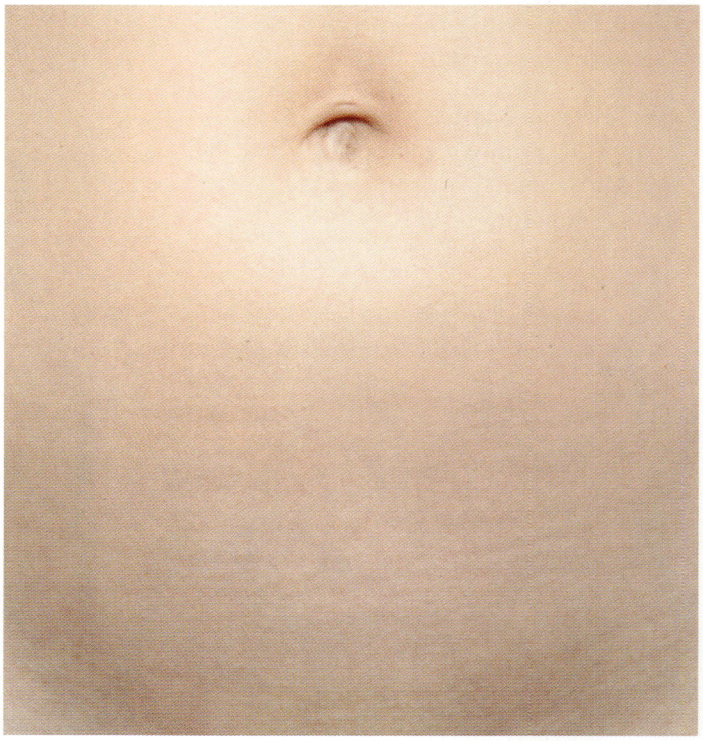

Esthetic procedures, particularly in the abdominal region, are taboo during pregnancy.

2.5.2 Relative contraindications

Age below 16 years, breastfeeding mothers, injection phobia, herpes simplex virus (HSV1) load (preventative treatment with an antiviral agent (acyclovir or valaciclovir) is advisable), coagulation anomalies or anticoagulation (only for deep injection techniques), existing or suspected destruction of anatomical structures, e.g. the hair roots.

Dysmorphophobia/dysmorphic syndrome
(Distorted perception of one's body)
Occurs in c. 15% of consultations in esthetic practice. This syndrome is characterized by the patient's disproportionate or unrealistic ideas or perceptions about him- or herself. It is difficult or impossible to please these patients. They often demand countless sessions and procedures. This is a psychiatric disorder, though sufferers regularly deny this. It requires a great deal of experience and instinct from the therapist. While countless sessions and procedures are often requested, the treatment results are generally doomed to failure.

3 Documentation and organization

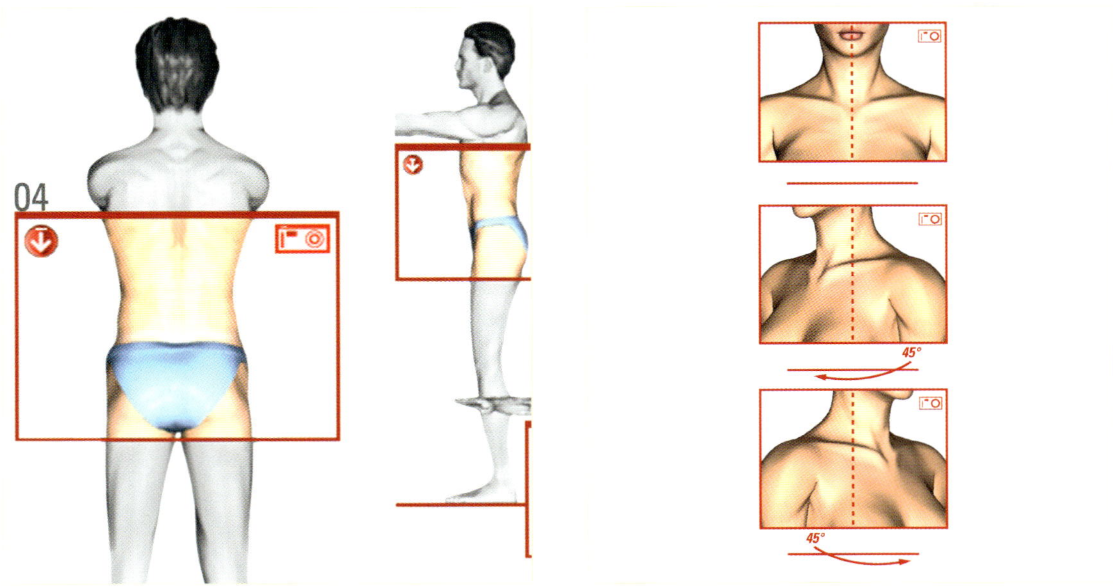

Positioning templates show the right image sections for each type of treatment, along with the corresponding pose and the correct angle.

3

Documentation and organization

Documentation involves the collection of all the relevant patient data such as age, medical history, relevant concomitant illnesses, medication history and previous esthetic treatments. All the treatments carried out are also recorded in the patient's file. Digital photo documentation provides a suitable before, during and after record of the treatment. An information session needs to take place before any treatment takes place and must be evidenced by means of a written informed consent signed by the patient (see Chapter 10).
The only convincing way to demonstrate the success of the increasingly non-invasive treatments used in medical esthetics is through expressive images. Professional, standardized photos charting the course of the treatment therefore play a key role in this specialist area. Photo documentation of a treatment is not only an important communication medium during the consultation, but also increases patient loyalty over the course of a long-term treatment. Professional follow-up images are part of a practice's quality management procedure and, last but not least, provide a safeguard in the event of a dispute.

3.1 Photo documentation

Photography plays an important role in dermatology and esthetics as a simple and objective recording method. This section provides an outline of how documentation can be introduced into the practice and how the quality of photographic documentation may be optimized.

3.1.1 General requirements for medical photography

Digital photos have long since superseded conventional analog photography. The before-and-after images used in many publications are not suitable for proper, comprehensive documentation. These images are often neither informative nor comparable. A professional image system should fulfill the following requirements:

- Standardization of the baseline and follow-up shots
- Ease of use and user-friendliness, allowing the picture-taking process to be delegated
- Patient-referenced archiving
- Inter-patient evaluation
- Analysis of the images
- Report writing
- Suitability for publication
- Cost-effectiveness.

3.1.2 Prerequisites for standardized follow-up images

Several points need to be taken into consideration for standardized treatment course follow-up images:

1 Suitable room
It is advisable to plan to take the pictures in a dedicated room or, at least, in a separate area without direct sunlight. A standard, single-color background should be used, for example blue.

2 Background
The background must be free of extraneous objects that distract the eye from the subject, such as books, plants or other people. Furthermore, the patient being photographed for documentation purposes should not simply be placed into the middle of the room, as this makes the image background impossible to control, so that it cannot be reproduced for subsequent photos. The optimum way is to set up a fixed documentation spot within the practice premises, with a uniform, neutral background – e.g. door, wall or room divider. For example, good photographs of the head, arms, legs and feet can be taken against the neutral surface of a patient couch, so that no extraneous, distracting objects are visible in the background.
The ideal background is homogeneous in a single, neutral color. Colors that are too bright and glaring or too dark are best avoided.

> **Practice tip**
> Homogeneous areas in single color hues such as grey, cream or, best of all, blue, make a suitable background for photographic subjects.

3 Standardized camera settings
It is virtually impossible to achieve comparable images by setting the camera up manually. For this reason, a very good option is to use suitable software to control camera settings, both for baseline and follow-up shots. The mediscope solution from FotoFinder® is one example of easy-to-use, efficient software. In this system, camera and computer are linked by a lead and controlled using the "CamControl" program. The user can use the program menu to select the required photograph profile, e.g. face shot. This action calls up the optimum camera parameters stored for this profile in the software. For subsequent shots, the program automatically selects the same settings as those used when taking the baseline picture. However, profiles can also be modified individually.

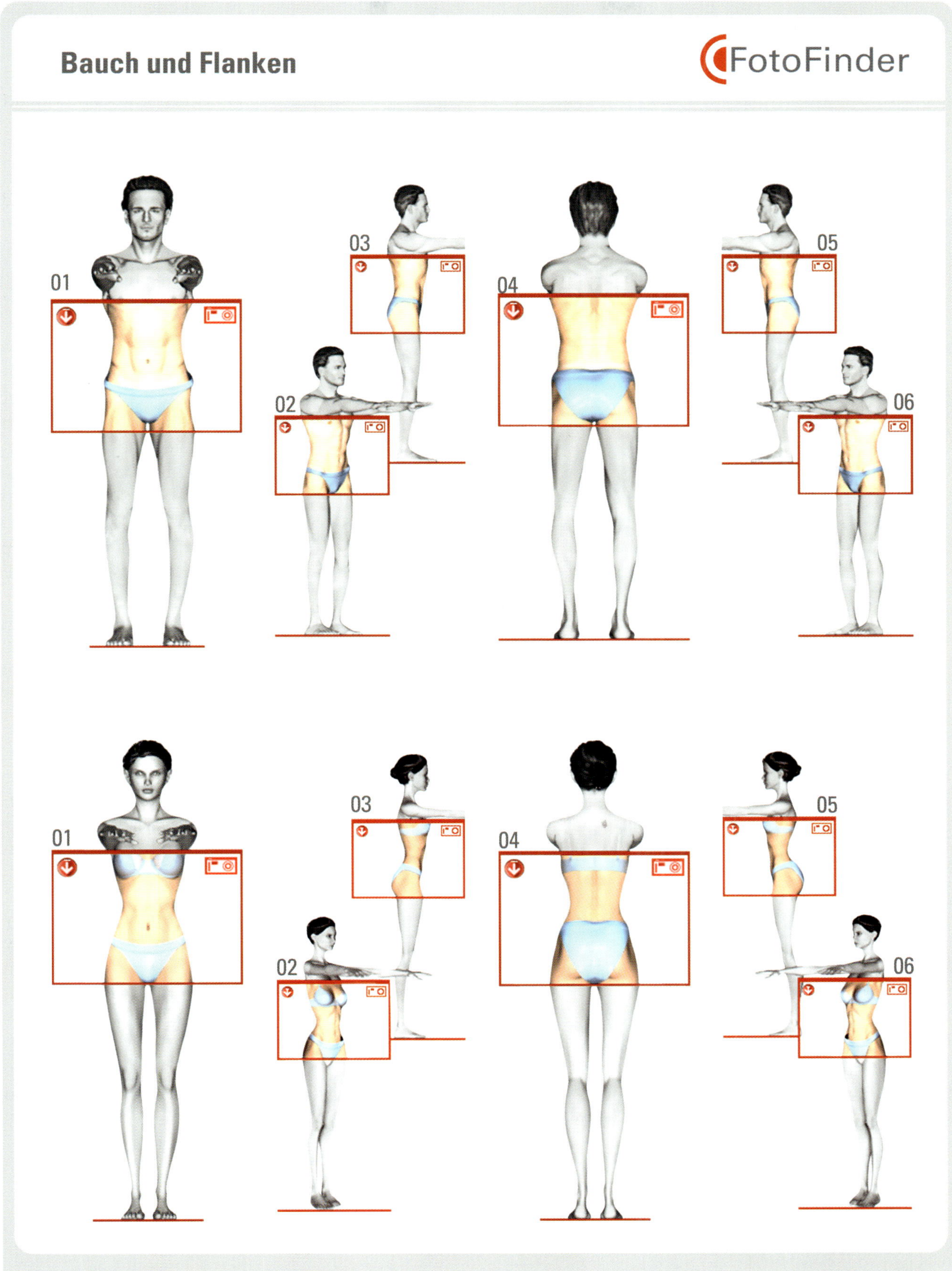

The positioning templates – in this case "abdomen and hips" – supplied with FotoFinder® Guided Photography show the right image sections for each type of treatment, along with the corresponding pose and the correct angle.

4 Suitable patient pose
Even the best photography is useless if the result of the treatment remains invisible because unsuitable image sections are used. The user-friendly software shows suitable positioning templates for every type of treatment, such as the right image sections, the corresponding pose and the correct angle of shot. The software guides the user through the entire picture-taking process. As soon as one image is stored, the program shows the next position. This easy-to-use software can therefore not only help the therapist, but also relieve him or her of the work, as picture-taking with this program can easily be delegated.

5 Patient pose and image detail in follow-up shots
A key point in producing photo documentation that is clear and comprehensive for both the treatment and the patient is to ensure an identical patient pose in the follow-up shots. Suitable software helps achieve this, as the transparent "ghost" outlines of the last shot are shown in the background of the live image. This means that the patient can be positioned with millimeter accuracy, and the same image sections are consistently selected. Special tripods with positioning aids ensure reproducible angles and distances. The precise results of the photography support the reliability of the treatment concept and consolidate the patient's confidence in the therapist's work.

Face shots
A portrait tripod with a chin rest, for instance, allows esthetic procedures to the face to be documented reproducibly, through accurate positioning and complete congruence between shots. The tripod can be tilted by 180°, so that patients can be photographed from 9 angles, whether frontally or in half or full profile. Optimum lighting without glare or shadow is achieved by bouncing the flash off two reflectors. The chin rest can be removed for shots of the chin and neck (see FotoFinder®).

Full-body shots
The adjustable-height tripod for full-body shots can be used to document total body treatments (body contouring etc.) from head to foot. To do this, the camera is moved up or down 5 cm at a time. A laser positioning system, with a red laser line, ensures that the patient's pose is standardized and that the distance between camera and subject is always the same.

Special photographs of certain skin conditions
Certain skin conditions are best documented using special lenses or filters.

Reddening and veins
Acne, allergies, couperose, spider-burst and varicose veins, etc. can be shot using a cross-polarization filter. This eliminates any reflections, showing the skin condition in its true colors.

Lines
Parallel polarization is suitable for the documentation of lines and wrinkles. Extreme side lighting ensures that even the tiniest, finest lines are strikingly visualized.

6 Lighting
Every light source has different color temperatures, with differing effects on color reproduction. Artificial light sources pose particular problems, because mixtures of different light sources do not provide good follow-up documentation due to the color variations involved.
Mixed light situations (daylight, various fluorescent lamps or other artificial light sources) almost always occur in practice, which makes color reproducibility of the condition more difficult and/or requires time-consuming post-processing with associated poorer quality. Mixed light situations can be avoided by using a bright, artificial light source for the shots.
This allows reproducible results to be achieved regardless of daylight and also, in most cases, regardless of any existing ambient lighting.
Lighting with a flash offers a few advantages, provided that the ground rules are followed. There are two variants: direct and indirect flash. For a direct flash, the adjustable reflector is directed at the subject. In the indirect technique, the reflector is directed onto a large white surface, e.g. the ceiling or wall of the room. The flash bounces off this surface, lighting the subject indirectly.

3.1.3 Archiving, analysis and publication

1 Archiving
Ideally, the shots should be taken and stored directly into the patient's digital file, and labeled with the relevant information (treatment etc.). The archiving process needs to differentiate between baseline, follow-up and processed images, and allow the photographs to be sorted according to the treatment (e.g. all Botox shots), visit (all shots taken on one date) or chronologically.

Maintaining the correct distance from the area being photographed

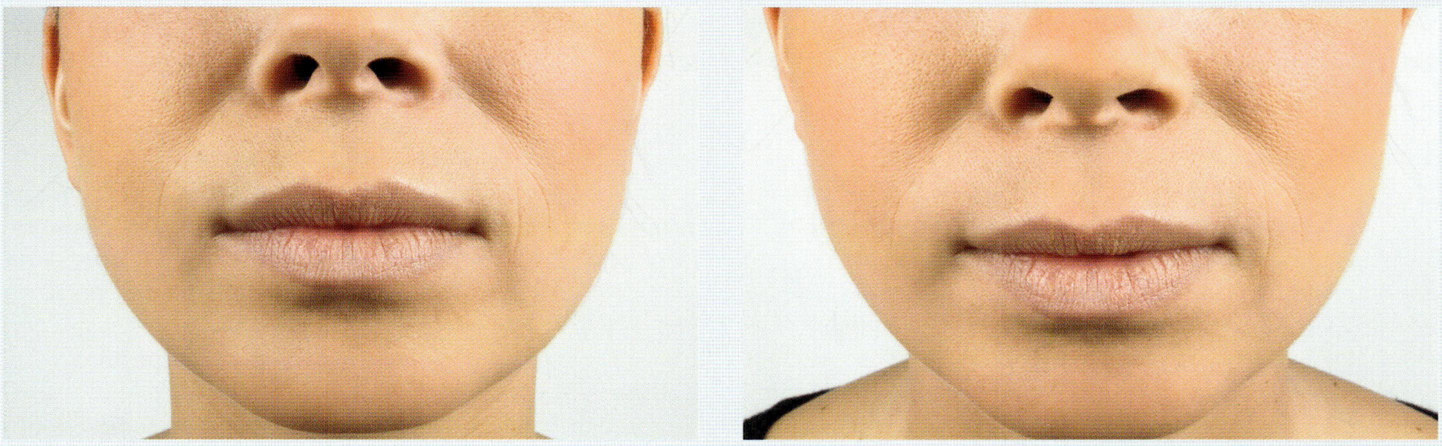

Distortions caused by moving the camera too close to the shot area

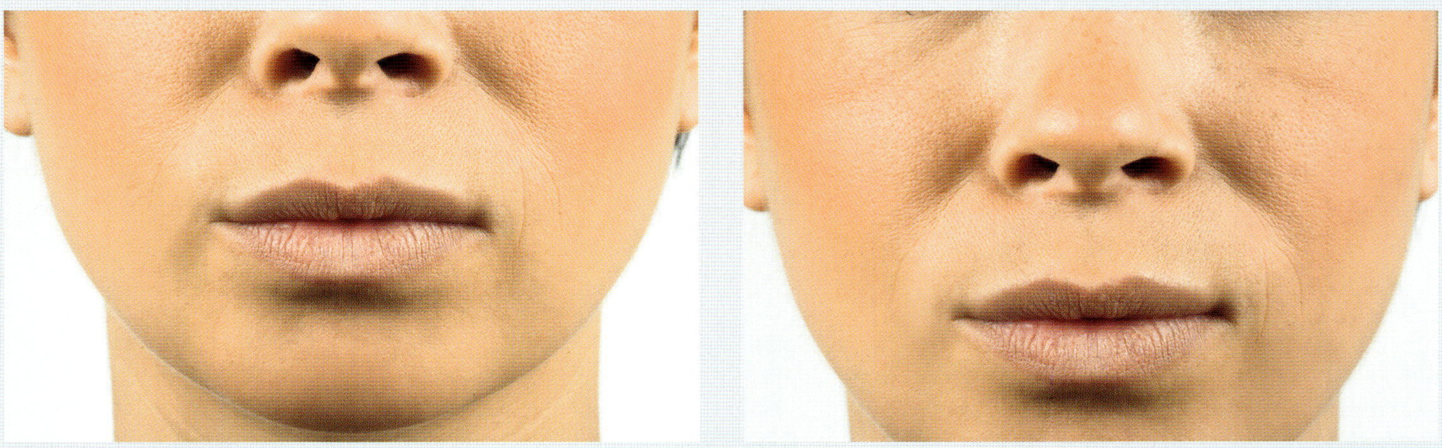

Better: shot taken by zooming in from a distance (100 mm focal length)

Correct camera angle

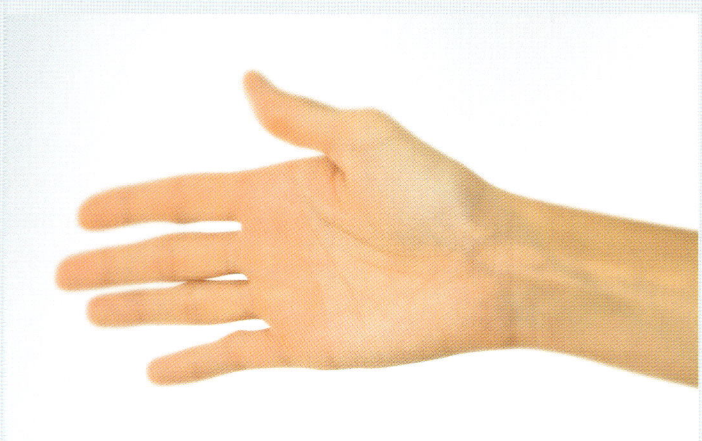

"Tipping" the camera causes some areas to be out of focus.

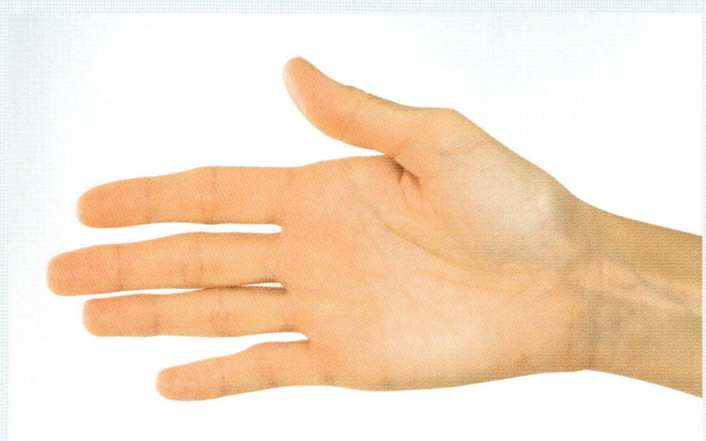

Ensuring that the camera is parallel to the imaging plane delivers a sharply focused image.

2 Analysis
Image comparison allows the course and outcome of a treatment to be shown on the monitor with outstanding quality. Good, functional software also provides inter-patient search criteria.

3 Publication
Images can also be post-processed; however, it is important to ensure that the original is not touched up. For example, FotoFinder® can be used to produce treatment plans using arrows and text. These amended shots are then added as a new image file and marked with an orange frame. Treatment plans and before-and-after reports can be printed out or stored as PDF files. Full image comparison series can be presented in PowerPoint for lectures and when presenting conference papers.

3.1.4 Analysis of the skin

Digital color images may be analyzed using a variety of expert systems. This is very helpful when drawing up specific treatment plans, and also improves communication between doctor and patient.

3.1.5 Key points

The use of a software-controlled image system forms part of a modern practice's process optimization and quality management. This form of highly simplified photographic process requires no specialist know-how and can be fully delegated to the practice assistants.

Practice tip

The company FotoFinder® kindly provided us with the standardized photo documentation system and suggestions for functional archiving. FotoFinder®'s mediscope software and its Guided Photography System help ensure smooth, trouble-free and easy operation.

3.2 Tips for photography and practice organization

Since photo documentation of both the course and outcome of the treatment is of key significance in the overall treatment concept, it is very important for the patient to have a consultation preparing her or him for the photo documentation. This includes an explanation of the photo documentation process.

3.2.1 The patient's posture and position

For optimum results when taking photographs, the basic requirements include ensuring that the patient stands still in an appropriate pose, and that the FotoFinder® system is operated correctly. If a tripod is not used, the camera must be held close, with the photographer's elbow pressed tightly against the body. Ensure that any measuring instruments and sensors are not covered with a finger or any other objects. The lenses and viewfinder should be cleaned regularly with cleaning agents designed specifically for the purpose. The sensor must not be either cleaned or touched.

1 Baseline shots
The first or baseline shot of a documentation series should be taken very carefully and conscientiously, as it represents the reference image. All the images taken during follow-up will be compared with this reference.

2 Details
Before taking detail shots, it is best to home in on the desired location gradually. If some time has passed since the last photo session, it can often be difficult to recall which area was last photographed. Where this is the case, a general view helps to find the correct location for subsequent shots.

3 Shot area
A certain distance needs to be maintained from the area being photographed, as the shot can otherwise become distorted or out of focus. Every focal length has its advantages and disadvantages in this respect. For example, shots taken with a wide-angle lens of less than 50 mm produce undesirable distortions – rather like viewing someone through a spy-hole – which are not appropriate for documentation purposes.
It is better to zoom in on the subject from a slightly greater distance. On the other hand, one should also avoid zooming in too far, as this can cause blurring.

4 Measurement
For the sake of convenience, and if no photography and archiving software is available, any measurements in the image should be made using a ruler. If any features need to be documented with a "yardstick", a good option, for hygienic and practical reasons, is to use a disposable ruler. These are usually 10 cm long and 2 cm wide, self-adhesive and can be written on with a ball-point pen. Images obtained in this way can be used as a calibration template in the software and allow measurements to be made afterwards. This is a particularly good option for before-and-after shots, e.g. to demonstrate the reduction in size of a lipoma that is being treated.

3.2.2 Practice organization

It is well known that many of the treatments and services in esthetic medicine are provided on a private, direct-payment basis. Patients must be informed about these services. All staff members at the practice must be familiar with the range of services on offer and be able to provide preliminary information regarding any individual supplementary offers.

3.2.3. Appointment planning and information material

When planning appointments, an appropriate time slot will need to be factored in even at the initial enquiry stage, or if a patient merely expresses an interest in mesotherapy. This time slot is important as it allows the patient's requirements to be explored comprehensively and professionally. The benefit of this time investment is that patients are comprehensively informed, turning them into potential "regular customers". If patients at a practice are given all-round professional care, and if the treatment outcome matches the expectations of both sides, this sets up a solid and long-lasting patient relationship. Another aspect is that news of a cost-effective treatment with a good outcome tends to be spread by word of mouth – representing the ideal form of targeted advertising. The professional impression is further enhanced by well-designed leaflets and brochures, prominently displayed or handed out at the practice. This promotional material can be used to present and explain the individual procedures in a vivid and esthetic format.

3.2.4 Information events

Well-informed and sensitive practice employees, together with patient leaflets and brochures, provide one way of communicating what the practice has to offer. Another option is to hold presentation evenings on specific subjects. These can be advertised at the practice. Good promotional events, including case studies and treatment records, combined with a professionally delivered presentation, communicate competence and experience. These presentations also provide an opportunity for questions from interested parties to be answered, and for any preconceptions to be either put into perspective or swept away altogether. However, when presenting case studies, care must be taken to preserve medical confidentiality and discretion. Confidentiality is the top professional requirement in esthetic medicine, in particular. Even where there is a lot of interest, no photo documentations, films or live treatments can be shown in public without the express permission of the patient, preferably given in writing. This is a sensitive area, carrying a high risk of breaches of professional duty and violations of the patient's personal rights.

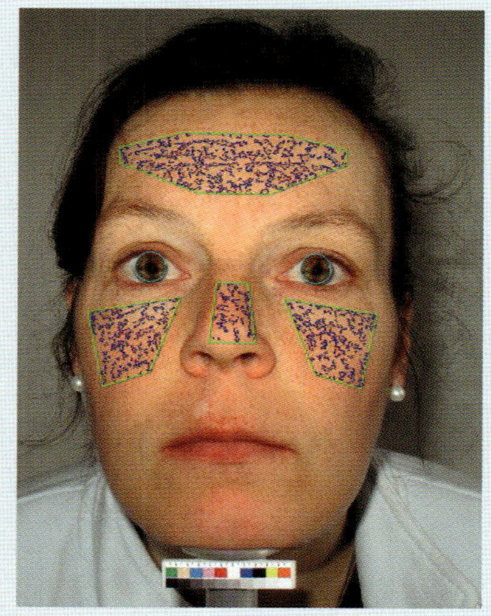
1

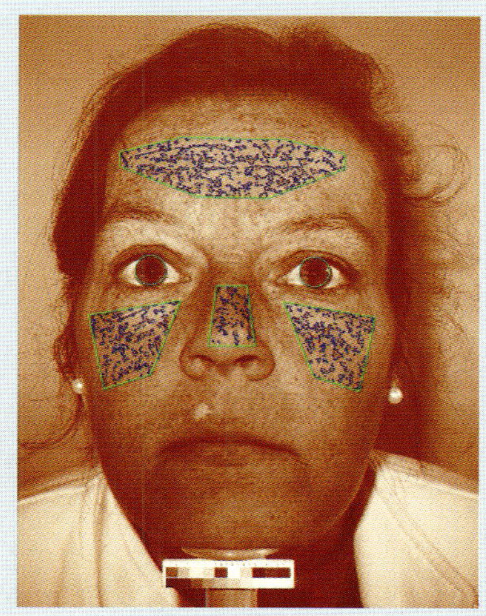
2

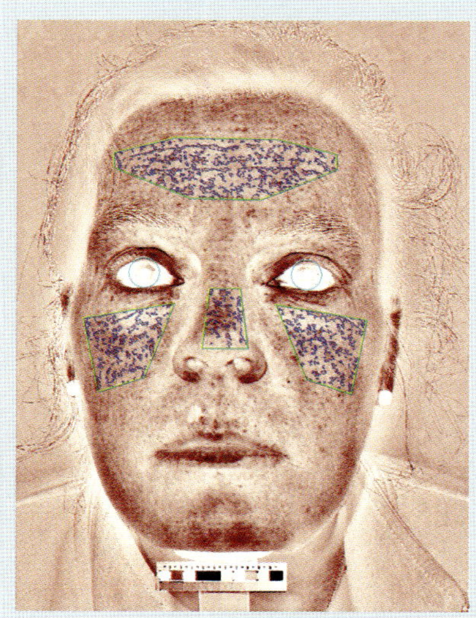
3

*Skin*Spector can be used to quantify both light-induced and vascular skin damage relative to age group. The program distinguishes between red and brown color skin values. This allows specific treatment plans to be drawn up and improves doctor-patient communication.

3

Detail shots

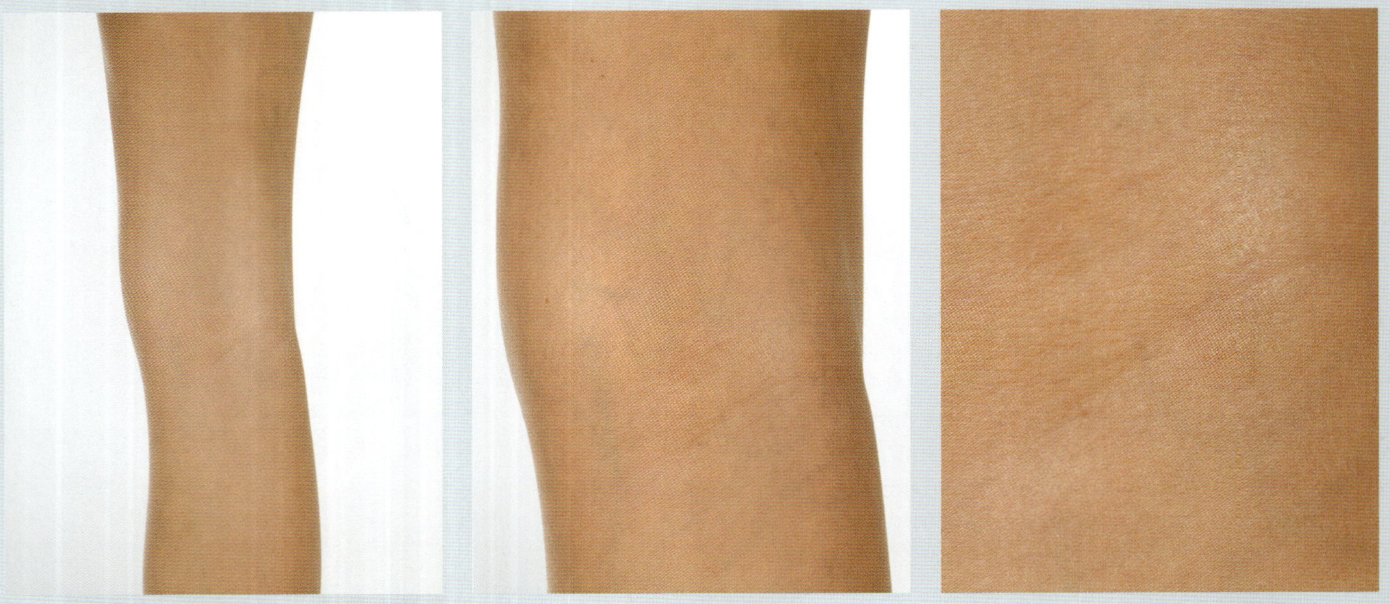

First take a general view and then zoom in on the area of interest in several stages.

Follow-up documentation: using the reference image as a guide

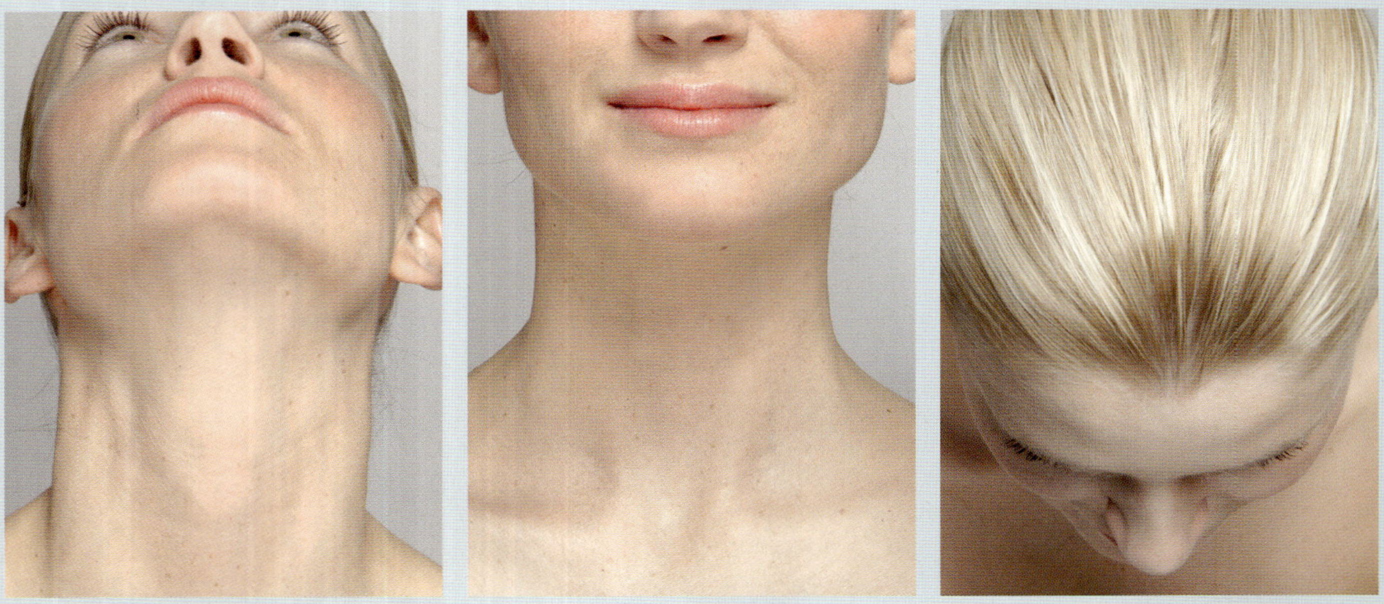

Before taking the shot, it is advisable to draw up a list of images detailing the image sections and details to be shot as precisely as possible. The treatment areas can be drawn into these images afterwards.

Tip

All interventions and procedures, starting with the information session, followed by the patient's consent and all through to the findings of the assessment and the treatment, must be documented. Special documentation templates are recommended for this purpose; these can be kept in the patient's file. Merely handing out an information sheet does not replace the explanation which needs to be provided verbally by the doctor. Those wishing to use pictures of their patients for presentations or publications must obtain an additional consent to do so from the patient.

4 Side-effects

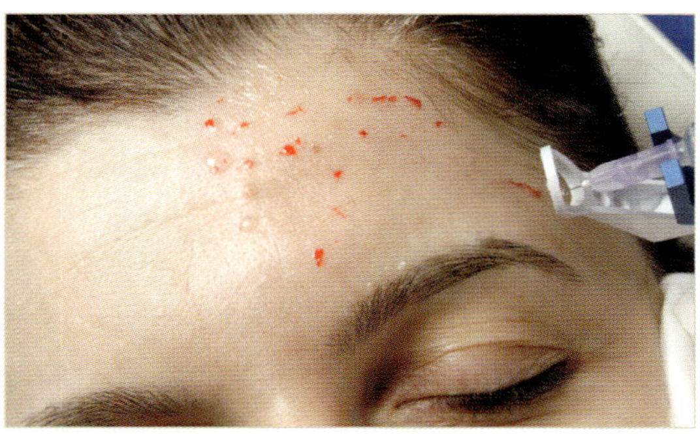

No more than a tiny drop of blood should appear when performing epidermal Mesolift.

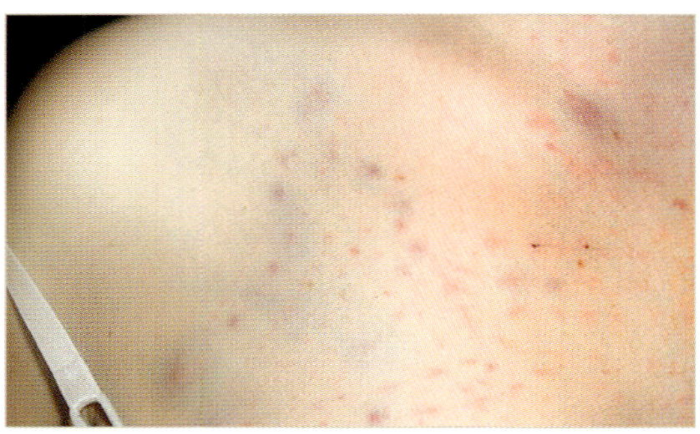

An incorrect injection technique leads to scratches, hematomas and a dissatisfied patient.

Side-effects

Side-effects can be caused either by the active substances used or by the injection technique. It is essential to refer to the package insert leaflet when using allopathic agents, and to the manufacturer's information with ready-mades. The general rule with low-dose local administration is that no systemic effects are likely, particularly with epidermal application. The greater the amount of active substance, the more potent the product and, the deeper the injection, the more likely it is that local and systemic side-effects will develop. Regardless of all the above, allergies need to be expected at any practice, and the appropriate precautions taken. However, typical reactive (dermographism) or drug-induced erythema (e.g. following Buflomedil or PPC) should be universally familiar and must not be confused with an allergic reaction. The same applies to sensitive tissues such as the lips and the area around the eyes, which can swell up considerably in response to physical irritation alone.

The safety of mesotherapy was demonstrated many years ago in the French studies ENATOME I and II. Systemic vegetative reactions are possible, but rare. The literature also contains very few reports of side-effects, caused mostly by incorrect or unhygienic techniques.

4.1 Local side-effects

The local side-effects of mesotherapy are reversible, short-term and occur particularly at the first treatment: mild pain, bleeding, small hematomas, mild reddening, swelling, peeling of the skin, discrete scratch marks, dermographism. These so-called initial reactions are well-known phenomena in naturopathy and should be explained to the patient as follows: This is a deep-seated cleansing and repair process in the skin and connective tissue. It is the only way that we can achieve long-term rejuvenation and beautification.

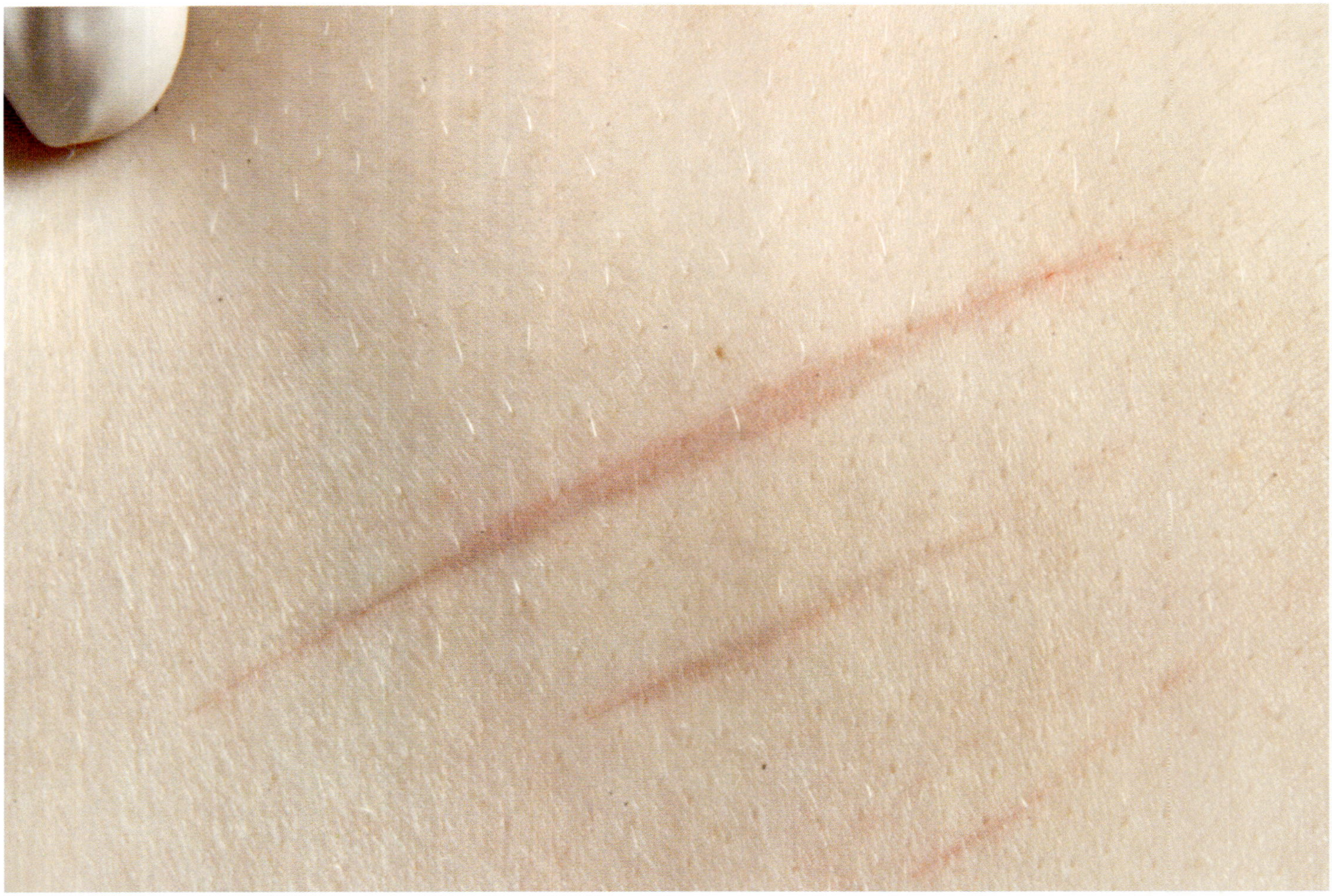

Short-term red dermographism along epidermal lines created at different times with the addition of Buflomedil. The capillary vasodilatation fades within minutes.

If there are any skin reactions, these can be touched up after the treatment using a suitable concealer, powder or make-up. Camouflage make-up may also help in extreme cases.

4.2 Rare side-effects

Even if all the precautions are carefully followed, allergic reactions may still occur in rare cases. Patients with a known predisposition can be given an antihistamine before the treatment as a precautionary measure. Some mesotherapists also add a few drops of Tavegil® (clemastine) to the mixture. The activation of latent herpes infections can be prevented with suitable medication. Pigment disruptions usually occur following unauthorized exposure to sunlight. Extremely rare side-effects include (aseptic) necroses, granulomas, keloids and infections.

4.3 Specific side-effects of lipolysis

The active substance PPC+DC, when used in lipolysis, regularly causes local irritation: reddening of the skin, tissue swelling and itching develop immediately after the injections. This immediate reaction persists for about 3 days. Pain caused by the local inflammatory reaction and any hematomas may be perceived for up to 2 weeks. It can be controlled by cooling, special taping methods or by taking an ibuprofen tablet on the evening of the treatment. More persistent tenderness, nodules or indentations, diarrhea or breakthrough menstrual bleeds in women occur in rare cases. Potential circulatory reactions which may range through to collapse are a possibility after high doses. Where that is the case, the patient should be instructed to drink plenty of fluids.
However, these side-effects are generally harmless and completely reversible.

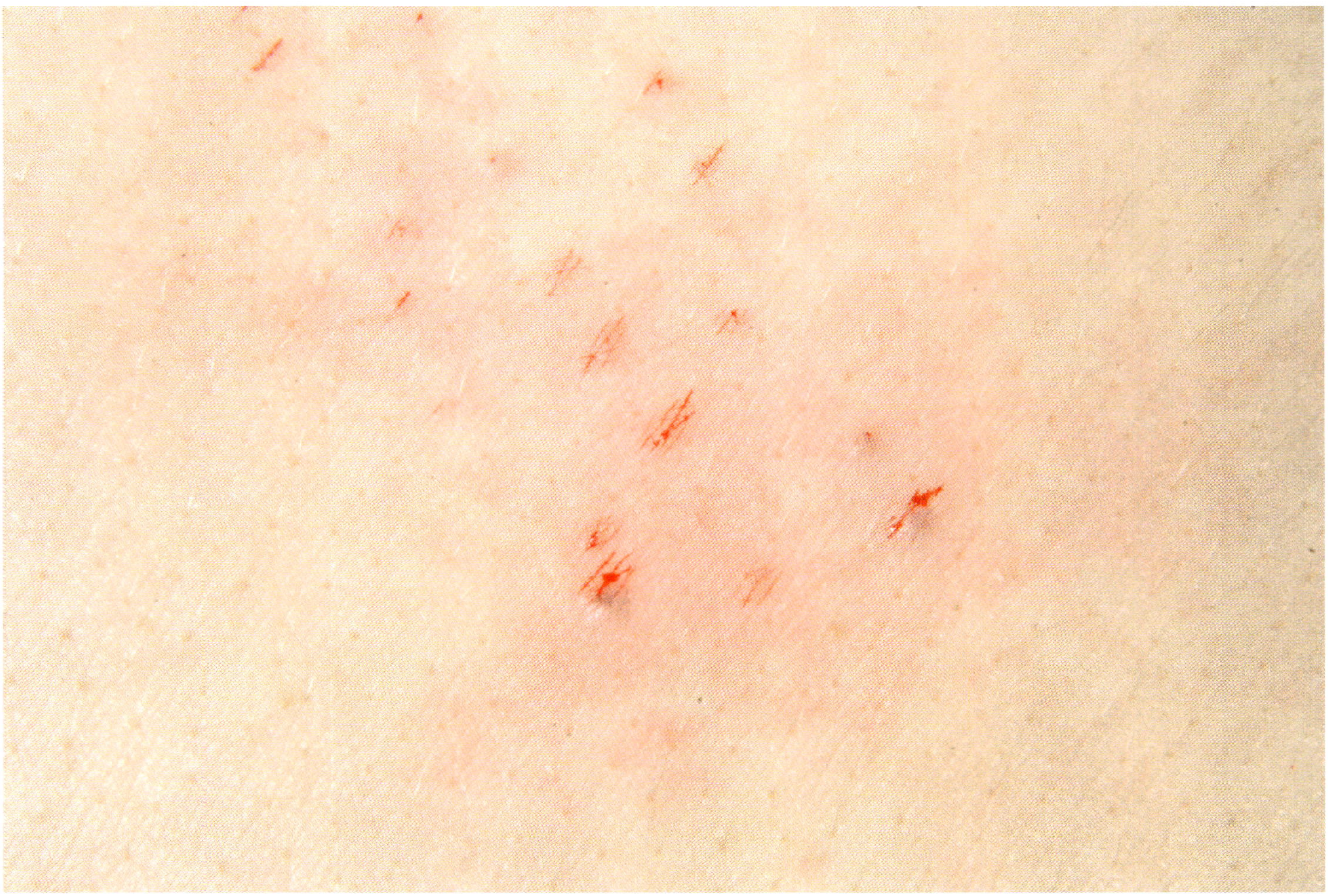

A bit of blood regularly seeps from the fresh microinjury created by intradermal or subcutaneous injections. The deeper the injection, the greater the risk of a hematoma. Any bleeding must be staunched by immediate compression.

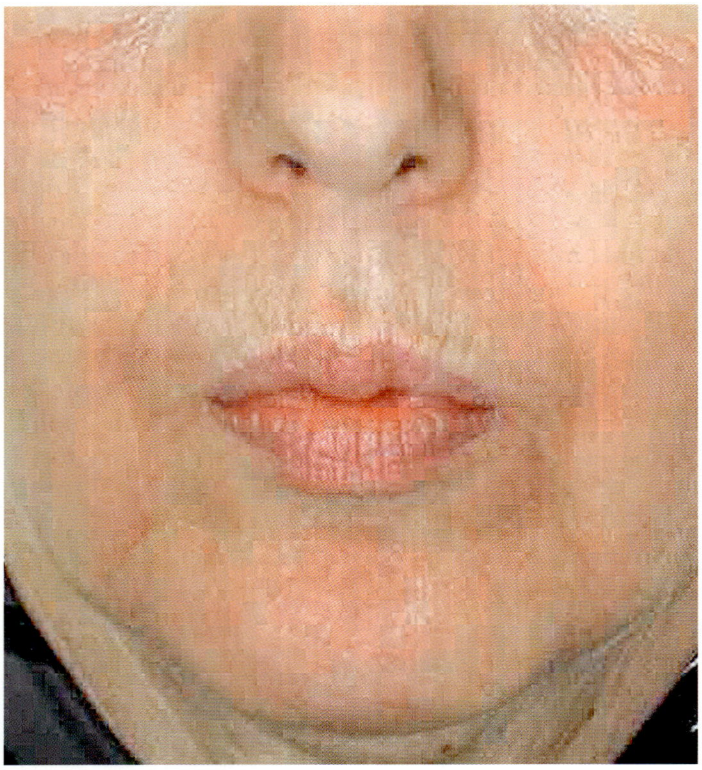

Allergy following Mesolift

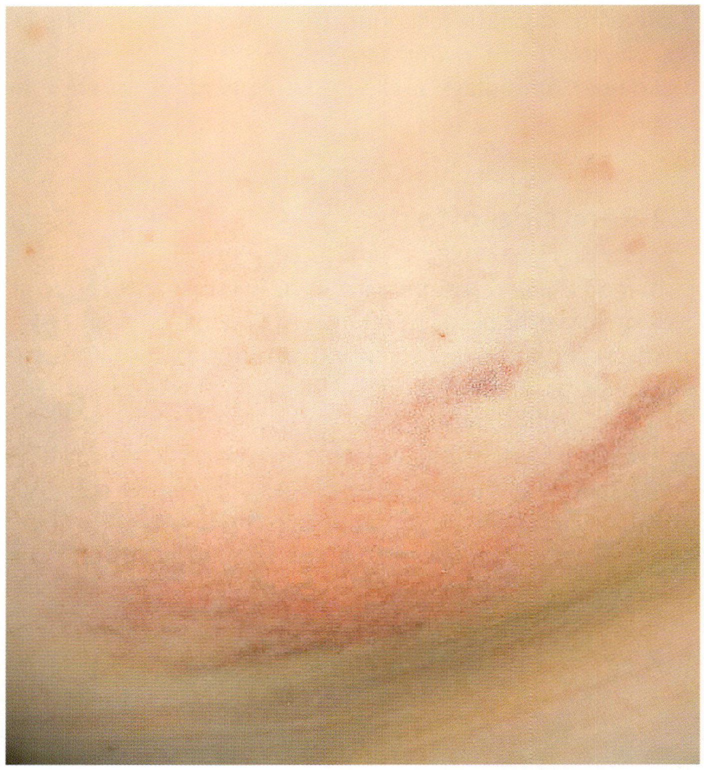

Hematoma on the abdomen

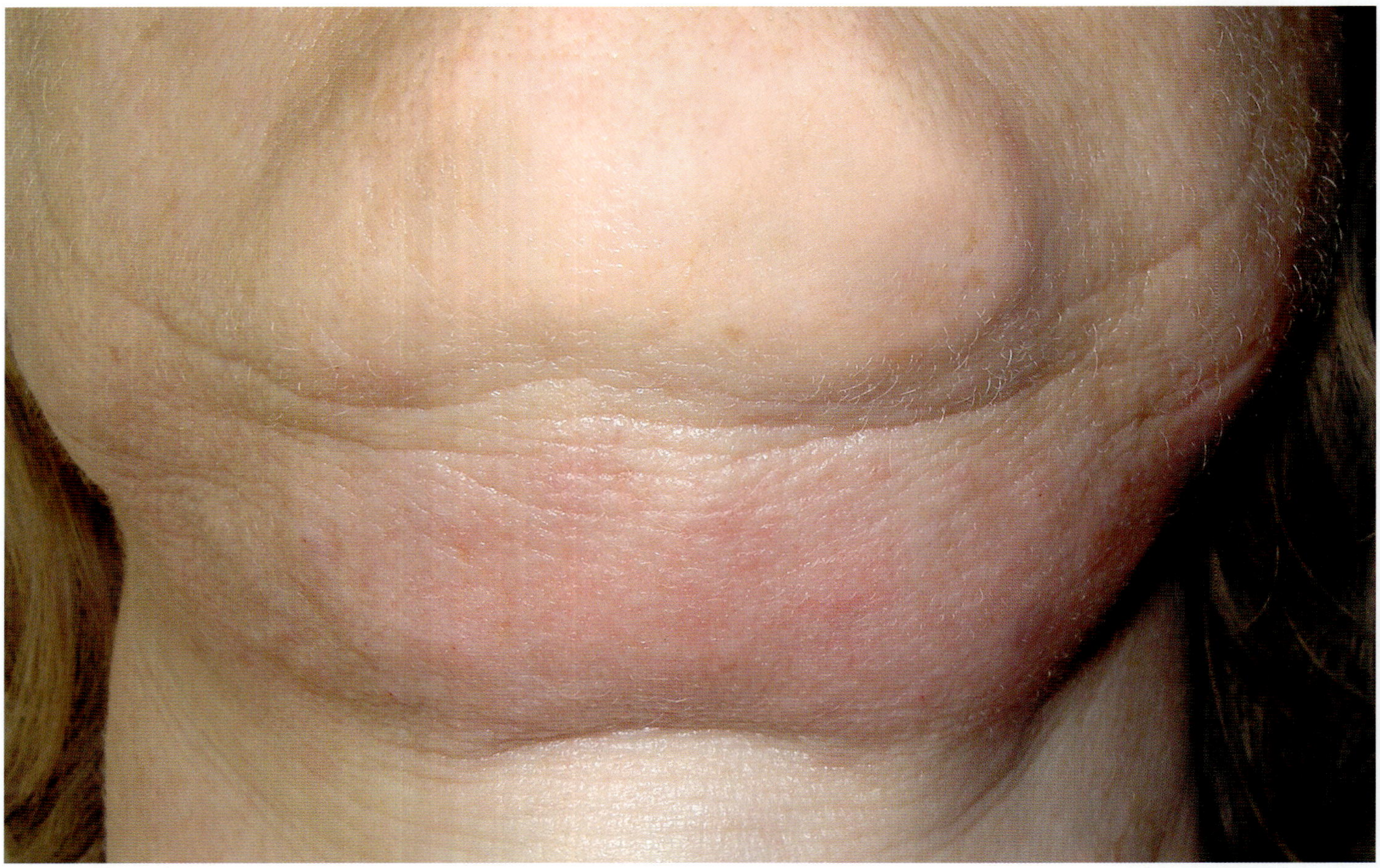

Typical submandibular reddening and swelling following lipolysis

5 Materials and techniques

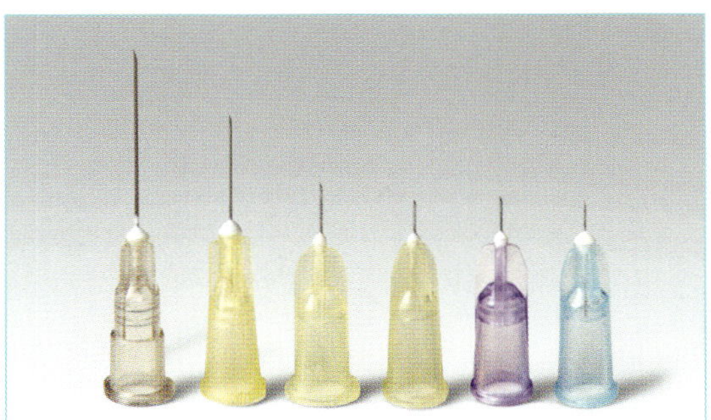

Various hypodermic needle formats may be used for mesotherapy and lipolysis

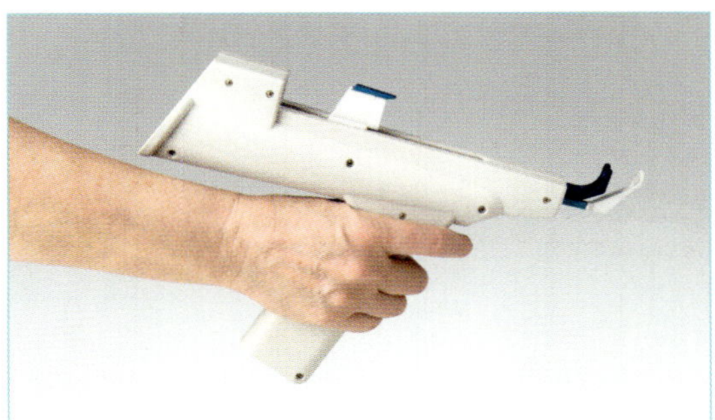

This injector is activated by pressing the trigger button with the index finger. The injection is always directed downwards.

Materials and techniques

5.1 Syringes and needles

Even though mesotherapy only involves microinjections, these should still be administered as non-traumatically and as painlessly as possible. Decisive factors in this respect, apart from the active substances, are the injection technique and the quality of the syringes and needles. All the materials should be silicon- and latex-free. Available syringe formats include the 1 ml, 2.5 ml, 5 ml and 10 ml sizes; it is important to ensure that they consist of three component parts (i.e. that the plunger is topped with a rubber seal which ensures easier, smoother delivery). If an electronic Mesogun is used, the correct syringe formats are important to ensure complete evacuation of the contents (suppliers listed in the Appendix, Chapter 11).

Short 4-mm and 6-mm needles are available especially for mesotherapy (Mesoram, Mesorelle, Mesojet). The Mesojet needles are distinguished by their special 5-sided bevel, which considerably reduces bleeding from the skin. However, they should only be used with an electronic injector, as the 5-sided bevel makes skin penetration slightly more difficult compared with the 3-sided (triangular) bevel. Although the needles listed here are high-quality, high-performance products, they still need to be changed several times when administering multiple injections. The needle can bend or become blunted, particularly when using the nappage (also known as gust or salvo) technique. In addition, the patency of the needle needs to be checked before every treatment. Each needle must be disposed of immediately after use, using a dedicated, securely sealed sharps container (Quick-box), which is disposed of via normal waste. Needles must never be recapped due to the risk of injury.

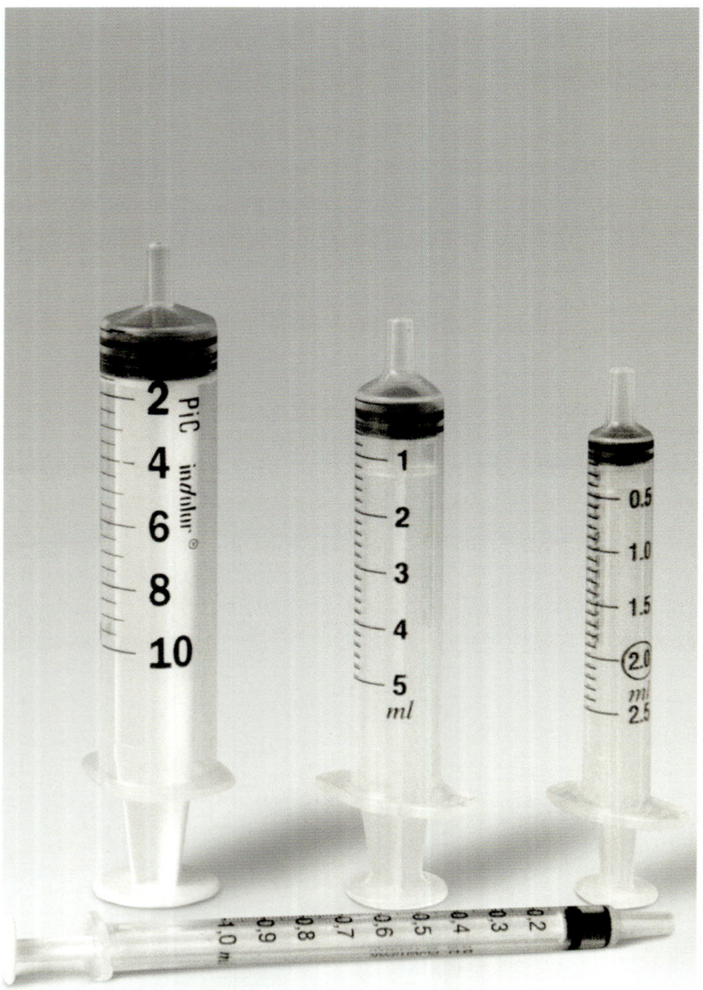

The syringes should be of high quality and fitted with a rubber seal for smoother glide during the injection.

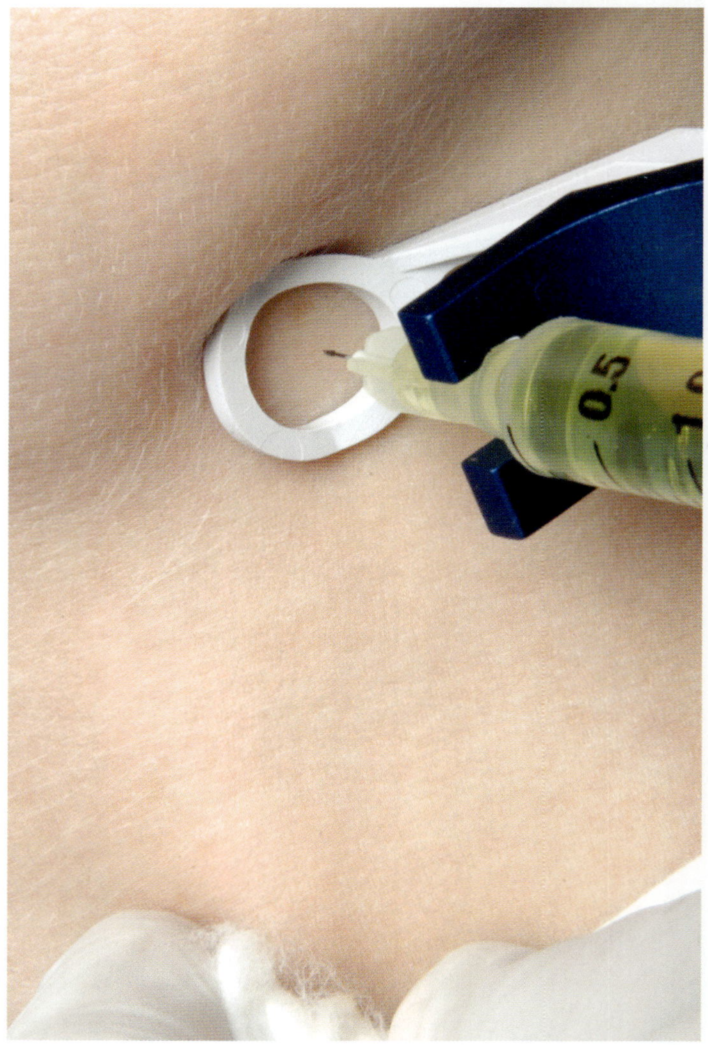

The injector enables the therapist to work with precision, even in anatomically problematic areas.

5.1.1 Mesotherapy needles and their uses

1. Microlance BD 0.3 x 13 mm: cellulite, lipolysis, hair loss, point-by-point technique, linear tunnel technique, manual epidermal technique, one-by-one injection technique, infiltration.
2. Mesoram 0.3 x 4 mm: Mesolift, hair loss, cellulite, Mesobotox, nappage and epidermal technique, one-by-one injection technique, for universal manual use or with the Pistor 4 or 5.
3. Mesojet 0.29 x 4 (also 6) mm, 5-sided bevel + polish: special needle for cellulite with venous and/or connective tissue weakness, in patients with increased susceptibility to hematomas or bleeding.
4. Mesorelle 0.26 x 4 mm: finest needle with a low flow rate, for the point-by-point and epidermal technique in sensitive patients or on sensitive areas, e.g. hands, feet, perioral or periorbital region, causes significantly less pain.
5. Sterican or Terumo No. 20 0.3 x 20 mm or BD Hypoint 0.4 x 13 mm: lipolysis for bigger fat pads and larger syringe volumes, for subcutaneous infiltration.

5.2 Injectors

The mesotherapy injector, also known as the mesogun or meso-pistol, is an indispensable tool for a practice specializing in esthetics. Firstly, it enables injections to be delivered

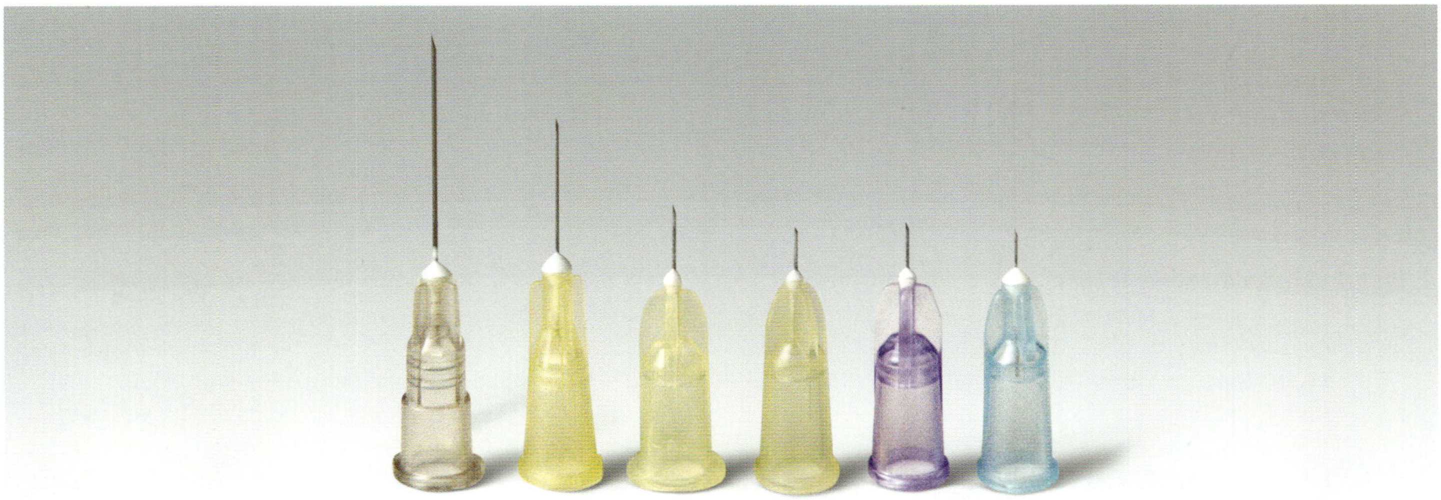

The needles differ in length, diameter and bevel. A suitable format can be selected according to treatment goal and skin characteristics.

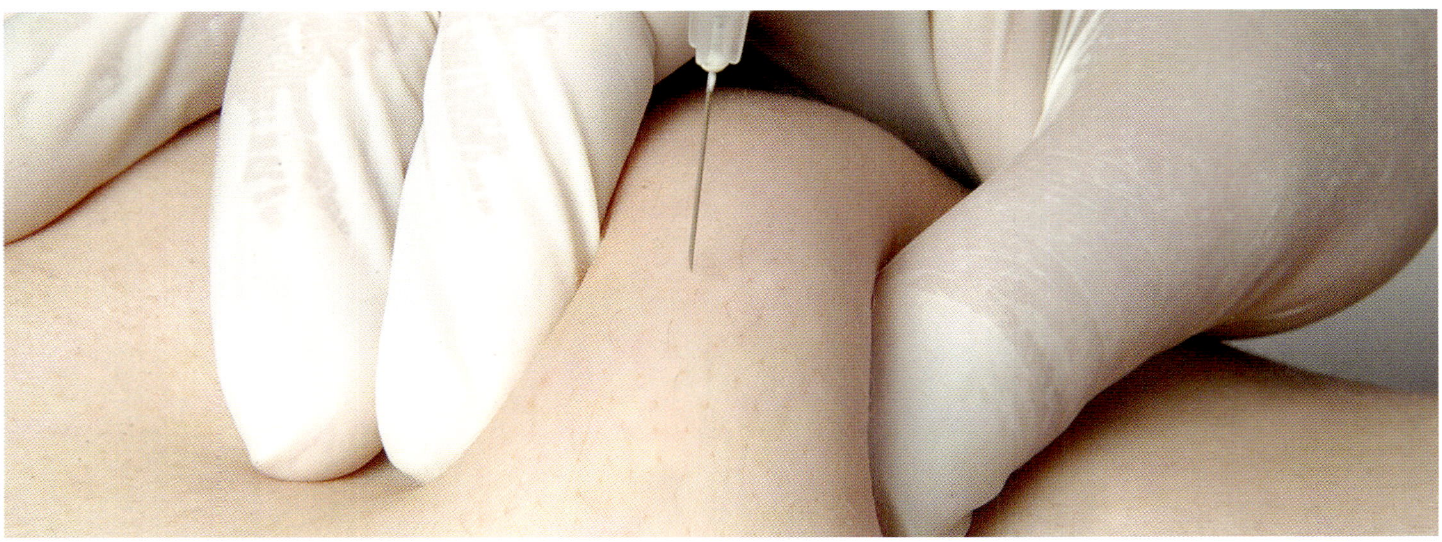

Pinching (raising a fold of skin) prevents injury to the deeper underlying structures, e.g. blood vessels or muscles, and stops unwanted injections into these tissues.

in a standardized and reproducible way; secondly, it prevents unwanted effects caused by a manual injection technique which may be rather short of perfect. However, the key advantage to the patient is that the injections are less painful. The reason for this lies in the speed of the electronically guided injections and in the skin tension maintained by the skin stabilizer. This is particularly important in delicate areas, e.g. in cellulite treatment, on the face (Mesolift) or in patients who are highly sensitive to pain. Furthermore, it is essential to avoid scratches on the face in particular. However, working manually is better for treatments within the brow ridges, on the hands and feet or inside the mouth (periodontosis treatment), because this ensures a better feel in these delicate regions. Apart from that, the general rule is that the luxury of an injector gun should always be offered to private payers. The cocktails used in esthetics are often expensive, and wastage of material should be kept as low as possible. Injectors are also superior to the manual technique in this respect.
The French-made injector *Pistor 4* and its successor *Pistor 5* have become established over a number of years, due to their reliability and versatility. Dr. Pistor was closely involved in their development, and the innovative modifications of the Pistor 5 offer even greater ease of use. The only consumable material required for each treatment is a single sterile, disposable skin stabilizer. Any maintenance or troubleshooting is provided promptly by the French manufacturer. Several compressor-driven devices (e.g. Dermatic 1, U 225 or Mesalyse) are available for large-scale use; these are capable of injecting even undiluted, non-cross-linked HA or large quantities at high pressure, especially in lipolysis.
All these devices must hold a CE certificate in Medical Device Class 2a.

5.2.1 Differences between Pistor 4 and Pistor 5

The Pistor 4 has been developed and refined to produce the Pistor 5, with its new electronic display that can be used to program the individual injection parameters. Syringes of 2 or 5 ml and needles 4 mm in length have been programmed

Pistor 4 information in brief

1. The injection is always directed downwards, so that no fluid can get into the injector. Regularly remove and clean the skin stabilizer mount.
2. Never allow the injector to fall.
3. When inserting the syringe (flaps point outwards), the lever needs to engage gently; it may be moved slightly to help lock it, but it must never be forced.
4. Work only with aqueous or slightly viscous solutions; exactly one drop per "shot" (trigger actuation) must be ejected in nappage mode.
5. When carrying out Mesolift using the epidermal technique (nappage mode), the potentiometer regulates the injection rate. In continuous mode (C), it regulates the dose injected. Starting the gun in C mode at the beginning of the treatment builds up pressure in the syringe, allowing the patency of the needle to be tested at the same time. In rare cases, the needle may be occluded due to a manufacturing fault.
6. To avoid scratch marks when using the epidermal technique and to ensure the correct surface absorption of the active substance, hold the gun at an angle and use the skin stabilizer (without a scale) for adjustment. In this mode, the skin is touched more than penetrated. The resultant liquid droplets must on no account be wiped off. The skin behaves like a sponge, actively absorbing the active substance. Use the Mesoram needle (0.3 x 4 mm) for this purpose. When applying the gun to the skin vertically (with a scale), ensure that your hand moves in step with the gun (i.e. rapid up and down movements).
7. For the lipolysis of smaller fat pads or when treating cellulite with the 4 or 6 mm Mesojet needle or the Microlance needle (0.3 x 13 mm), inject vertically without the skin stabilizer, using the point-by-point technique in C (continuous) mode, setting the potentiometer to maximum.
8. Do not leave the battery in the device for longer periods, e.g. overnight or over the weekend, as it will lose its charge. To ensure slow (complete) charging, remove the battery and plug into the wall power supply. Only use the plug for connecting and disconnecting, i.e. do not pull on the cable.
9. For quick on-the-job charging, plug the injector into the wall power supply with the battery inserted (the green light on the gun and the battery comes on).
10. Release mode: if a syringe jams, the slide bar can be pushed back by simultaneously pressing the On and Release buttons.

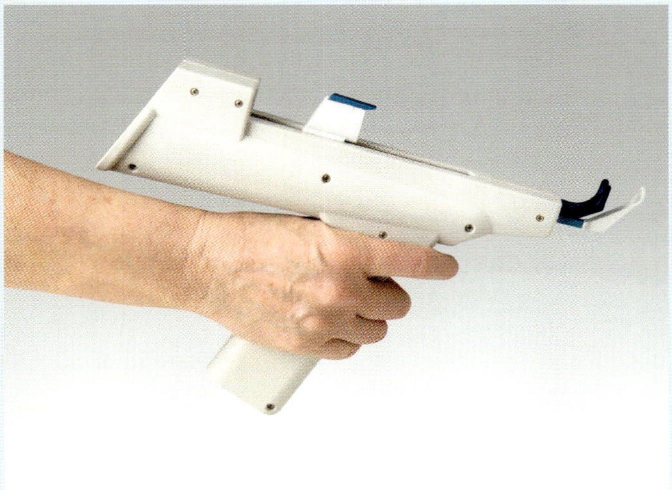

The Pistor injectors are light, allowing smooth, strain-free operation.

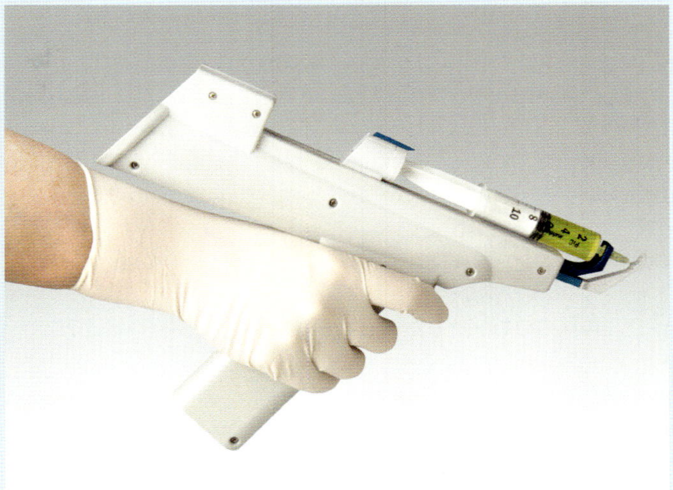

To build up pressure in the syringe, always start in continuous (C) mode, until the first few drops emerge.

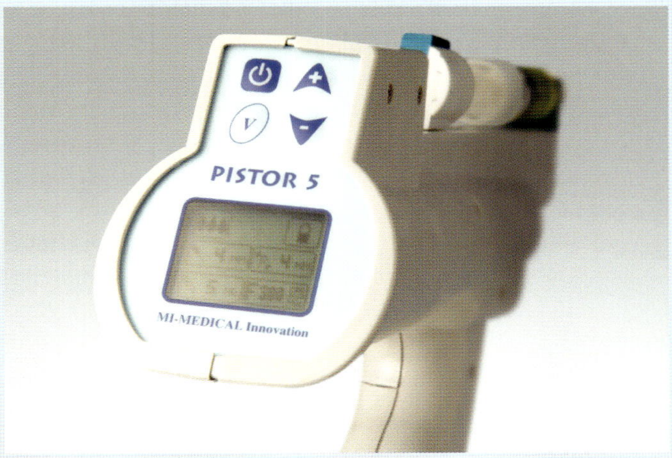

The electronic display of the Pistor 5 in nappage (gust) mode.

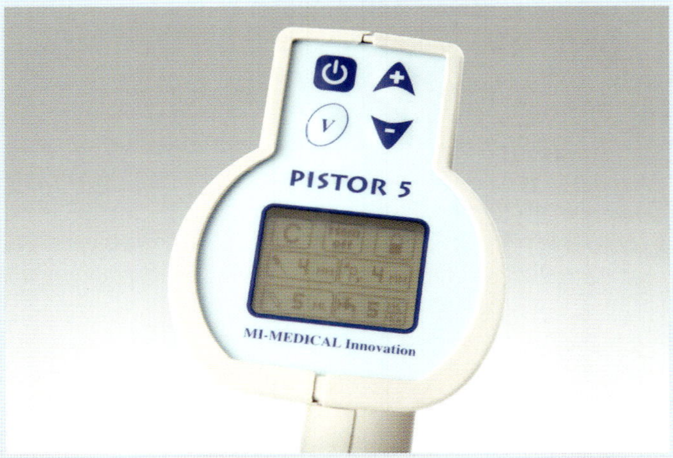

The electronic display of the Pistor 5 in continuous mode

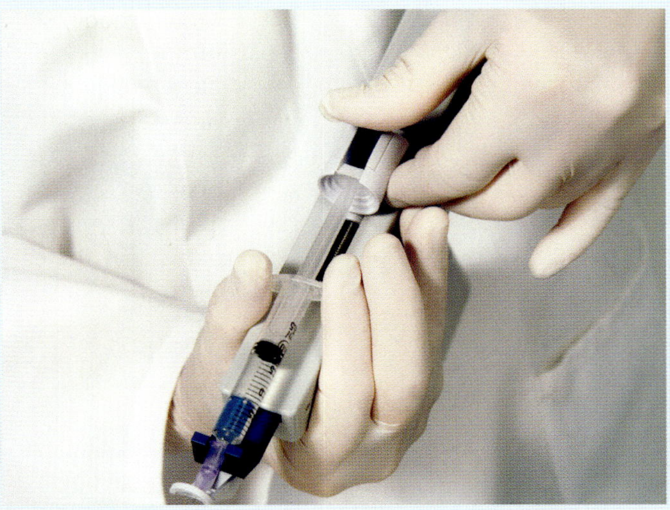

How to position the hands when inserting the syringe

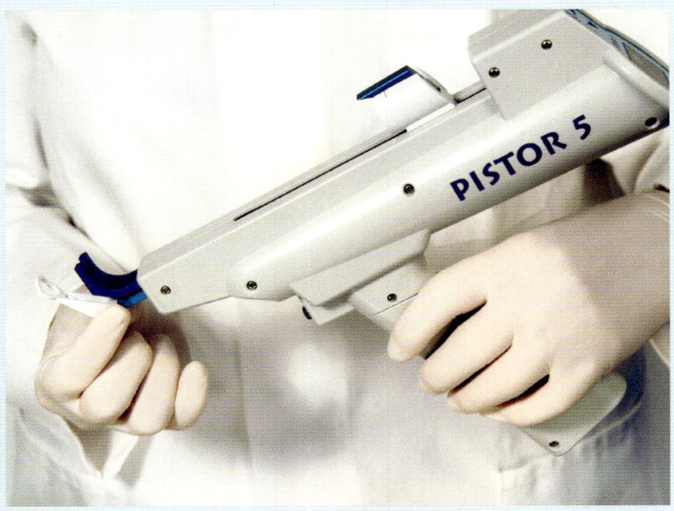

Fitting the skin stabilizer

in for the standard setting. The pressure is built up on continuous mode (C) and the injector then switched to nappage mode for Mesolift. The maximum rate is 300 injections per minute. For infiltration treatments, the machine is left in C mode, which allows parameters such as the injection depth or flow rate to be set. The Pistor 5 is much lighter and quieter to use and also has considerably improved battery technology.

5.3 Mesotherapy injection techniques

Injection techniques in mesotherapy differ from other techniques, and their practical application must therefore be learned. The injections are given either manually or with injector guns; the latter should be given preference, particularly for use on the face in Mesolift. The angle of entry of the needle determines the penetration depth. In Mesolift, the skin is merely touched, and the skin stabilizer used only as a visual guide. If the skin stabilizer is fitted vertically, it will not be possible to use the nappage technique, but only one-by-one injections or infiltrations.
Linear or round multi-injectors or Dermojet® devices (in which the liquid is shot into the skin with the aid of compressed air) must never be used in mesotherapy. Work only with sterile, single-use materials.

5.3.1 Intracutaneous injection (depth of injection ≤ 1 mm)

Doses of ≥ 0.1 ml produce a welt (see Figure). Welts cause pain due to overstretching of the epidermal skin layers. They take several hours to several days to subside fully.

5.3.2 Epidermal injection (depth of injection ≤ 1 mm)

In the epidermal "dragging" or point-by-point technique, doses of only 0.01 ml (single drops) are applied per injection, i.e. no welts appear.
The ultrafine Mesorelle needle makes it possible to administer almost painless injections and it is used particularly on fine, sensitive skin areas, e.g. lips, skin around the eyes, fingers and feet. In sensitive individuals, it is also the preferred needle for Mesolift of the face and neck/cleavage region.
In the epidermal dragging technique, the needle (a BD Microlance 13 mm in length is best) is only dragged across the skin with a quivering, "Parkinsonian", linear movement. The elastic oscillations of the needle are exploited when doing so. This filigree-like technique allows quick coverage of larger areas.
The network-like distribution of injections is another option. This results in a long-term effect of the active substances, e.g. in cellulite treatment or Mesolift.

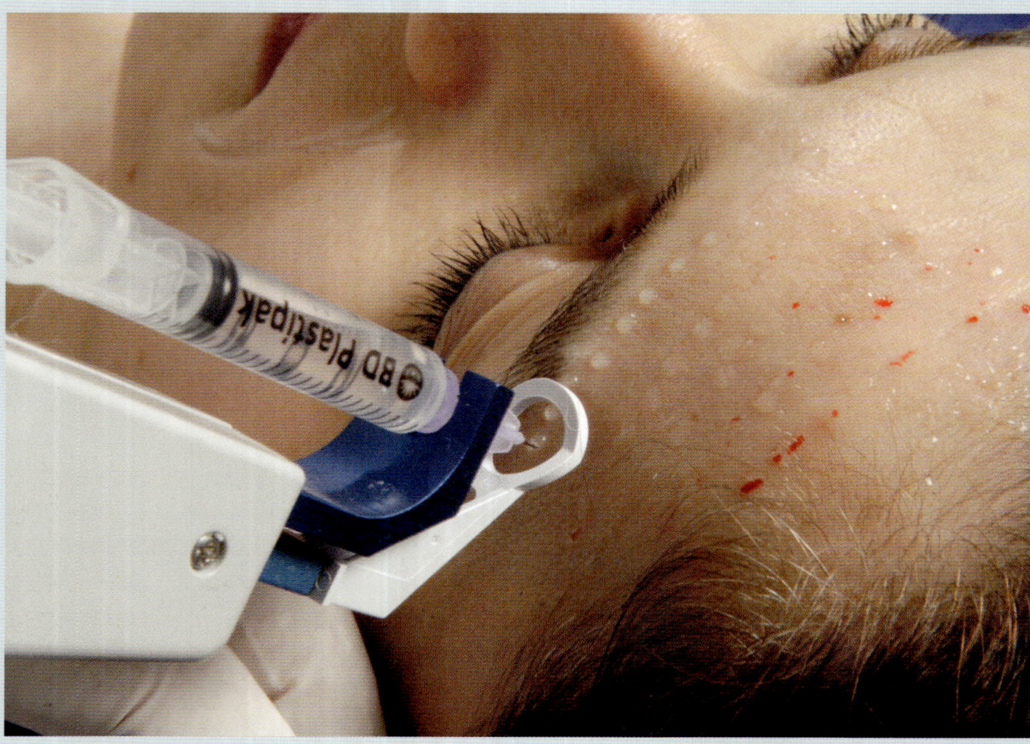

Epidermal mesotherapy injection technique using an injector gun: the fine droplets are actively absorbed by the skin and disappear within minutes.

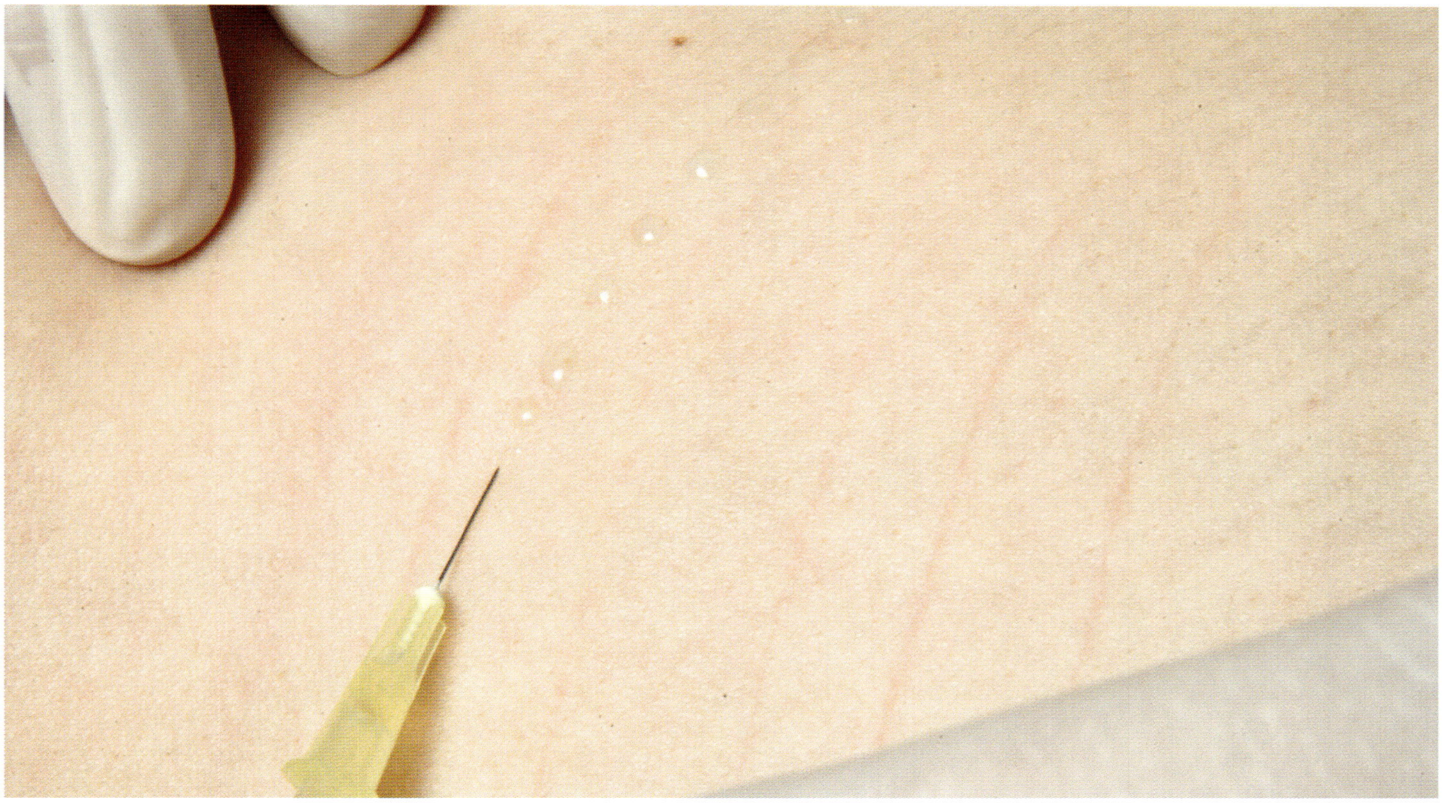

Manual epidermal technique: the needle is stroked across the skin with very little downward pressure. An even pressure on the plunger applies the liquid uniformly, drop by drop.

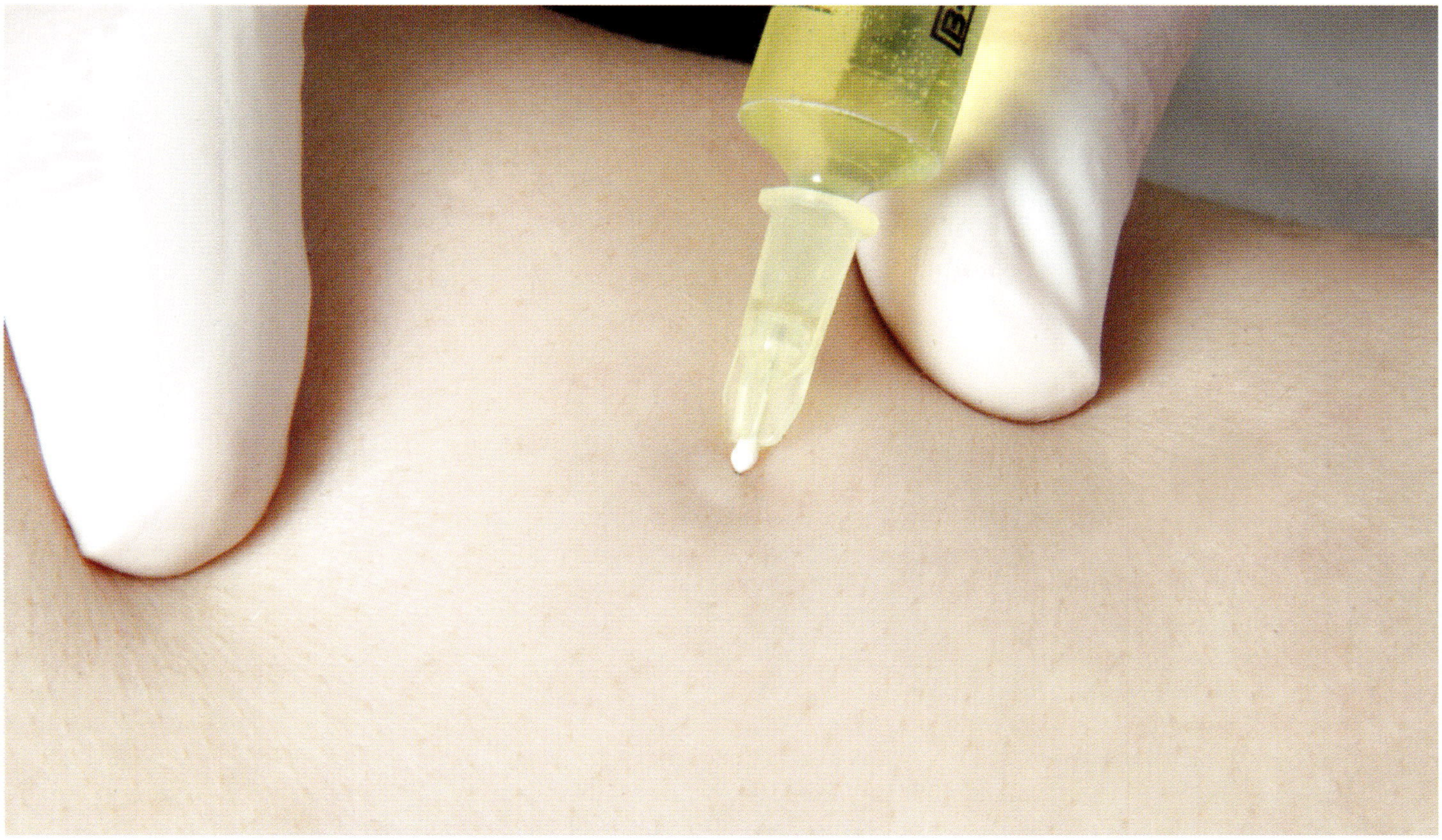

The welt represents a superficial skin depot. Active substance transport away from the welt takes place slowly by diffusion.

Injection techniques		
Technique	**Depth**	**Characteristics**
Epidermal technique	≤ 1 mm	Painless, no blood, large areas, skin stimulation, long-lasting effect, slow diffusion. Important e.g. when using non-cross-linked HA
Nappage	1–4 mm	Superficial to deep dermis, quick and linear injections, volume ≤0.1 ml (single droplets). Distance a few mm
Serial	2–4 mm	Point-by-point technique, as well as targeted delivery to acupuncture points, quick-acting, but also rapid diffusion, volume < 0.2 ml. Distance 5–10 mm
Infiltration	≥ 4 mm	Subcutaneous, higher volumes can be delivered, though these can have a systemic effect. One-by-one injection technique, but a local depot is created by larger volumes (≥0.2 ml). Distance 5–10 mm
Mixed technique		Combination of superficial and deep techniques in the same session and the same zone

The angle of entry of the needle should be almost tangential and the pressure on the plunger gentle but continuous. There should be no bleeding, as this would mean that the needle has already penetrated too deep into the skin. This injection technique is not painful.

The bevel of the needle should always face *upwards*. The droplets of liquid lying on the skin are not removed; instead, the skin is given time to absorb them. The skin is like a sponge. It actively absorbs the active substances if given time to do so. This means that there is no wastage of these expensive mixtures.

When working with electronic injectors in nappage mode, they are held at a slight angle, with the injection always directed downwards. Whether using a manual or assisted technique, the skin should always be held tightly stretched with the other, free hand. This also helps greatly to ensure non-traumatic application with minimum pain.

5.3.3 Intradermal injection (depth of injection ≥ 1 mm)

Intradermal injections are also given with the 4-mm needle, injecting to a depth of 1 to 4 mm, as required. The volume per injection is 0.1 to 0.2 ml; larger volumes are painful as they cause overexpansion of the tissue. Here, we talk of serial injections or the nappage technique, i.e. multiple injections are given linearly, one after the other, e.g. to treat hair loss or in Mesobotox. The quicker the work, the less pain it causes. Mesojet 6-mm needles can also be used for deep intradermal injections delivered to the body, e.g. for cellulite treatment. Here, the special needle bevel considerably reduces the risk of bleeding and hematoma. However, because of the higher skin resistance, the Mesojet needles should only be used in injector-assisted treatment.

In regions with thin, delicate skin, such as the face and neck, injecting to a depth of 4 mm would mean the needle reaching the subcutis or even bone or a blood vessel. Therefore, the angle of entry and the depth of injection need to be adjusted to local requirements. Another option is to pinch the skin with the free hand and to inject into the resultant roll. Doing so avoids injuries to deeper underlying structures. This technique is also used in creating "tension columns" in the skin to increase traction forces in Mesolift, injecting volumes of up to 0.5 ml per point.

The deeper techniques sometimes produce visible bleeding on the skin, which requires immediate compression. If this is not done, some patients may be disfigured by hematomas for days. These carry the risk of permanent pigmentation, particularly in non-white patients. It is also essential to remember never to inject into an existing hematoma.

5.3.4 Subcutaneous injection

In lipolysis in particular, the compound is administered in the form of deep infiltration, also at a rate of 0.5 ml per point. The target structure here is the adipose connective tissue. Injecting into muscles or tendons must be strictly avoided. When using injectors, the work should be done in C mode. When injecting manually, the syringe plunger should be depressed with the palm, for better ergonomics.

The depth of injection and the angle of entry determine the length of time that the active substance remains in the skin: the shallower the injection, the longer the agent's residence time (for a prolonged effect) and, the deeper the in-

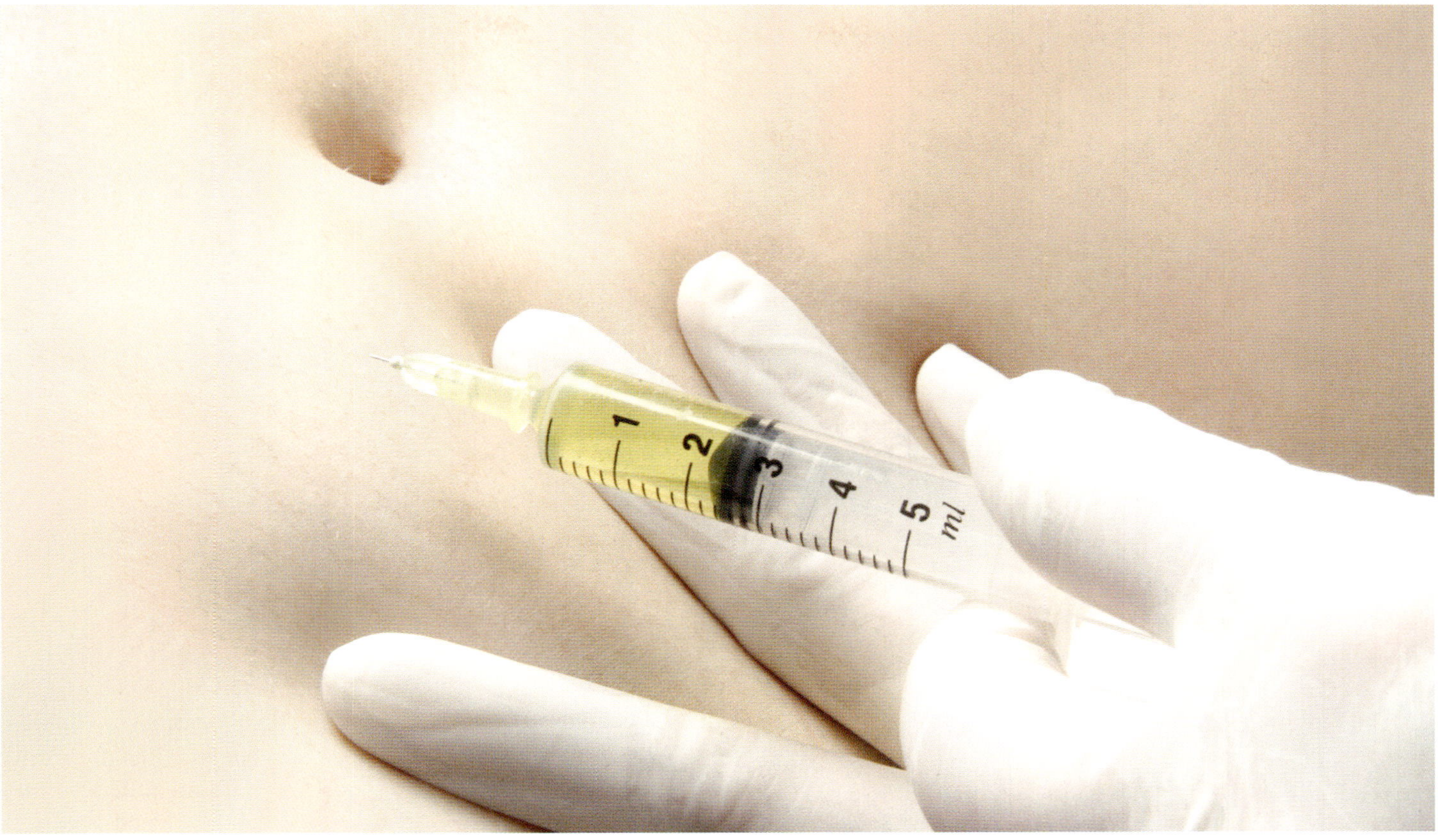

Intradermal injection with an angle of entry of 45 degrees

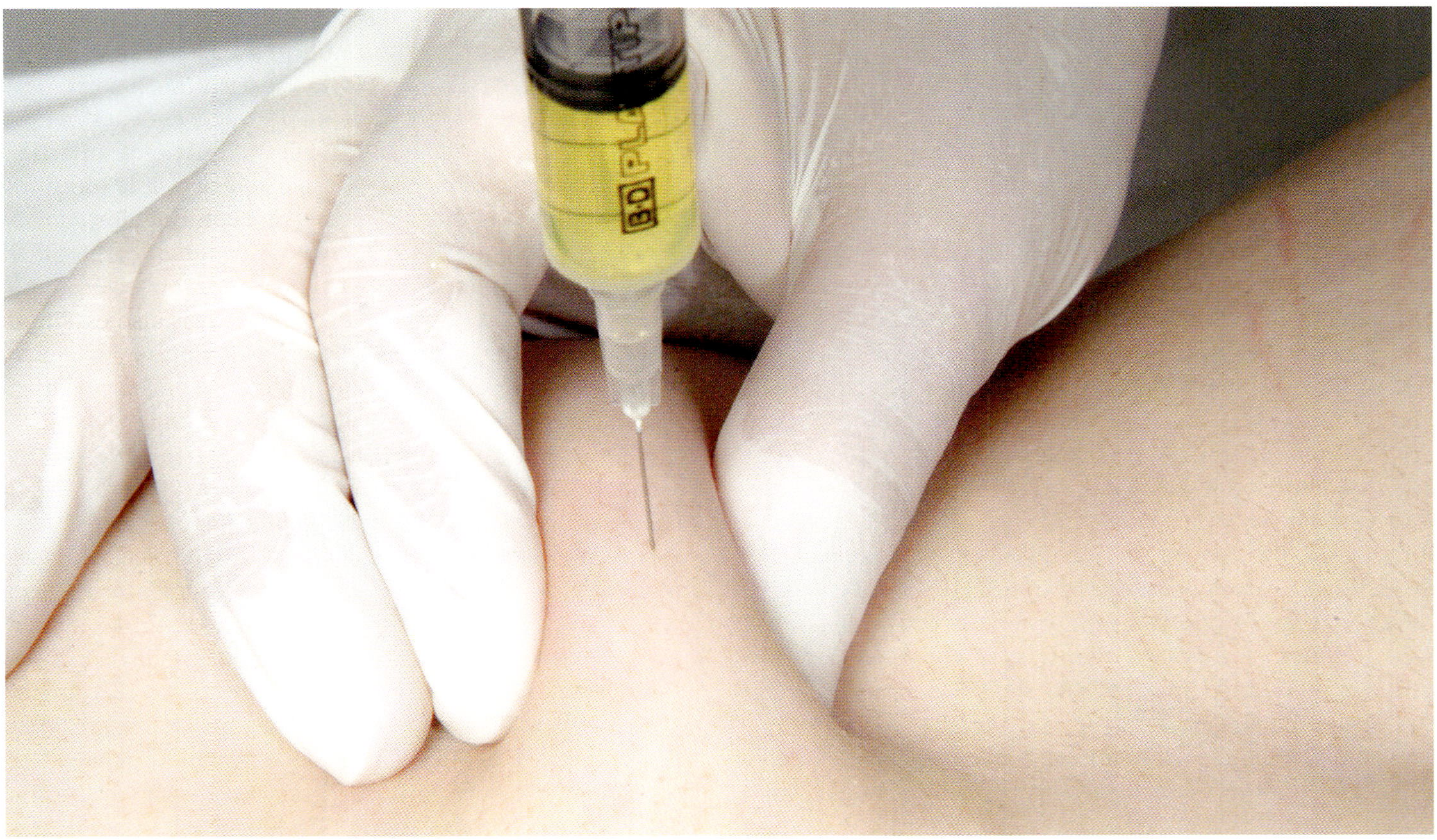

Subcutaneous injection with an angle of entry of 90 degrees

Schematic diagram showing mesotherapy injection techniques and depths

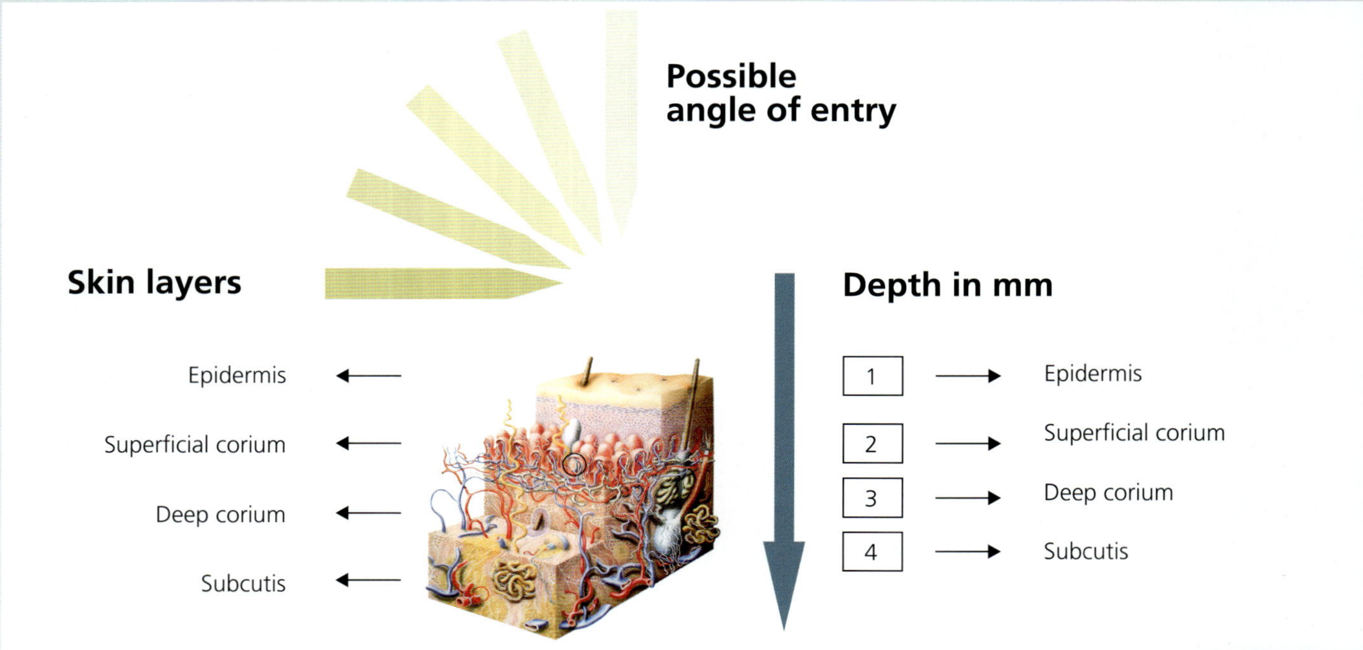

Angles of entry from tangential to vertical: the angle of entry and the depth of injection determine the active substances' residence times in the skin.

jection, the more quickly the substance is transported away from the administration site.

The skin's anatomy and physiology form the basis for the effects of mesotherapy.

The *epidermis* consists of a hydrolipid protective film with a pH of 5.0–5.9, topped by a physiological bacterial layer, which is not destroyed fully even by the most thorough cleansing. The skin-lipid barrier lies below this, made up of keratinocytes built up into a multi-layered squamous epithelium. The basal membrane contains the immune system's Langerhans cells, together with the melanocytes, responsible for the body's own protection from sunlight. Pressure receptors, hair follicles, sebaceous glands, nerve endings, small skin muscles and a network of capillaries are all embedded in the matrix of the *corium*. At its junction with the subcutis, there are vibration and heat receptors, blood and lymph vessels, sweat glands, nerves and, deeper down, an increasing amount of adipose connective tissue. The most important physiological functions of the skin are microcirculation, neurovegetative regulation, immune defense and the molecular sieve function of the extracellular matrix.

The epidermis and corium are separated by the basal membrane. The cell layers of the stratum germinativum show the highest level of biological activity. They are the target area for Mesolift. The skin's basal membrane represents the boundary between the inside and outside of the body, between blood-perfused and non-perfused tissue.

It is well known that this natural skin barrier represents a distinct boundary for all skincare products and treatments by the beautician. Penetration of the skin's basal membrane, paving the way to more intensive and, indeed, medical effects, is the sole preserve of healthcare professionals. This applies equally to mesotherapy, HA filler treatments and micro-needling (e.g. with the Dermaroller™).

In micro-needling, numerous micro-wounds are produced on the skin by highly invasive means, a procedure which can trigger side-effects in some cases. In the 1950s, this purely mechanical process, involving multiple, dry punctures in the skin, was already described by Pistor as "Mesothérapie sèche". Its esthetic benefit comes from the wound healing processes and the stimulation of the dermis, and is manifested as collagen and elastin induction after six weeks. The Fraxel® laser works on a similar principle, so that people describe mesotherapy as having a *fraxel-like effect*. However, the additional administration of pharmacologically defined preparations into the skin brings added benefits. The successes which have been achieved with the Mesolift methods have led to interested parties advertising the totally different method of electroporation as mesotherapy or Mesolift.

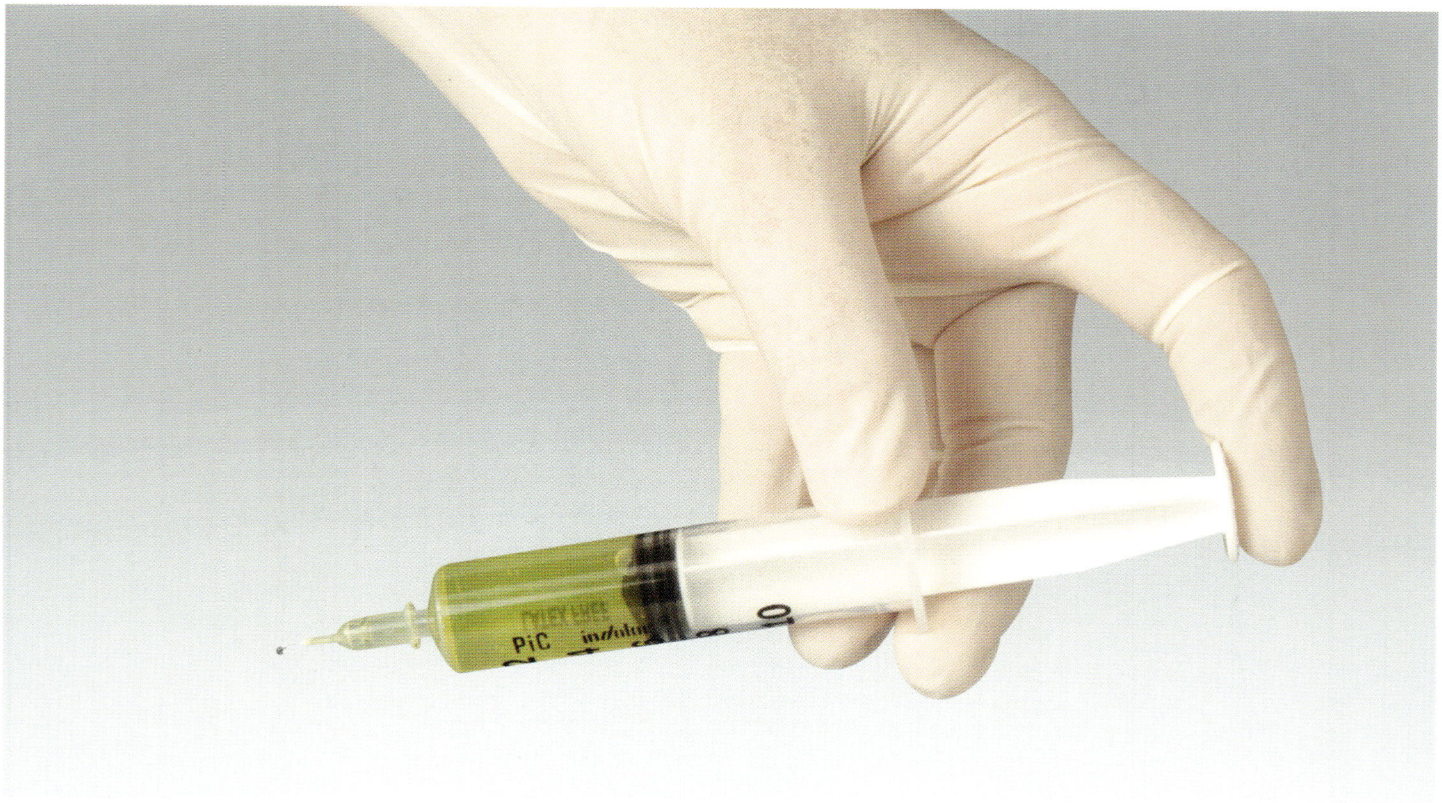

Retrograde tracing technique (nappage, epidermal technique): gentle pressure on the plunger with the index finger; linear hand movement.

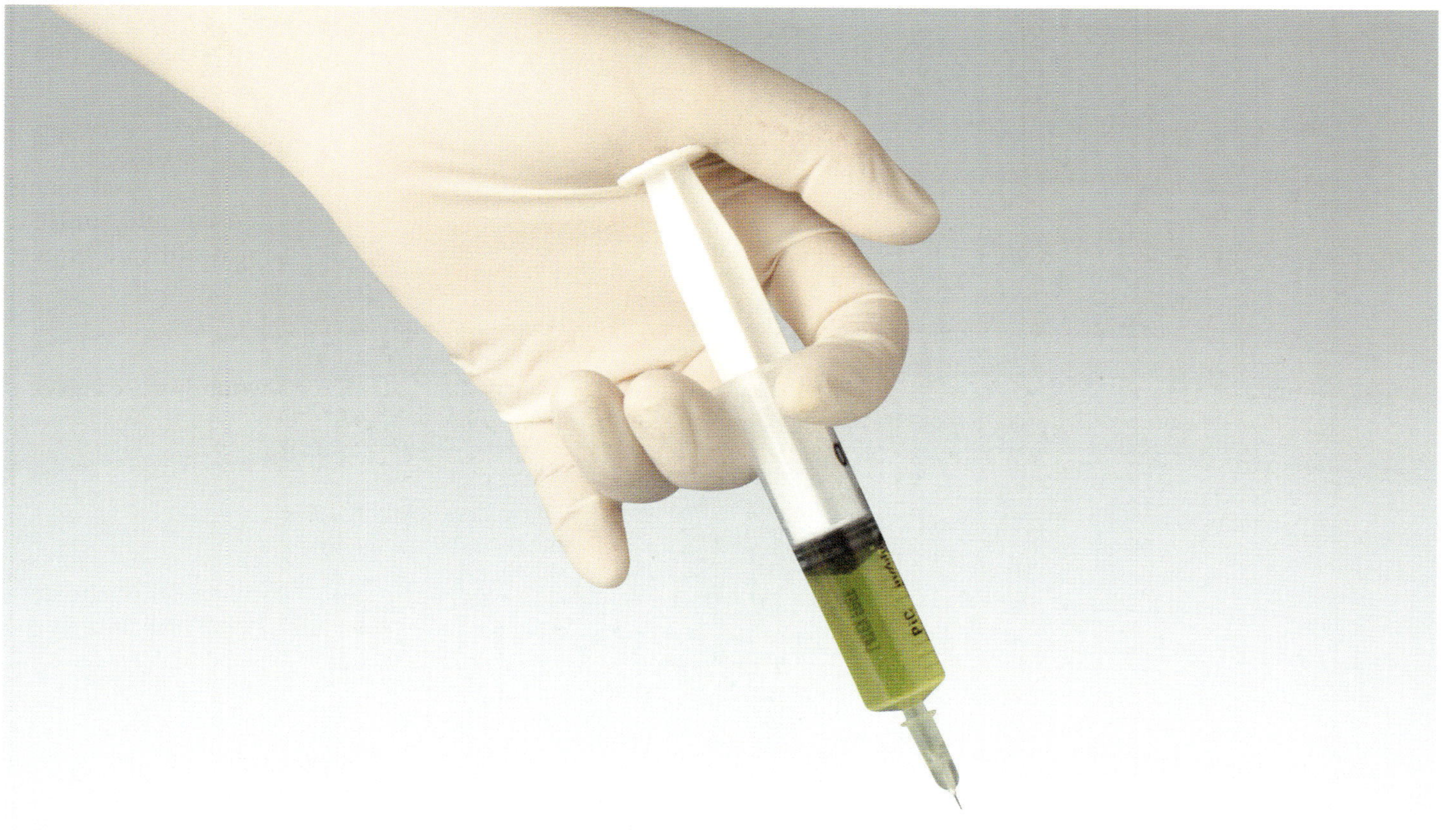

Series of infiltrations using the one-by-one injection technique: firmer pressure is applied to the plunger using the thenar eminence or palm.

Selection factors: which technique to use?

The choice of injection technique in each case depends on the following factors:

- Location
- Indication
- Specific pathology of the tissue being treated
- Active substances used
- Condition of the skin
- Age, medical history and the patient's individual sensitivity.

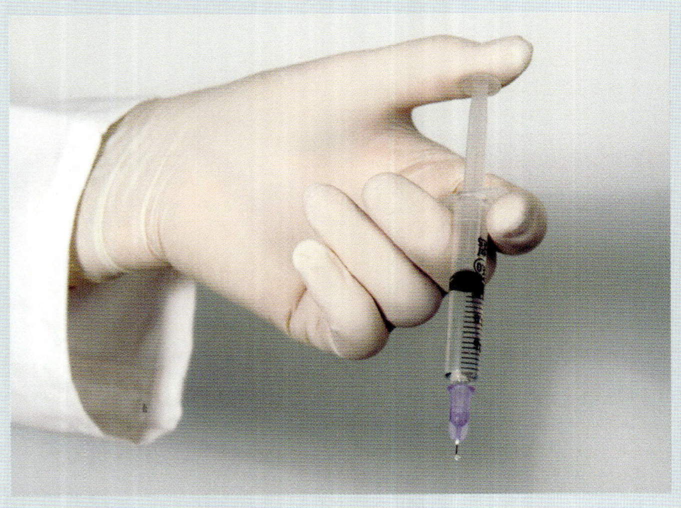

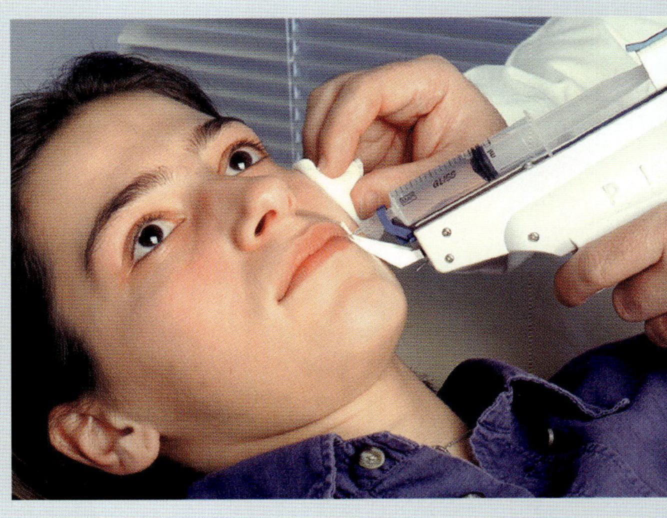

Technique – administering the injections:

1. Nappage (network-like distribution, for larger areas)
2. Series (single injections, inject for c. 1 sec)
3. Infiltration (inject for c. 3 sec per injection)
4. Mesoperfusion (with electronic devices only)

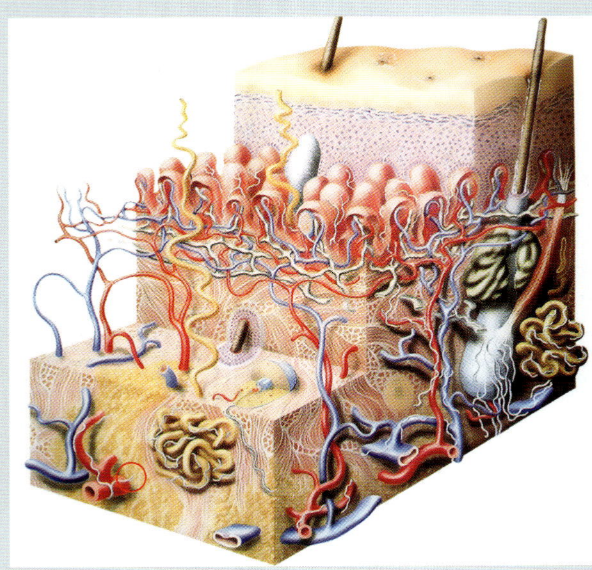

	Uses (indications)
1 mm	Mesolift, Mesoglow, Mesodrain
2 mm	Nappage, salve, cellulite, mesobotox
3 mm	Intradermal mesotherapy, cellulite, hair loss, stretch marks
4 mm	Mesoperfusion, creating "tension columns" (Mesolift), cellulite
5 mm to 15 mm	local fat pads, lipolysis

6 The consultation

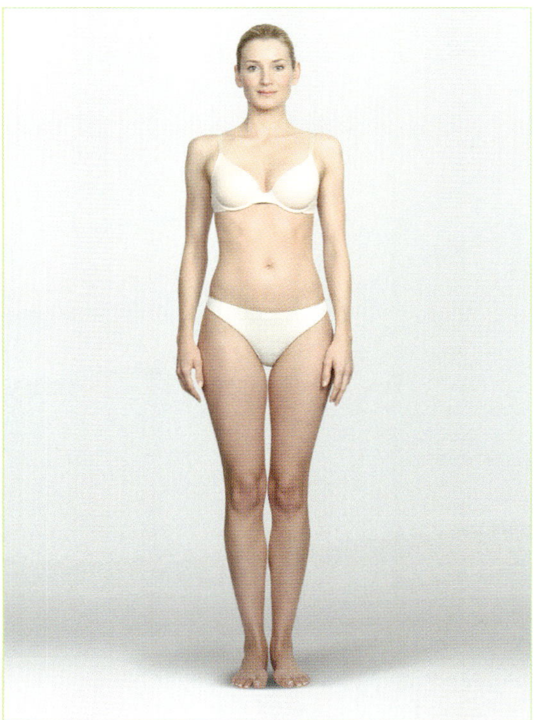

Examples of observation criteria include facial contours, fat distribution, the structure of the facial expression lines, any asymmetry, etc.

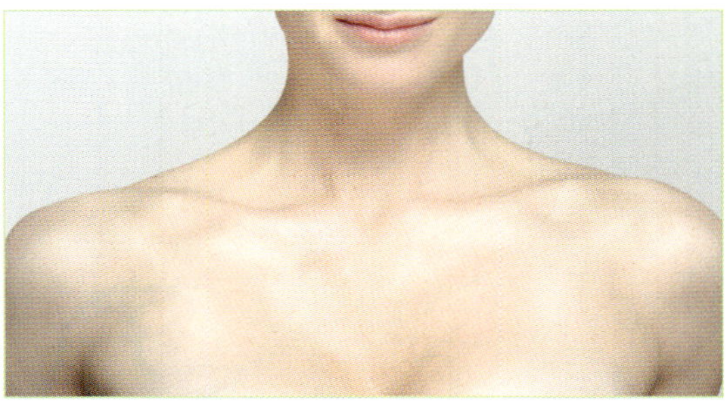

When inspecting and examining the patient, just as much attention should be paid to facial expression and body posture as to overall visual impression, for example of the neck and cleavage region.

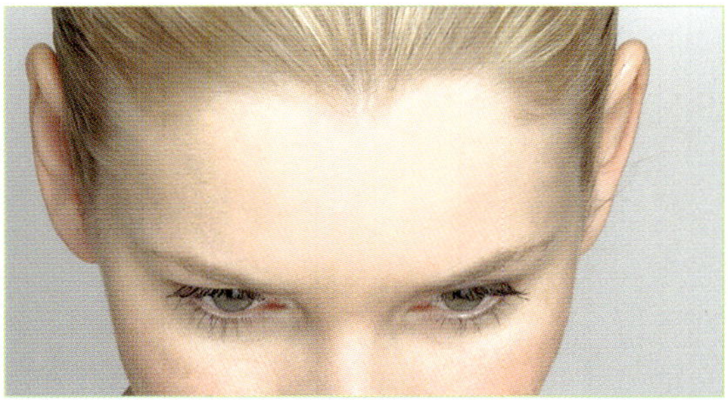

When assessing the status of the hair, it is particularly important to determine the type of hair loss: is it diffuse, androgenetic or autoimmune?

The consultation

6.1 History, inspection, palpation, marking the skin

When taking the patient's history, it is very important not only to include the usual medical history, but also the patient's particular esthetic history. Unfortunately, any previous treatments are often not documented in a cosmetic record, so that they must be actively elicited from the patient and recorded in writing. Duplication can be avoided if certain diagnostic procedures or laboratory tests have already taken place. Particular importance must be placed on determining if the patient is pregnant, on allergies or drug intolerances, and on any medicines or food supplements the patient may be taking. Thus, for example, aspirin or enzyme products can considerably increase an individual's predisposition to hemorrhages. Oral anticoagulant therapy is not necessarily an obstacle to mesotherapy, but the treatments should be limited to superficial techniques. An adverse family history, autoimmune disorders, HIV, hepatitis or herpes infection should also be considered in the consultation.

For body modeling treatments, it will be necessary to record height and baseline weight, as changes in weight have appreciable effects on the treatment outcome. Current BMI is a key factor in the therapeutic strategy, which should include clarification as to whether a local treatment is to be carried out alone or in combination with weight loss measures. The local treatment may help the patient achieve her desire to lose weight in her specific problem zone, rather than in the face or breasts.

$$\text{BMI} = \frac{\text{body weight}}{(\text{height in m})^2}$$

BMI 20–25	Normal weight	
BMI 25– 30	**Grade I**: overweight	Must be treated if there is high blood pressure, diabetes, osteoarthritis or an elevated cholesterol level
BMI 30–40	**Grade II**: obesity	Grade 2 and 3 must be treated (increased risk of diabetes and heart disease)
BMI more than 40	**Grade III**: severe obesity	

When inspecting and examining the patient, just as much attention should be paid to facial expression and body posture as to overall visual impression. The state and consistency of the skin, connective and adipose tissue and hair must be ascertained. This is followed by an assessment of skin type, perfusion status and any pathological changes. In some cases, there may be some prior damage, e.g. as a result of previously used permanent fillers. Dysmorphophobia (dysmorphic body disorder) may be present in a small percentage of cases, and the physician should be familiar with this syndrome. It is a false, psychopathological perception of one's own body. An esthetically successful treatment comprises all the aspects discussed above, and the better the patient selection process, the choice and the combination of the required measures, the more convincing the eventual treatment outcome will be.

6.1.1 Observation criteria

Face, frontal view

- Face shape and asymmetries
- Facial contours and fat distribution
- Assessment of structural and facial expression lines
- Skin quality, skin color
- Hairline and hair structure
- Is treatment of the neck and/or cleavage also necessary?
- Degree of elastosis
- Assessment of the hairline and hair structure.

Face, side view, profile

- Assessment of the profile
- Structural and facial expression lines
- Fat distribution
- Contours, particularly the transition between chin and neck (double chin, sagging?).

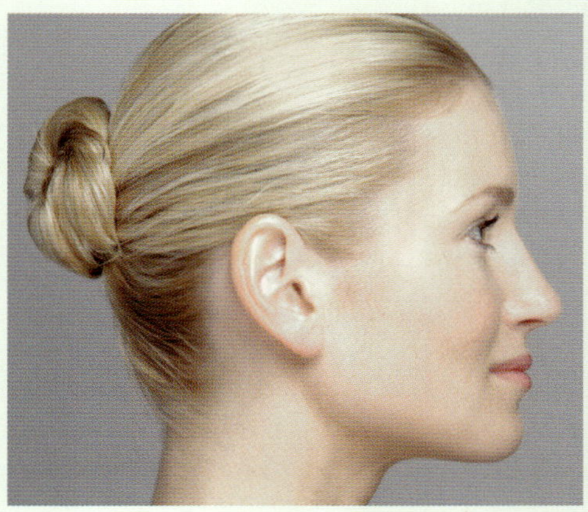

The blurred contours of the mandibular line and the transition between chin and neck only show up in profile.

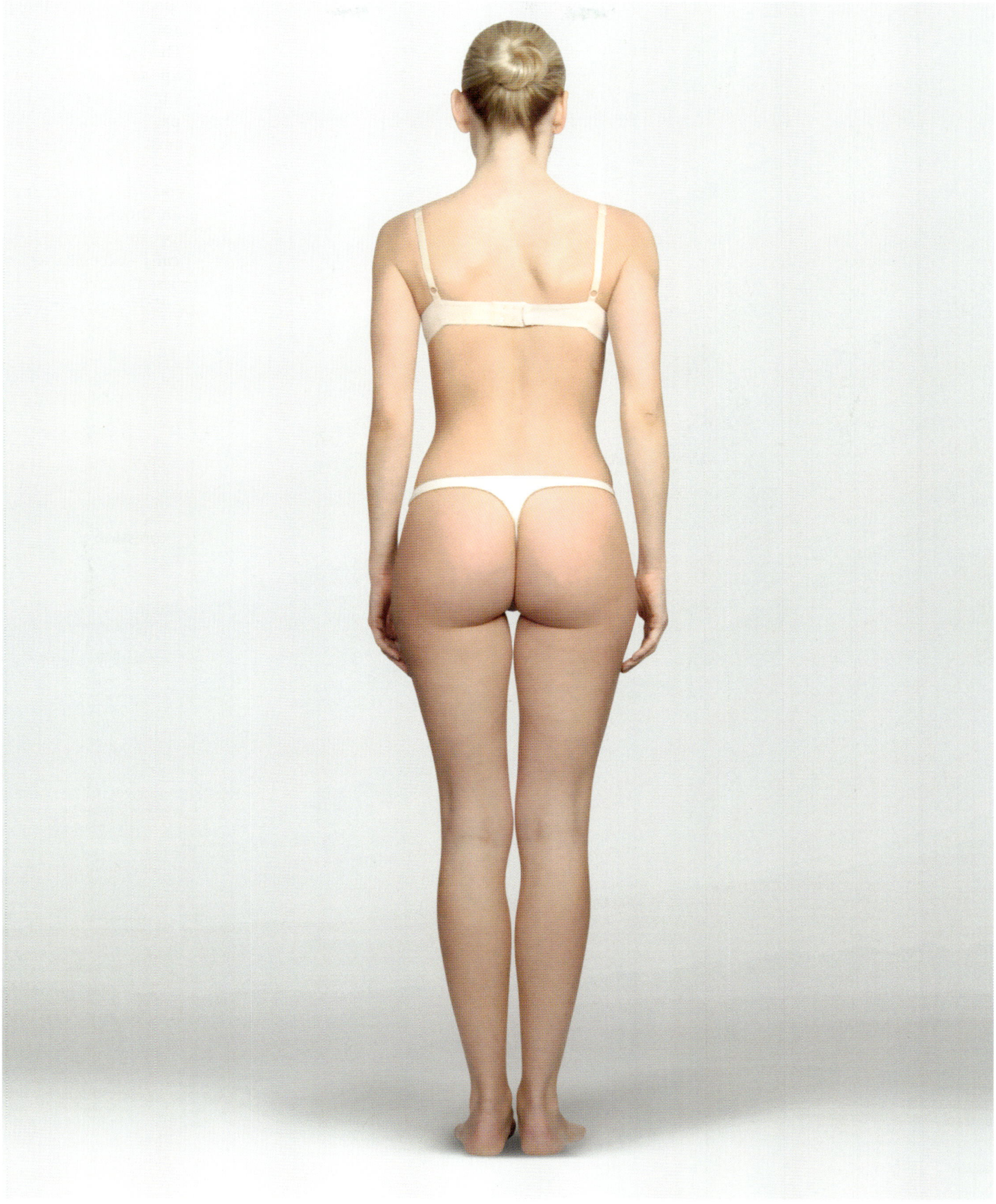

In the whole-body inspection, the zones to be treated are determined (with the patient standing) and the skin then marked (with the patient lying down) for the subsequent treatment.

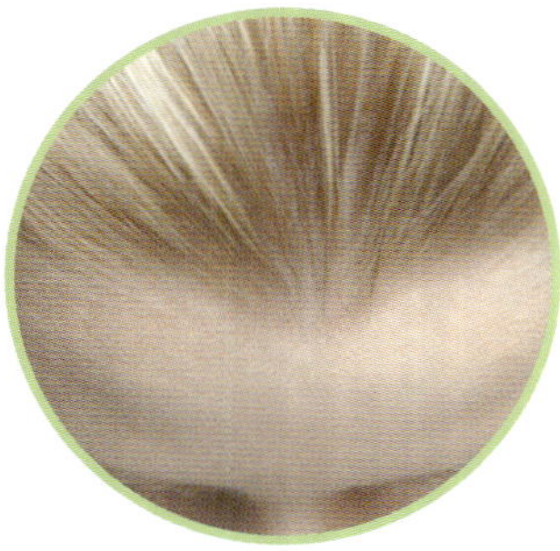

1 Hairline

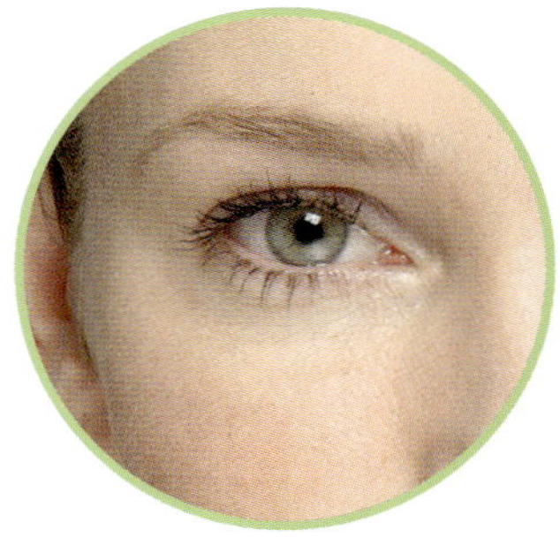

2 Eye region

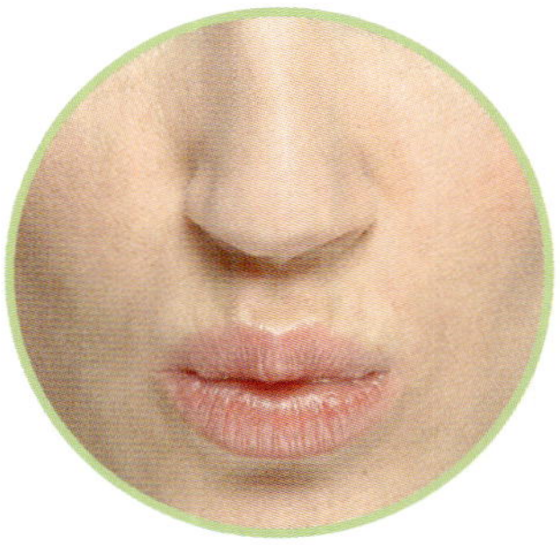

3 Lines around
the mouth

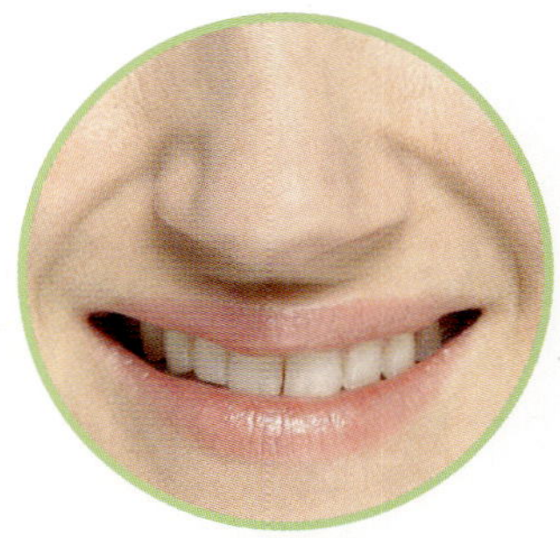

4 Nasolabial lines

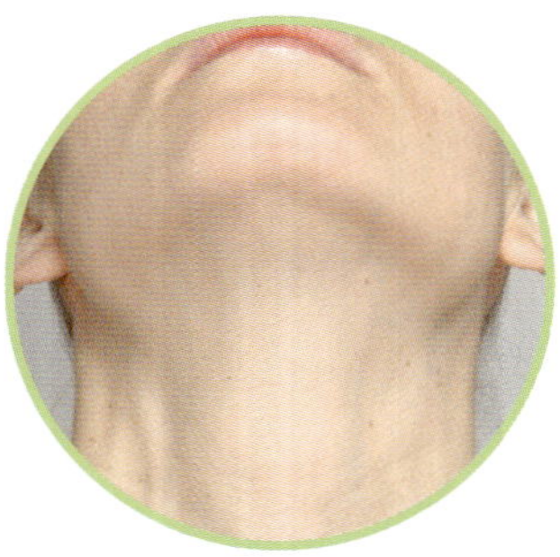

5 Chin

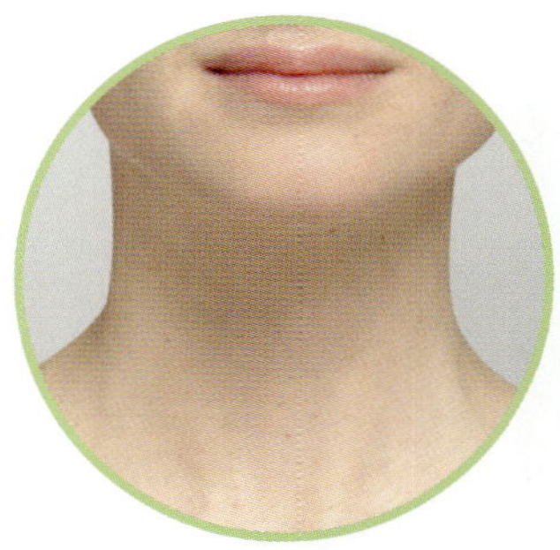

6 Neck

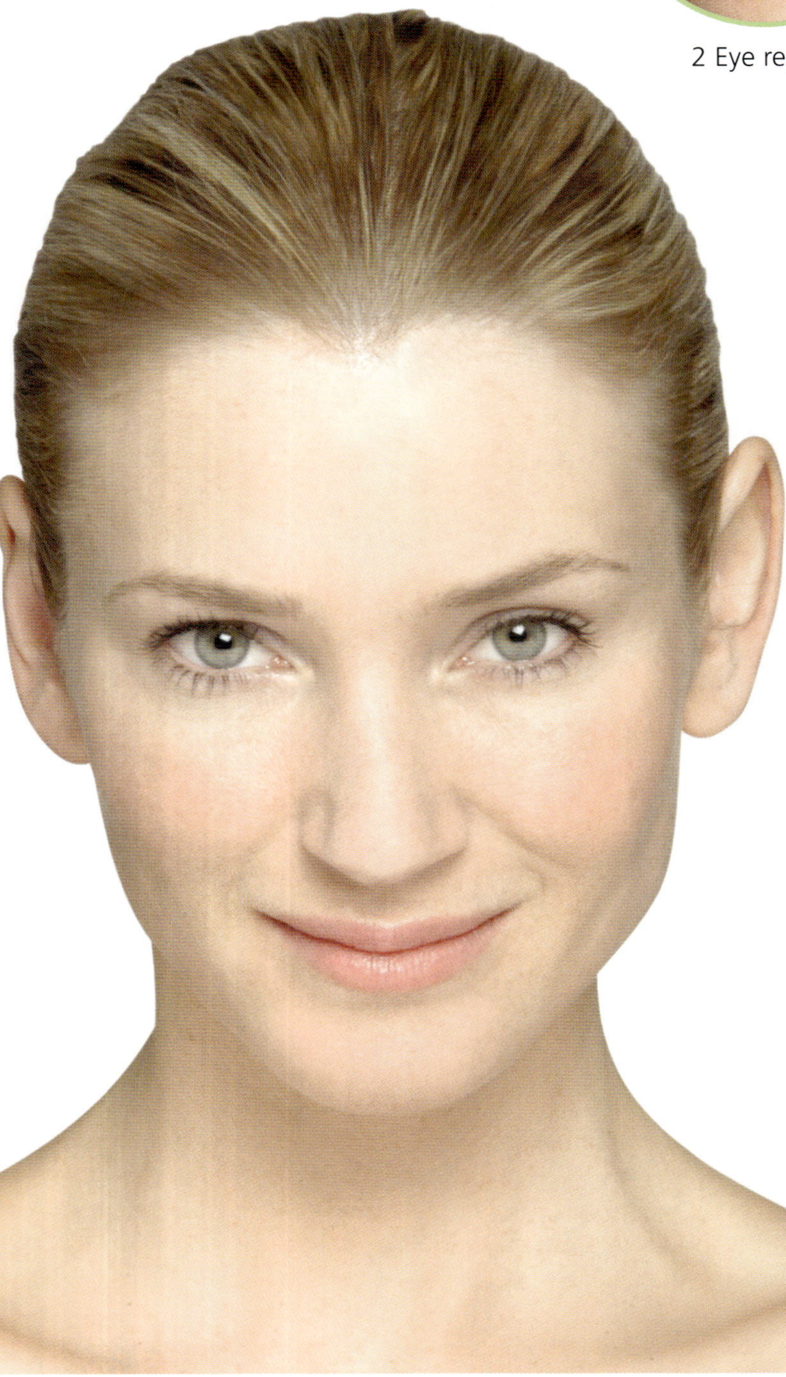

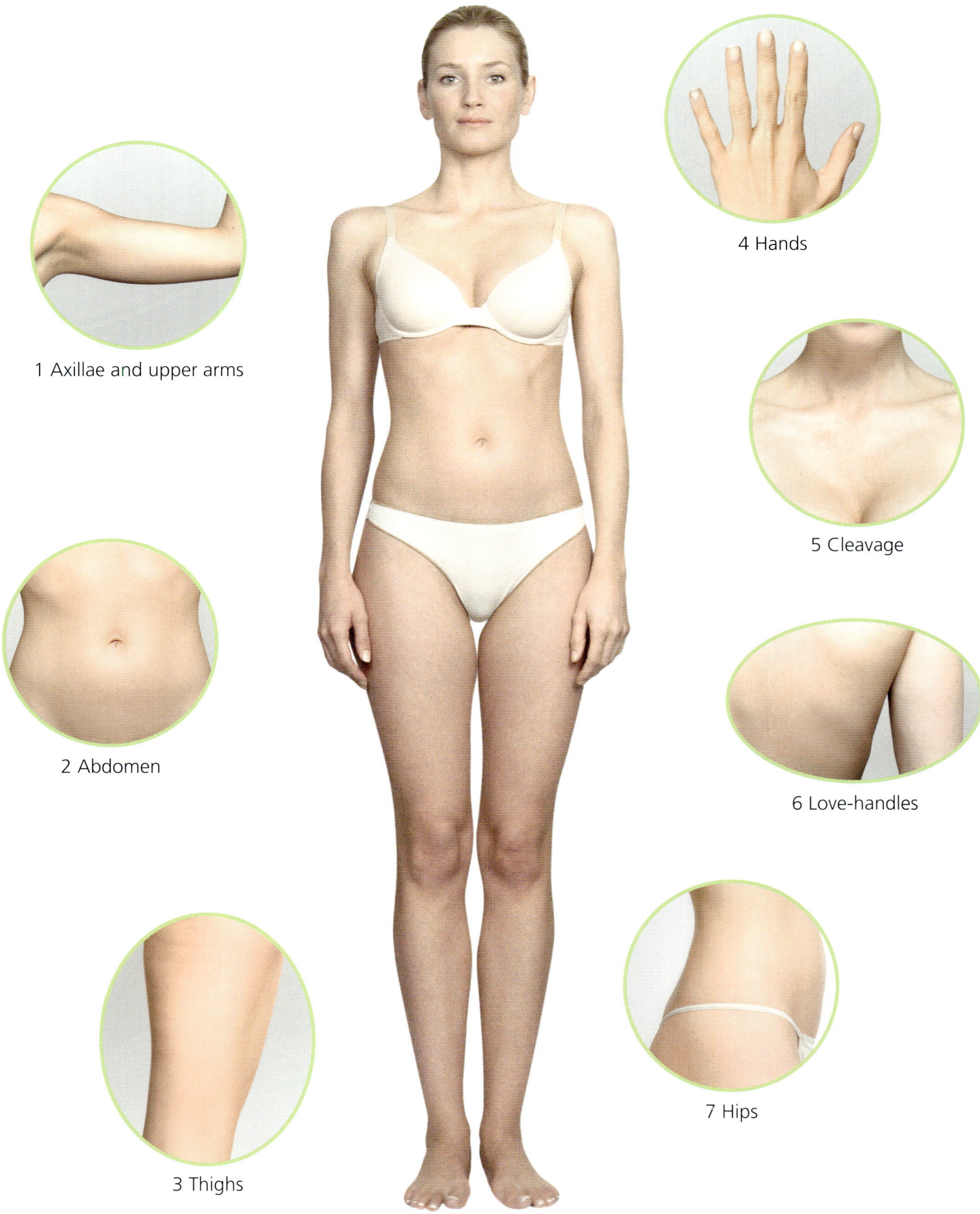

Overview: treatment areas on the body

Body, overall view, front, back, side views
- Evaluation of posture and musculature
- Fat distribution, metabolic or gynoid type
- Skin quality
- Adipose and connective tissue quality
- Venolymphatic insufficiency in the legs?

6.1.2 Key points of the first consultation

- Take your time
- Document everything
- Explain the alternatives (example: lipolysis or liposuction, Mesolift or facelift)
- Examine the patient and then summarize the results of the examination
- If necessary, draw up a global therapy concept (coaching, lifestyle counseling)
- Find a consensus – and motivate the patient!

6.1.3 Marking

It is often necessary to mark the area to be treated by drawing on the skin. The patient can also follow this process visually. Hand-held and/or wall-mounted mirrors are very helpful for this. The body's anatomy changes considerably with every change in posture. Marking is carried out with the patient sitting (face) or standing (body), as the effects of gravity become apparent in these positions. Facial structures (lines, too much or too little volume) are best evaluated with the face tilted forwards slightly. A white eye-liner pencil should be used to draw on the skin, to avoid causing persistent dark marks. Before doing so, the skin should be disinfected and anesthetic cream applied, if necessary.

6.2 Objectivization and documentation

As with any medical treatment, everything needs to be carefully documented in the patient's file. Apart from documenting the history and examination findings, the therapist needs to make an accurate record of the treatments provided (location, material or active substance mixture, injection technique).
At the first consultation, the baseline status is documented by means of a description, photographs (frontal and profile, target zone), measurements (manually with measuring tapes, rulers and gauges, or using special instruments, if available). This allows the treatment results to be verified.

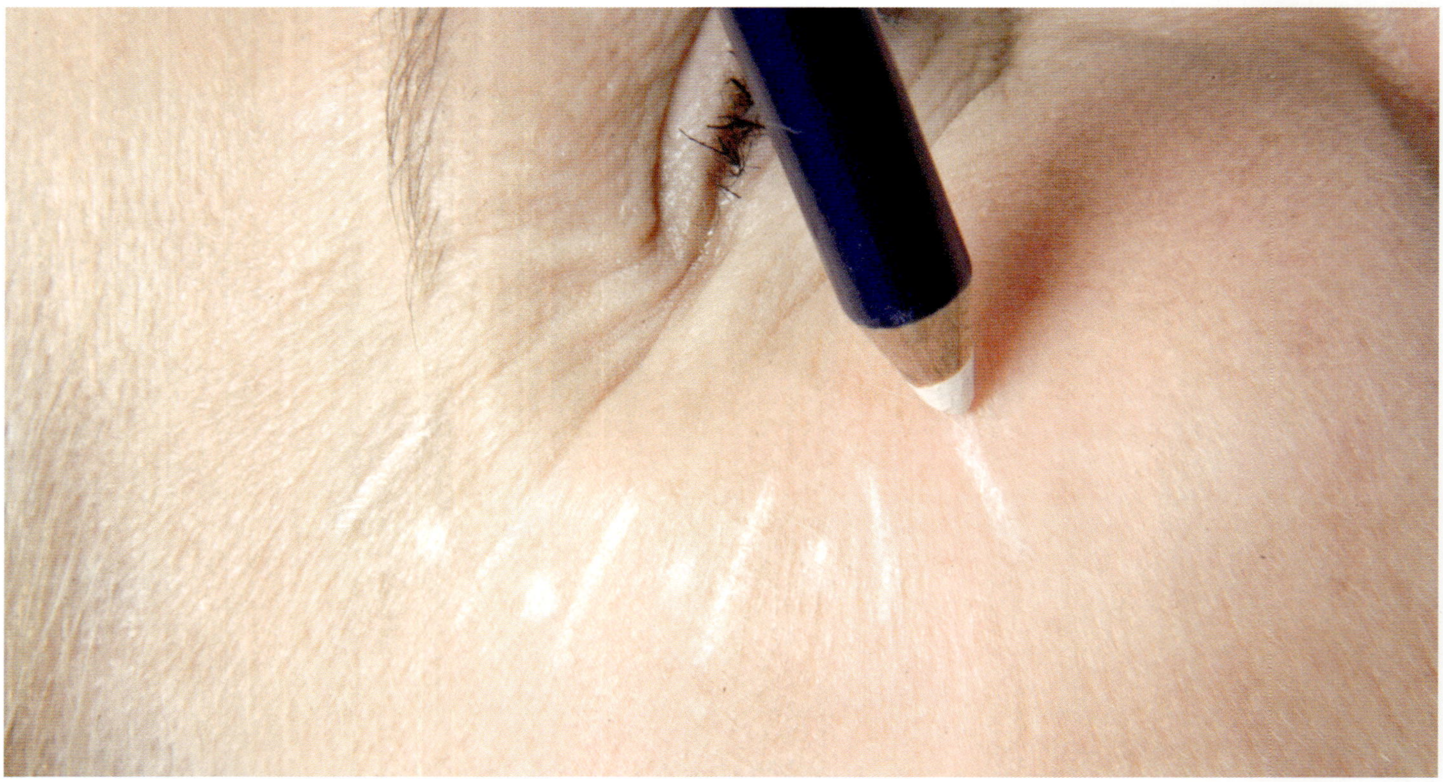

In Mesobotox, "hills" and "valleys" are marked with the muscles tightened. The injections are given intradermally into the "hills" (white dots). The higher the "hills", the more powerful the muscle and, consequently, the higher the dose.

Investigative biopsies tend to be unusual in esthetics. The signed informed consent forms and treatment cost agreements must be stored with the rest of the documentation for ten years. Tip: give the patients a printed out "before" picture. The following scales are helpful in recording the status of the skin, hair and adipose connective tissue.

Documentation of the findings – an overview			
Skin analysis	Fitzpatrick skin type	Glogau photodamage	Le Coz degree of elastosis
Hair	Hair loss type: diffuse, post partum, androgenetic, autoimmune, toxic	Ludwig Scale Hamilton Scale	Trichogram
Cellulite fat pads	Type, extent, location. Use identical reference points when measuring with measuring tape	Stage	Pinch test, calipers

Skin type/Phototype (Fitzpatrick skin type scale)		
	Reddening of the skin, sunburn	**Tanning**
I	Always	Never
II	Always	Sometimes
III	Sometimes	Always
IV	Never	Always
V Dark-skinned	Never	Always
VI Black-skinned	Never	Always

Photoaging of the skin (Glogau scale)			
Type 1	No lines	Age 20–30 years	Early stage of photoaging, minimal fine lines, minimal pigment changes, no keratosis
Type 2	Lines appear during movements involved in facial expression	Age 30–40 years	Moderate photoaging, moderate fine lines around the mouth when smiling, early lentigines, palpable but not yet visible keratosis
Type 3	Creases also at rest	Age 50–60 years	Advanced photoaging, structural and facial expression lines, visible keratosis and dyschromia, couperose
Type 4	Pronounced wrinkling	Age ≥ 60 years	Severe photoaging, the whole face is lined, skin atrophy, marked changes in color and pigment

Extent of skin elastosis (Le Coz)	
Stage 1	Skin sagging visible only in certain positions
Stage 2	Skin sagging can only be ascertained with the pinch test
Stage 3	Skin sagging always visible with marked hyperextensibility

Four clinical grades of cellulite	
Grade 0	No visible cellulite when standing or lying down, even when the skin is pinched
Grade 1	No visible cellulite when standing or lying down, but becomes visible when the skin is pinched
Grade 2	Visible when standing, but not when lying down
Grade 3	Visible when both standing and lying down

6

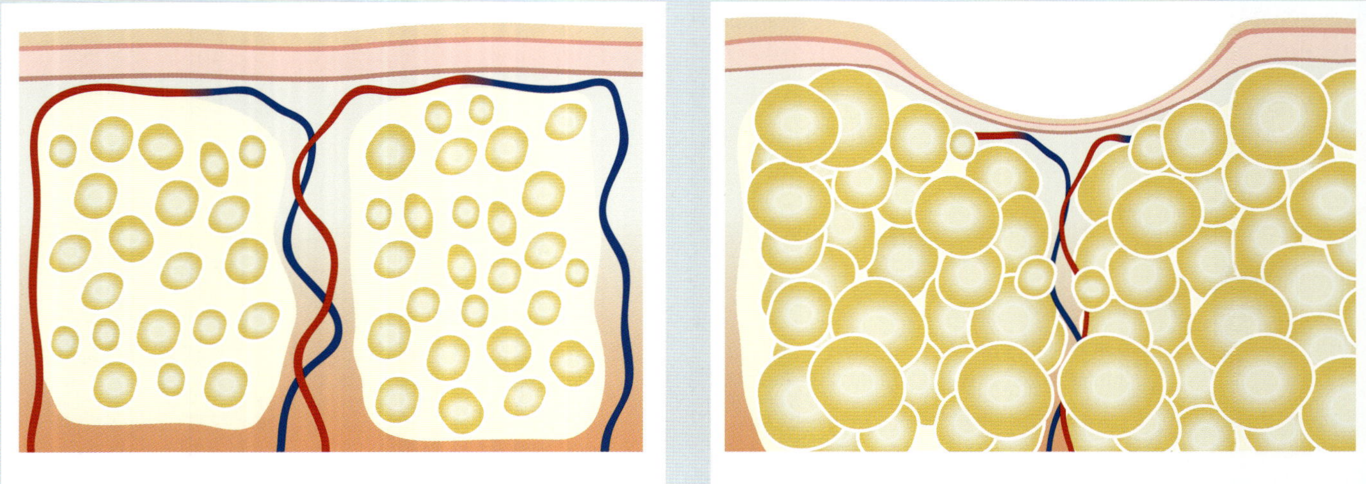

Pathophysiology of cellulite: the adipocytes are surrounded by fibrous tissue, with resultant disruption of the microcirculation and trophic disturbances.

6

6.3 Informing the patient and before-and-after rules

When treating healthy individuals, it is particularly important to ensure that they are provided with comprehensive information; this will need to be more detailed and extensive the more invasive the procedure. This information includes not only the nature of the chosen procedure – its effects and side effects, risks and special features – but also its expected consequences (e.g. any down-time), the likely duration of its effects and the expected outcome.
It is essential to respect the patient's wishes and goals. In this context, it is also necessary to determine whether there are any feasible alternatives and what these alternatives are. Patients should also be warned about the off-label use of medicines. The information is provided on a one-to-one basis and also in writing. The written information sheet must be signed by the patient. It is not enough to hand out a standard form. The information sheet explaining the treatment costs also requires a signature.
In addition, the information session includes formulation of the therapy goal together with detailed information for the patient regarding the courses of the individual treatments, the schedule, the number of sessions and the before-and-after rules.

6.3.1 Rules the patient needs to observe before the treatment

- The patient must not take any aspirin or enzyme products two days before the mesotherapy.
- He or she must inform the therapist about any regular medication (e.g. oral anticoagulants) and previous illnesses; women must also inform the therapist if they are pregnant.
- He or she must inform the therapist about all allergies or intolerances.
- The patient will also need to be asked about any predisposition to keloids or pigment disorders.
- The skin may only be cleansed with water and soap, without applying any skincare products or make-up on the area being treated. The hair must be washed before a hair treatment.
- No immunizations should take place one week before the mesotherapy.

6.3.2 Rules the patient needs to observe after the treatment

- Full baths, saunas, massages, mudpacks or lymphatic drainage must be avoided for 24 hours after the treatment.
- Sunbathing and visits to the solarium are not permitted for 48 hours.
- The patient should not wear any colored, new or very tight clothing which may come into contact with the treated area.
- No ointments, creams or powders may be used, unless prescribed by the physician.
- Radiotherapy or electrotherapy is not permitted for 3 days.
- The patient's usual skincare may be resumed after 24 hours.

Suggestions for the information sessions may be found under *Aids for the Therapist,* Chapter 10.

The Hamilton Scale

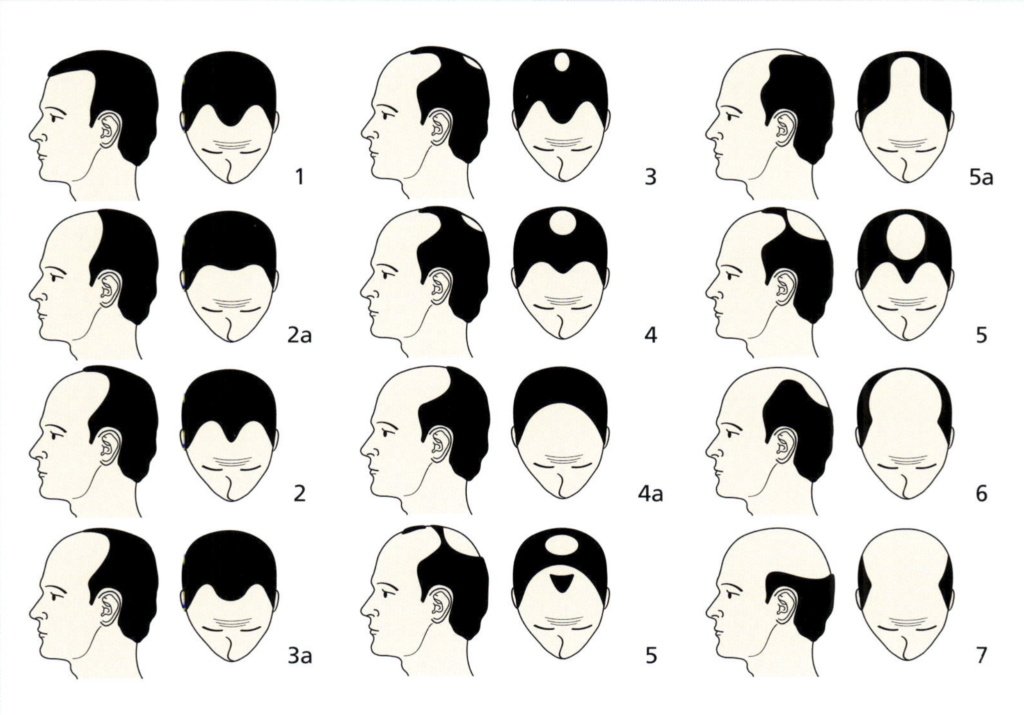

Diagram showing the stages of male hair loss.

The Ludwig Scale

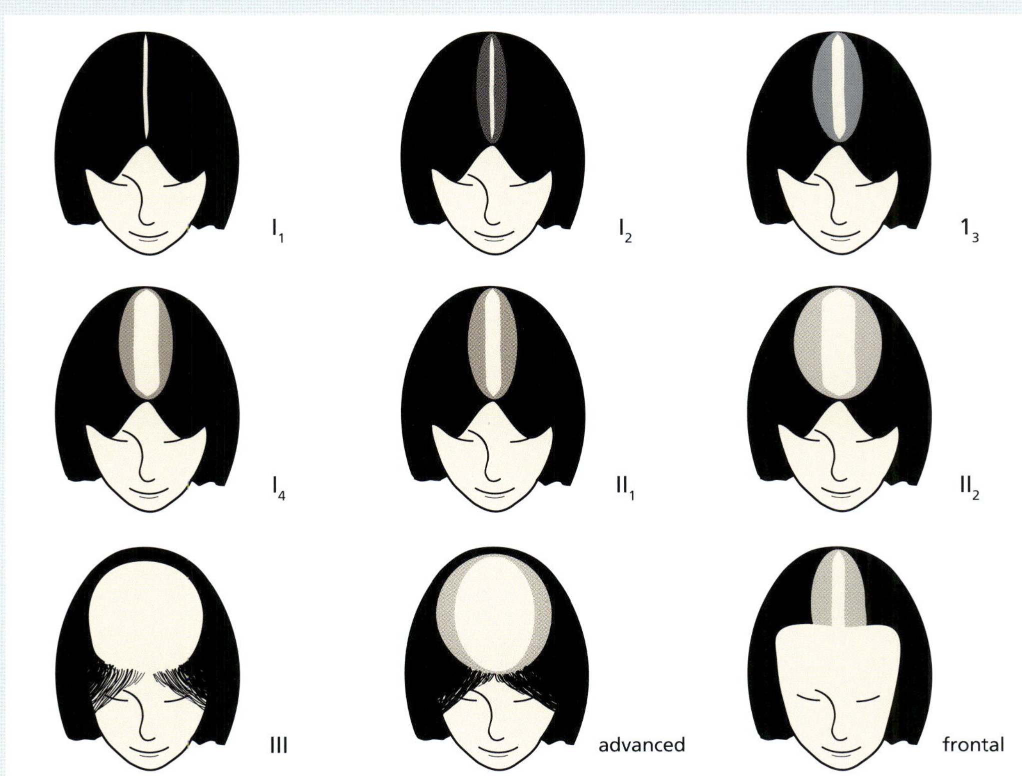

Diagram showing the stages of female hair loss.

6.4 Treatment strategy and therapy plan

The first stage of a high-quality esthetic treatment consists of a properly made diagnosis. This needs to take into account not only the local findings which are of particular interest to the patient, but also his or her overall constitution, skin type, previous and concurrent illnesses, a possible pregnancy and lifestyle habits. We must distinguish between the primary and secondary treatment strategies which are needed to achieve the desired goals

6.4.1 Primary treatment strategies

The following questions need to be clarified:
- Monotherapy or combination therapy?
- Which regions of the body, in what order?

Thus, for example, it is important for a planned lipolysis treatment of the face to be carried out first. The need for Botox or filler treatment can only be decided 6 weeks later. However, Mesolift can always be performed concurrently, as large-area regeneration therapy. If it is not possible to carry out all the desired treatments on one day, the most urgent problem zone is tackled first. An alternative treatment rhythm may also be offered. It is necessary to determine both the location and also the nature and number of the treatments, together with the intervals between them.

- Will a series of build-up treatments be enough?
- Or will maintenance therapy be needed?
- Is the outcome definitive?

The individual therapy plan can be adjusted to individual requirements as the treatments run their course. The patients need to be informed about waiting times, their own personal chances of success and the rules that they need to follow.

6.4.2 Secondary treatment strategies

A global practice concept includes simple anti-aging measures, e.g. the advice to restrict calorie intake with increasing age, while ensuring an adequate fluid intake and supply of micronutrients. Lifestyle has a 40% influence on skin aging. For this reason, I always advise smokers to undergo treatment to quit smoking during one of my mesotherapy sessions. Overweight patients should be provided with a specific weight loss program. Electronic toners and exercise machines (Ultratone®, power plate® etc.) are often helpful if muscles have become flabby or to remedy incorrect posture. Many working people need natural remedies to help them cope with exhaustion, burnout or stress. Stress is a common cause of hair loss, premature skin aging or cellulite. Mesostress can produce a significant improvement in psychosomatic disposition. Mesodrain is indicated in ede-

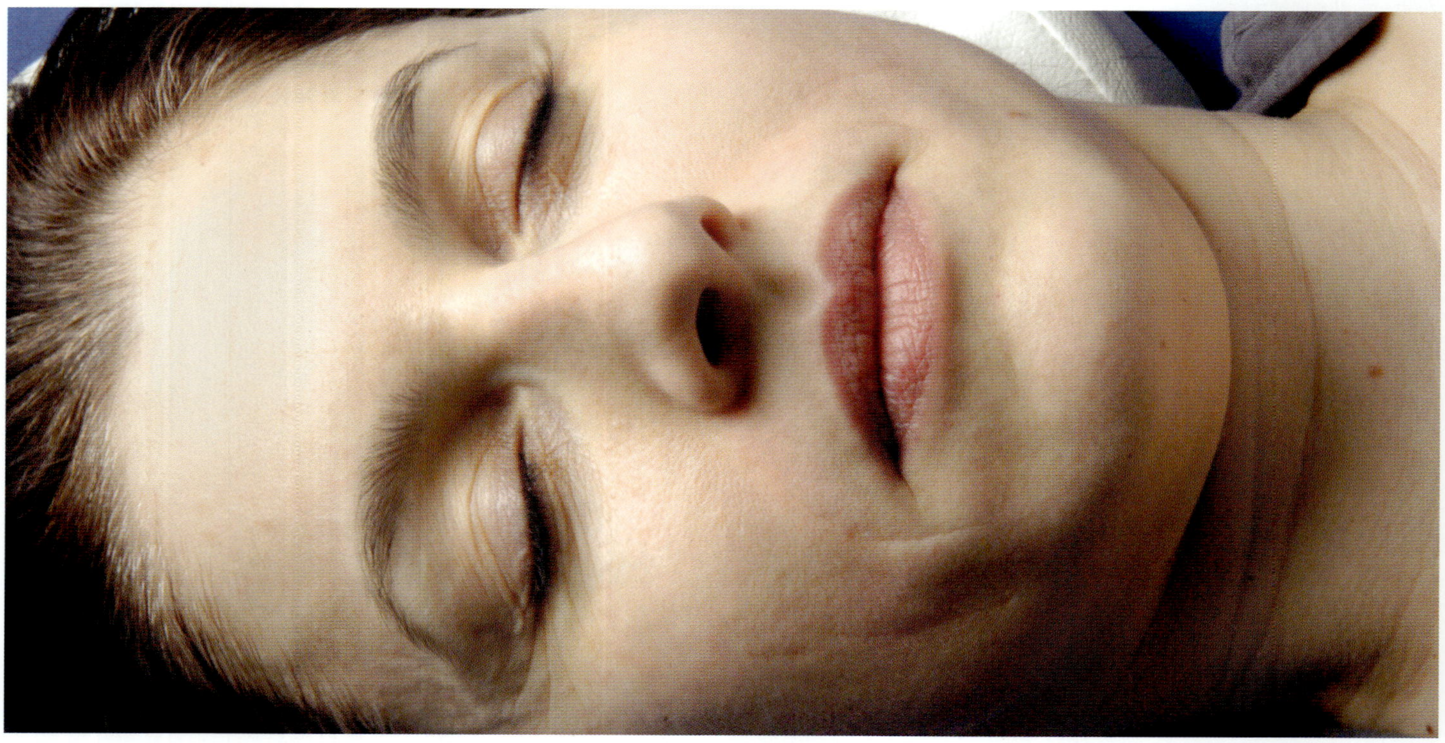

Changes in facial anatomy when sitting or lying down (cf. picture on the right). The effect of gravity becomes particularly apparent in the lower half of the face.

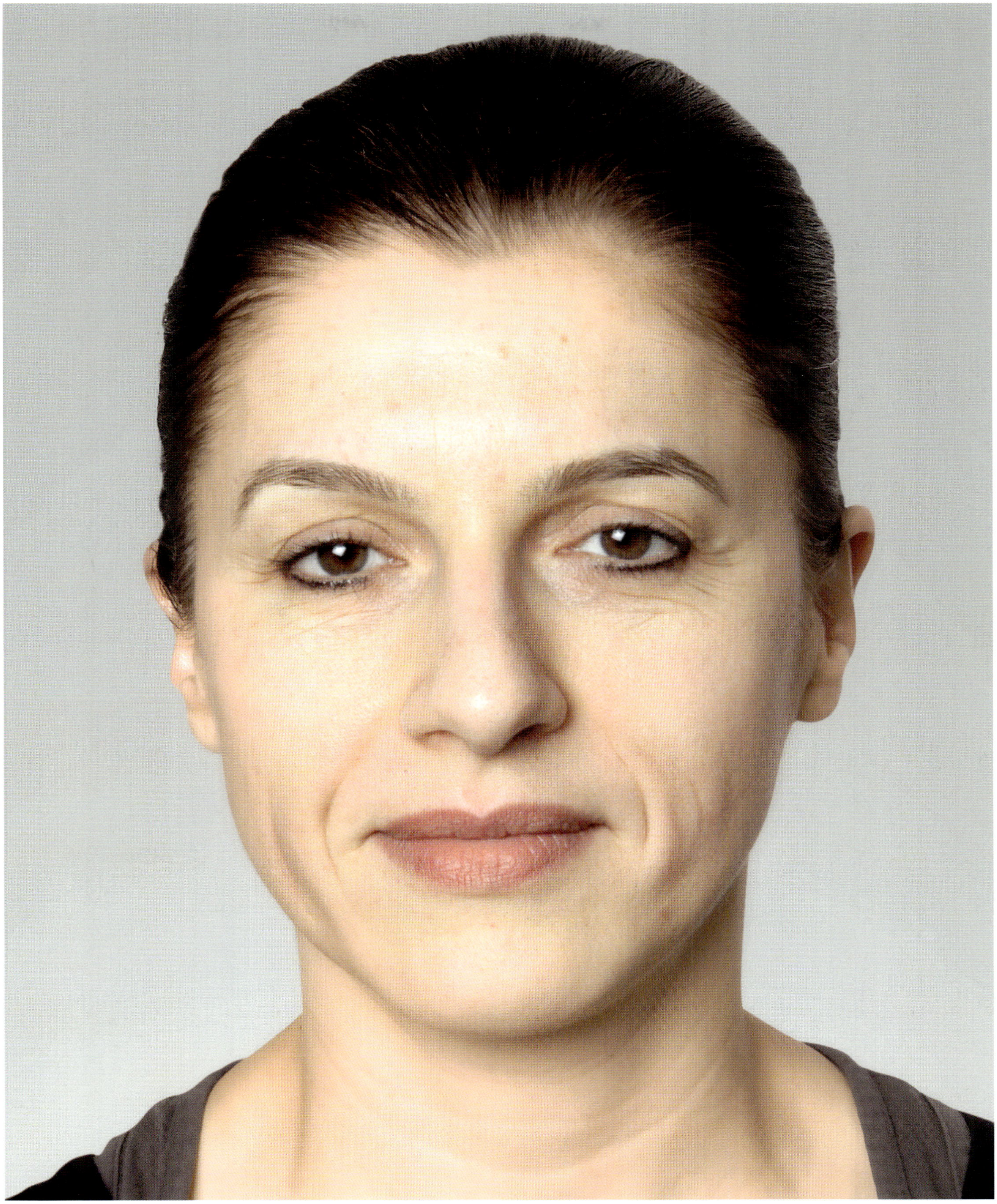

The effect of gravity becomes apparent with the patient upright (photo documentation of the baseline findings, with the patient wearing no make-up).

ma and/or venolymphatic insufficiency of the legs. In some cases, it may be necessary to call in other specialists, such as dermatologists, phlebologists, surgeons or anti-aging experts. Only a healthy patient who feels comfortable in his or her own skin can radiate beauty. At my practice, health and beauty are seen as a single unit, and a switch to curative medicine – and vice versa – is always an option, if necessary.

The first session and the consultation are time-intensive, and it is absolutely vital to take plenty of time in this delicate area of treatment. Doing so lays the cornerstone for a doctor-patient relationship which may last many years, and provides the motivation for consistent build-up and maintenance therapy. However, after this initial time investment, the treatment itself usually proceeds relatively quickly. Both – the consultation and the treatment – require a lot of experience from the physician and a bit of patience from the patient, as it can take days to weeks before the treatment reaches its full effect. In return, the patient then benefits from the typically long-term effects of the stimulated repair and regeneration processes.

Patients must be warned against "quick fixes" before important events, such as weddings, job interviews, etc., since the desired effects are not always apparent shortly after a first treatment, in particular; this is also the time when initial reactions or side-effects are particularly likely to occur.

7 The treatment

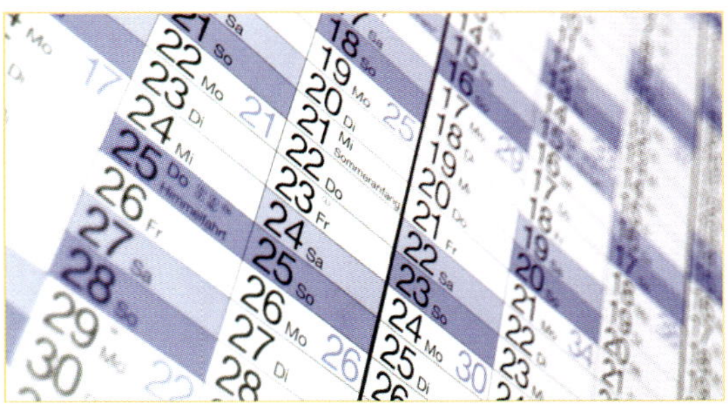

The treatment intervals need to be agreed with the patient.

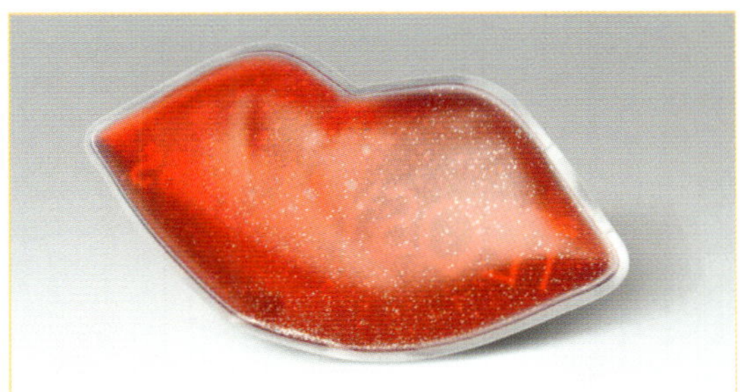

Single-use cooling elements, e.g. cool-packs, need to be available at the practice to control more severe reactive swellings.

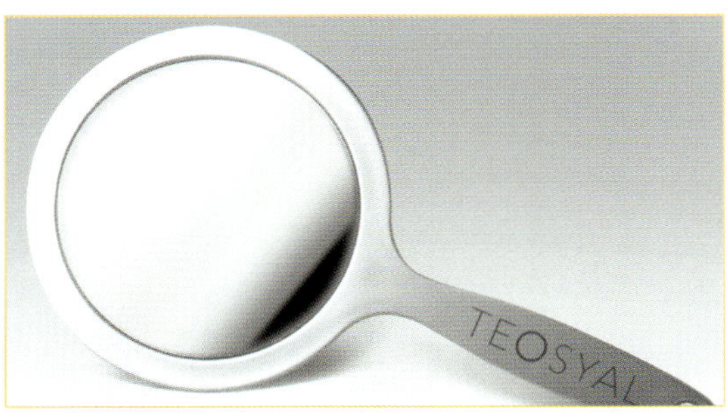

A hand-held mirror shows the signs of facial aging particularly clearly with the head tilted forward.

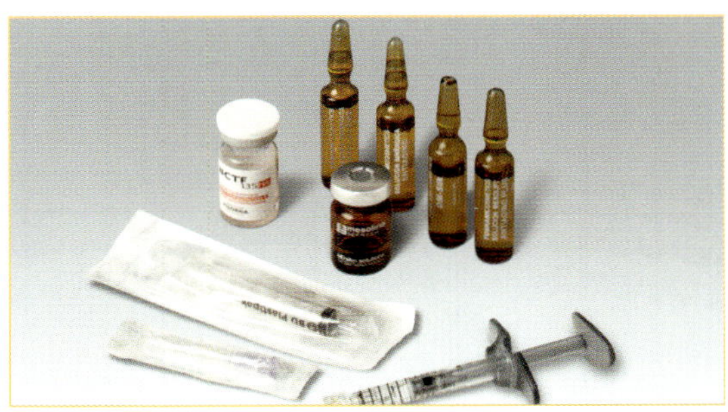

Materials used for the treatment need to be kept in sufficient supply and under the correct storage conditions. Always observe the use-by date.

The treatment

7.1 Treatment intervals

The minimum interval between two mesotherapy sessions is one week. For example: build-up phase in hair loss (6 sessions) then a transition – if needed – to the maintenance phase. The interval in Mesolift and cellulite treatment is 2 weeks during the build-up phase (3 to 6 sessions depending on baseline status). Intervals of up to 4 to 6 weeks are needed in lipolysis, which is a special case. This period represents the length of time that the lipid breakdown process in the connective tissue remains active. During the maintenance phase, it is usually enough to schedule monthly, quarterly or six-monthly booster sessions. In this respect, it is important to ensure that any traces of preceding treatments (e.g. hematomas) have disappeared. Existing hematomas must not be re-injected as this may cause permanent pigmentation.

7.2 Setting

A calm and relaxed atmosphere is as important for the patient as is a comfortable environment (correct room temperature, no disruptive phone calls, obliging staff). Patients need to be provided with facilities for make-up removal if they are having facial treatments. Hair bands should also be provided. The therapist him/herself will often need loupe glasses, together with professional lighting and hygienic surfaces of sufficient size where non-sterile gloves and drapes, cosmetic pads and cellulose pads can be put down. Treatments are always carried out with the patient lying down, except when treating hair loss, when the patient is seated. The patient is positioned with the aid of an adjustable treatment couch or beauty chair, draped with a paper cover or boilable fabric, with a knee bolster, neck support and thermal blanket, if needed.
It is also important to ensure that there is enough room in the treatment area for an assistant (if applicable) and also to allow the therapist to move around the patient's head during facial treatments.

7.3 Pre- and post-treatment

A gentle skin peel is a good way to prepare for and enhance a Mesolift treatment for skin rejuvenation and regeneration. This can be performed with e.g. 20 % glycolic acid (e.g. Glycopeel Filorga) or a mild TCA peel (TCA secure from Toskani). Peeling rids the skin of keratotic cell layers and improves the subsequent active substance uptake. For sensitive, thin skin, it may be necessary to include some ***down-time,*** which will mean two treatment sessions, i.e. first the skin peel and then, 1 to 2 weeks later, the Mesolift. Another way of supplementing Mesolift is the MesoMask treatment, which is used for additional skin ***brightening*** (e.g. Spot-Out mask from Toskani) and is performed during the interval between treatments. The importance of ***brightening*** procedures is still highly underestimated in Germany. They are used to produce a homogeneous complexion and have nothing to do with artificial ***whitening.*** Studies have shown that a face with age spots is perceived as being considerably older than the same face with lines.

7

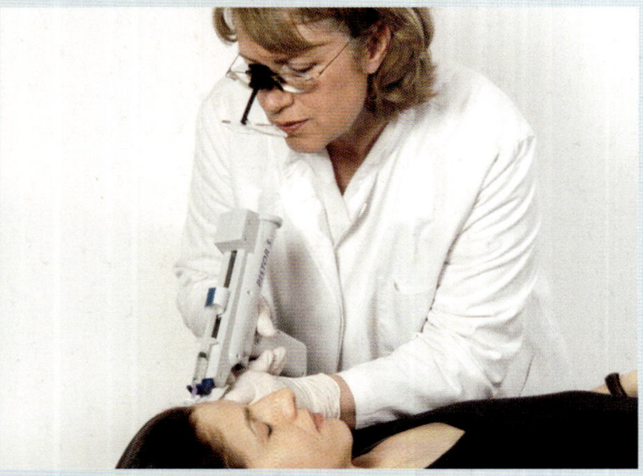

Maintain a calm and relaxed atmosphere during the treatment.

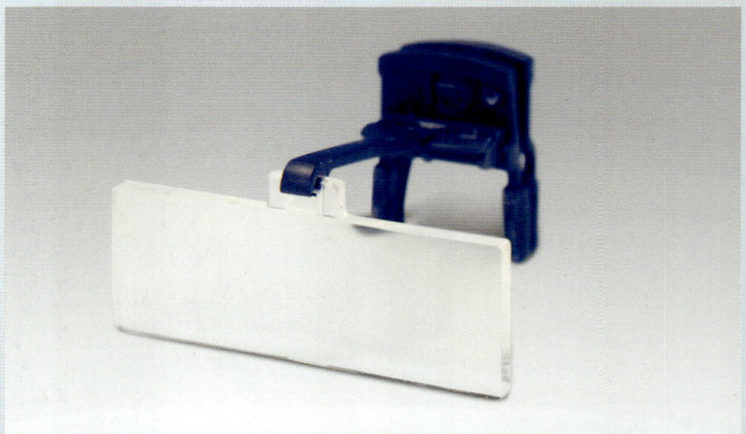

Loupe glasses are a substitute for the operating microscope. They magnify the skin surface two times. This makes it easier to identify skin impurities and superficial veins, so that injury to the latter can be avoided.

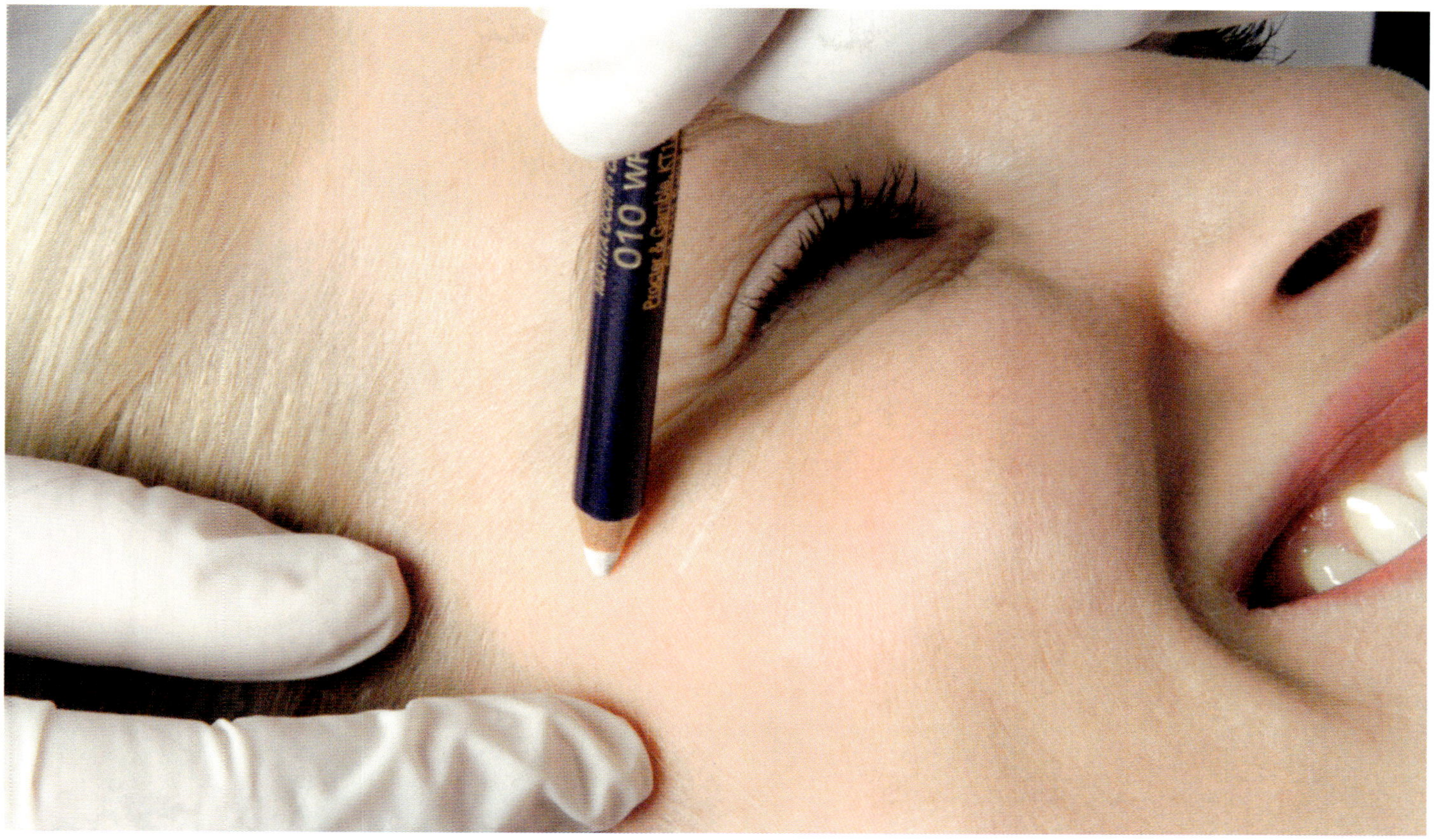

Good lighting is needed when marking and treating the skin.

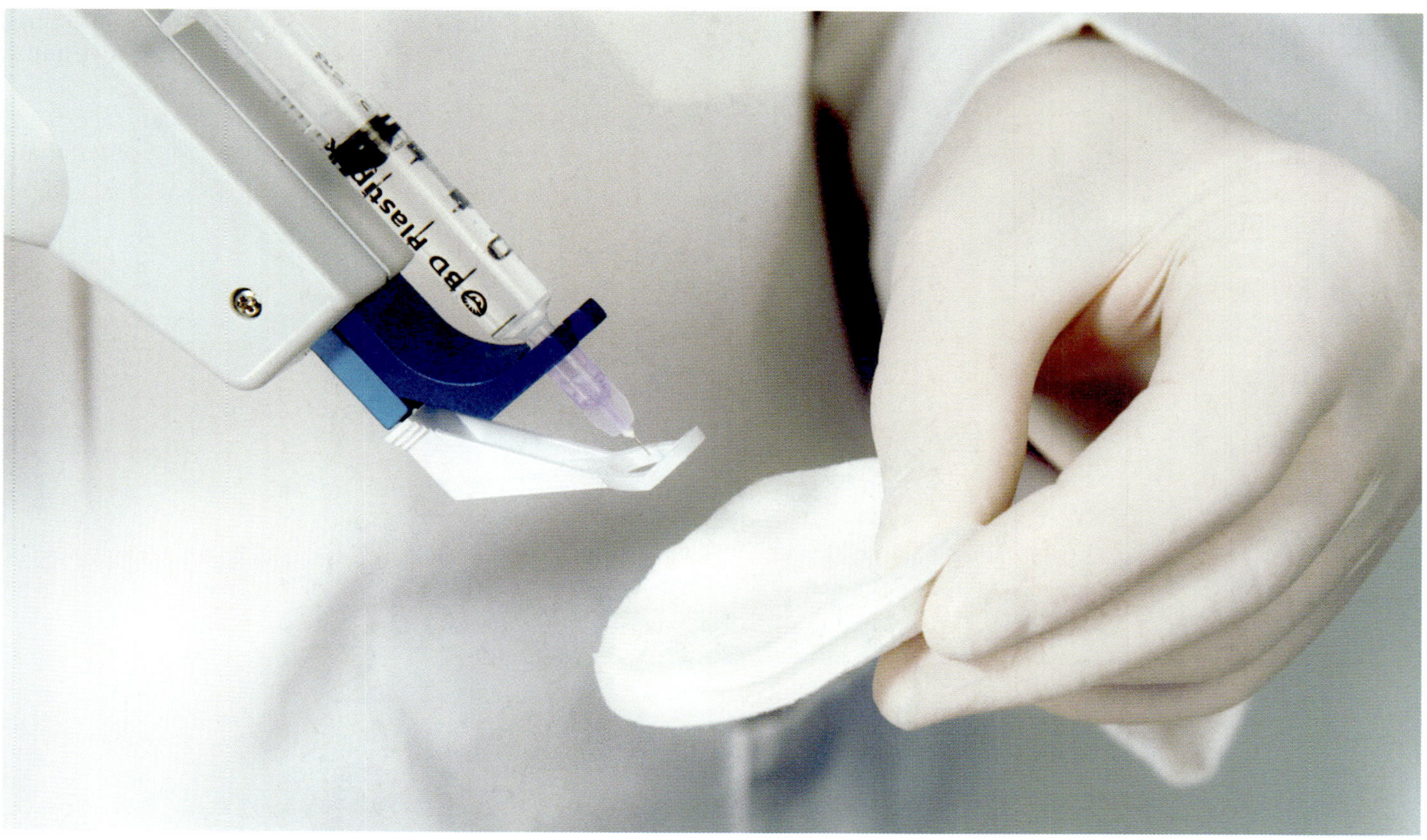

Test the patency of the needle and ensure that the viscosity of the liquid is correct before the treatment. A single drop should be ejected per trigger actuation in nappage mode.

Since mesotherapy is a very gentle and minimally invasive method, and is performed with microinjections, an anesthetic cream will only be needed in a few areas (forehead, mouth and eye area) and not for all patients.
Emla® cream needs quite a long time to take effect, and works best when occluded with shrink-wrap film. A more potent formulation containing high-dose lidocaine/tetracaine can speed up the process considerably. A great variety of products are also available for post-treatment. Examples worth mentioning include *Pre/Post-Injection* cream and the practical *Covering Repair* (tinted cover-up cream in various skin colors, with HA, Arnica extract and color pigments) from the Swiss company Teoxane. Other products suitable for immediate post-treatment use are Cicaplast® from La Roche Posay, Vitamin K Creme Toskani or the biological Rescue Gel from Living Nature™, containing manuka honey and manuka oil. Single-use cooling elements, e.g. cool-packs, need to be available at the practice to control more severe reactive swellings. More severe inflammatory reactions or hematomas, e.g. following lipolysis, can be treated by taping or with a compress soaked in the product Retterspitz® äußerlich. Another tried and tested measure is to give the patient D6 Arnica globuli to take home as a rescue treatment. Patients must be warned to get in touch immediately if they develop persistent skin reactions or any other health problems. It may also be a good idea to arrange a fixed follow-up appointment. Practices with retail outlets can offer medical care products for sale, e.g. the dermatologically developed and good-value Restar products, which can be obtained through www.mesotherapie-shop.de. It is important for all daily skincare products to have a sufficiently high sun protection factor.
If specialist hormonal cosmetics are required, e.g. with androstanolone against cellulite or estriol/17-alpha-estradiol against skin aging in women, these are usually available by prescription.
Receptura® also supplies a potent anesthetic ointment and delivers it on receipt of an appropriate private prescription. At the time of writing the price for 100 ml of Receptura® (see p. 128 for the supplier address) was c. €1.00.

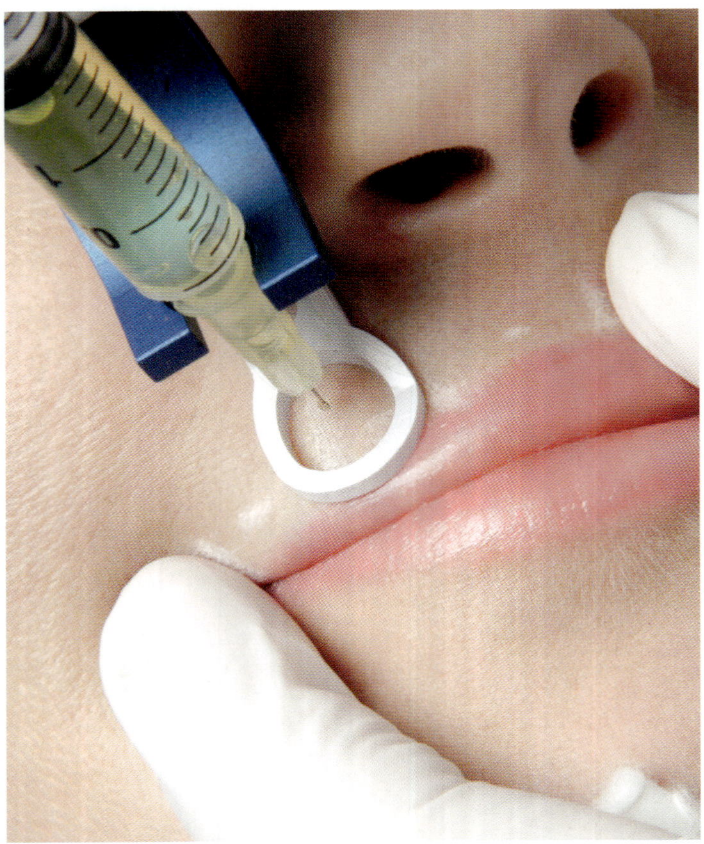

Sensitive areas of the face, such as the forehead, region around the eyes and lips can be numbed with anesthetic cream.

Anesthetic ointment for mesotherapy

- Lidocaine 23 % (POM)
- Tetracaine base 3.5 %
- Tetracaine HCl 3.5 %
- In 100 g of Lipothene 133™ base.

Properties
Highly potent anesthetic ointment for the relief of injection pain during mesotherapy, e.g. in the perioral region.

Special features
- Quick onset of action (five minutes)
- No occlusion required.

Cautions
- Do not use on large areas.
- Can lead to irritation and reddening of the skin in sensitive individuals.

Application
Apply thinly and sparingly following skin disinfection and wipe off any residues before the injections begin.

Storage conditions
Keep refrigerated as it
- has a limited shelf life
- is very economical.

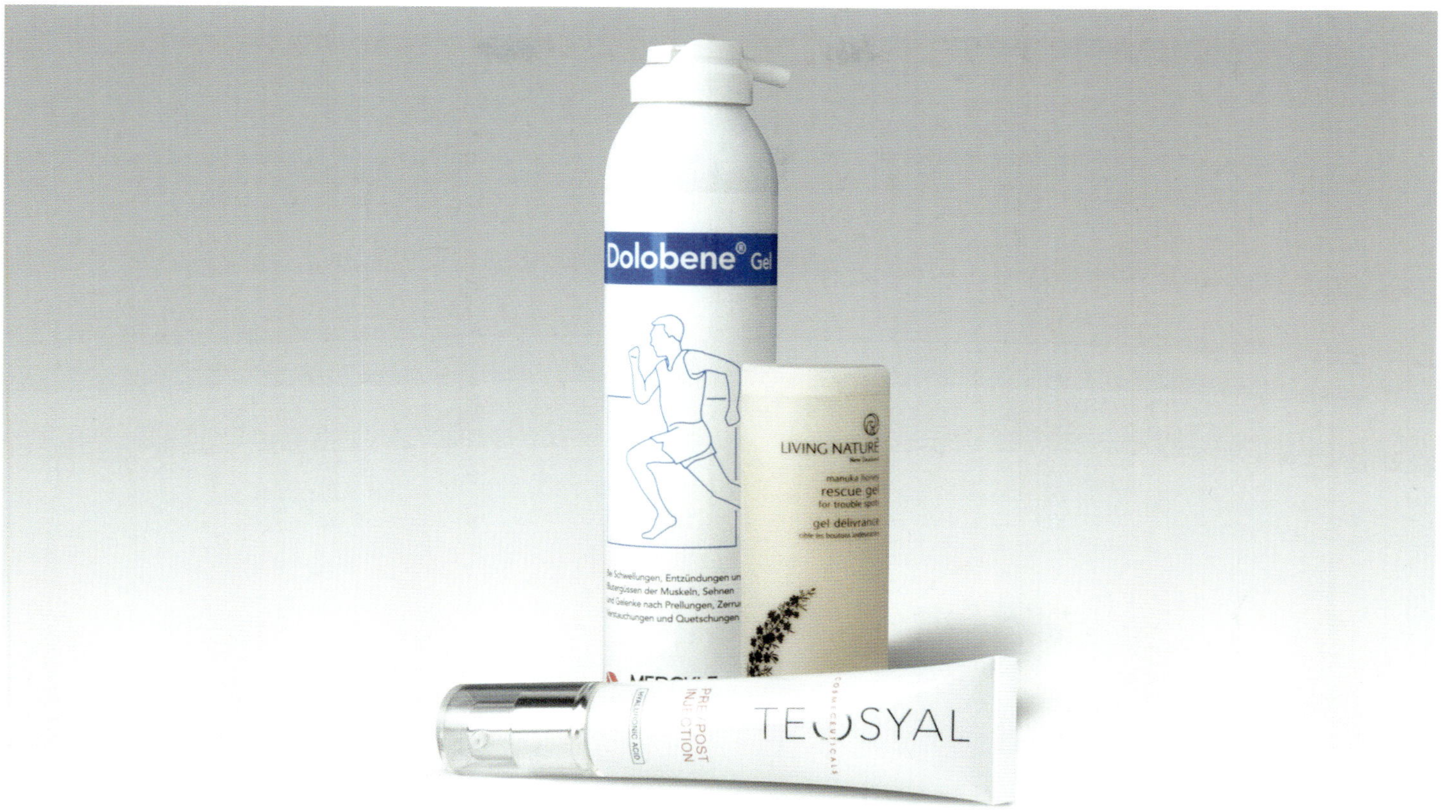

Various products for topical use may be used in the post-treatment phase.

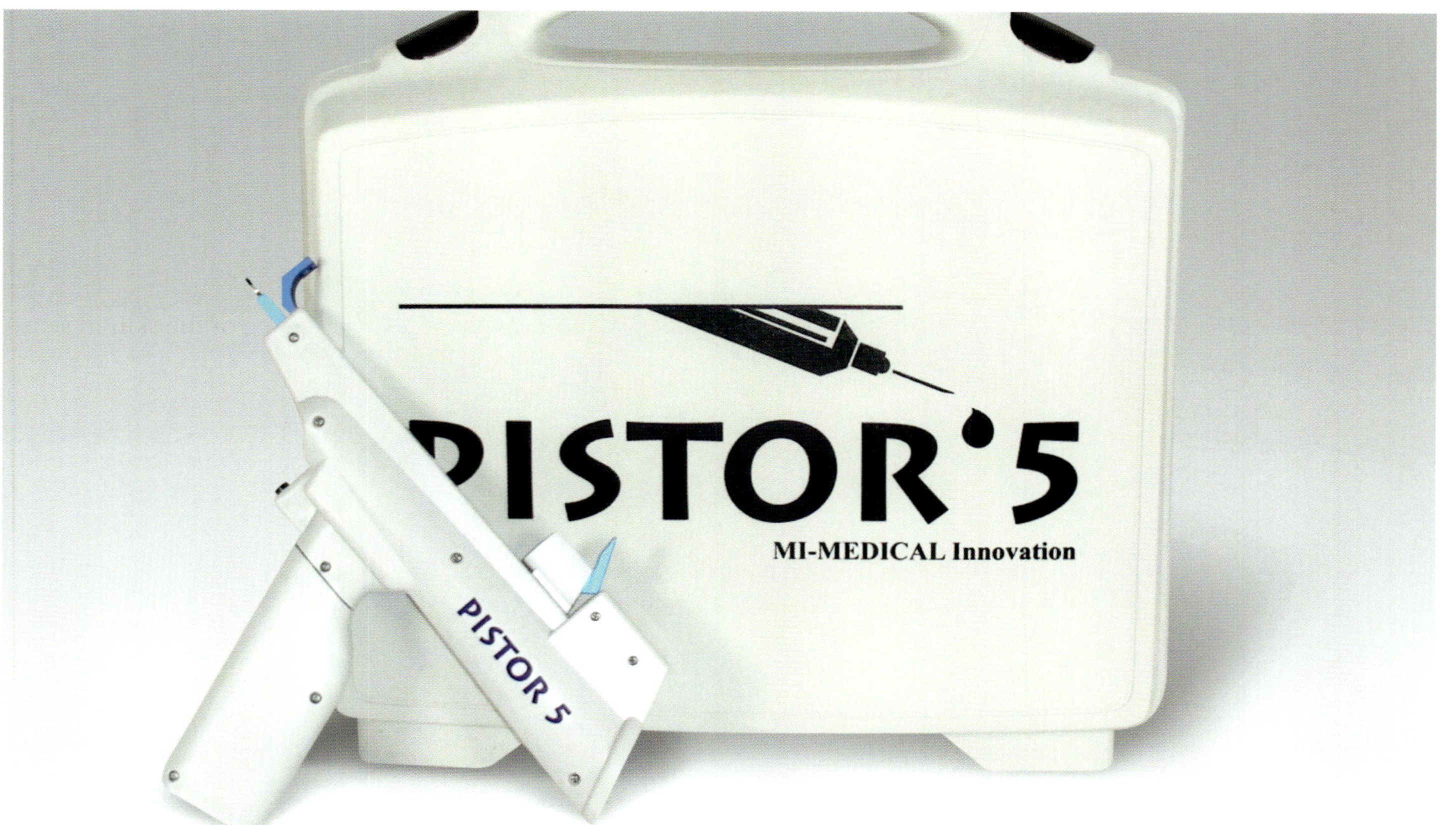

A few electronic mesotherapy devices are also suitable for mobile use in their transport packaging.

7

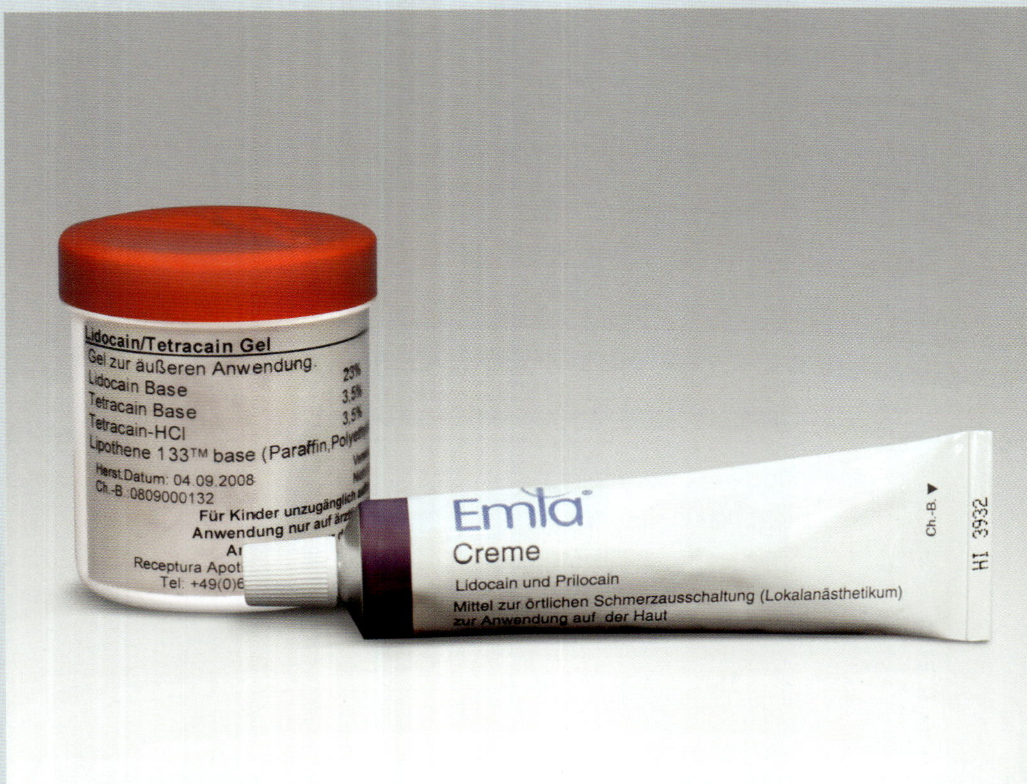

Lidocaine- or tetracaine-based local anesthetics can be used in sensitive patients.

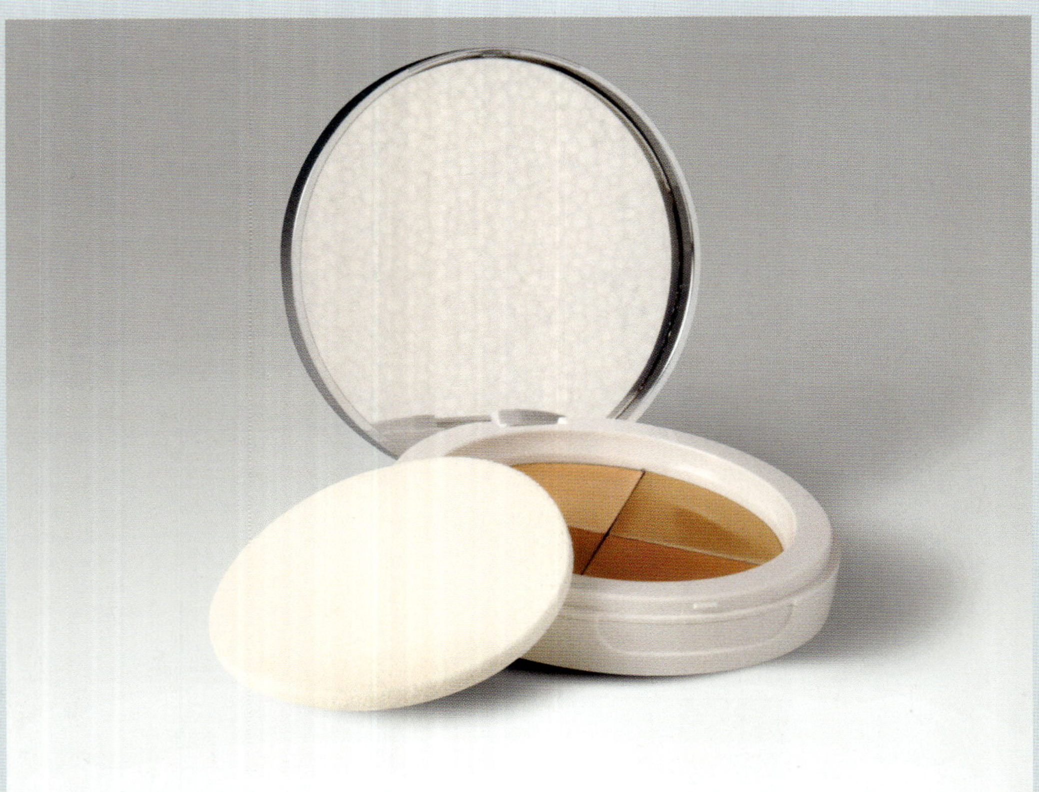

A medical concealer which comes in various skin colors can be applied with a Q-tip to cover up any traces of the treatment immediately after the session.

8 Regional treatments

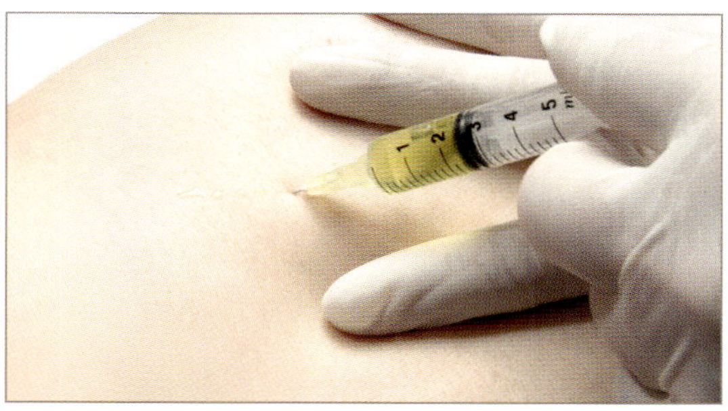

Mesotherapy for skin firming and rejuvenation.

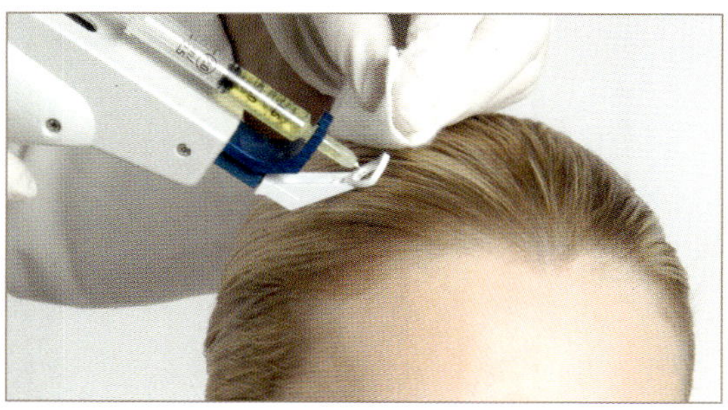

Mesotherapy to stimulate hair growth.

Note
The following symbols are used to mark treatment areas in the photographs in this chapter:
Dotted lines = epidermal technique
Large light gray dots = serial one-by-one injection technique
Large dark gray dots = infiltrations

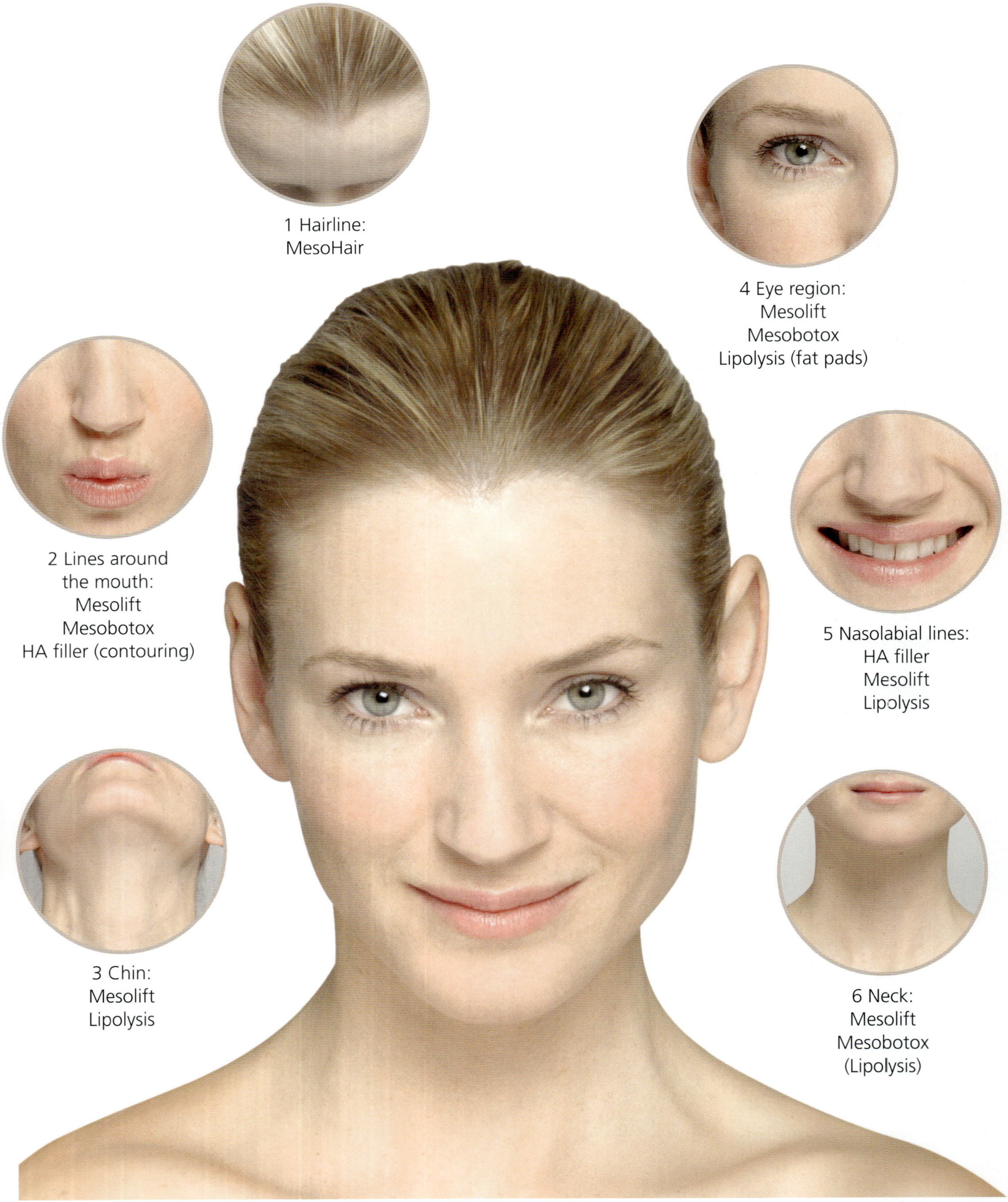

Overview: Treatment areas on the face and the possible therapy combinations.

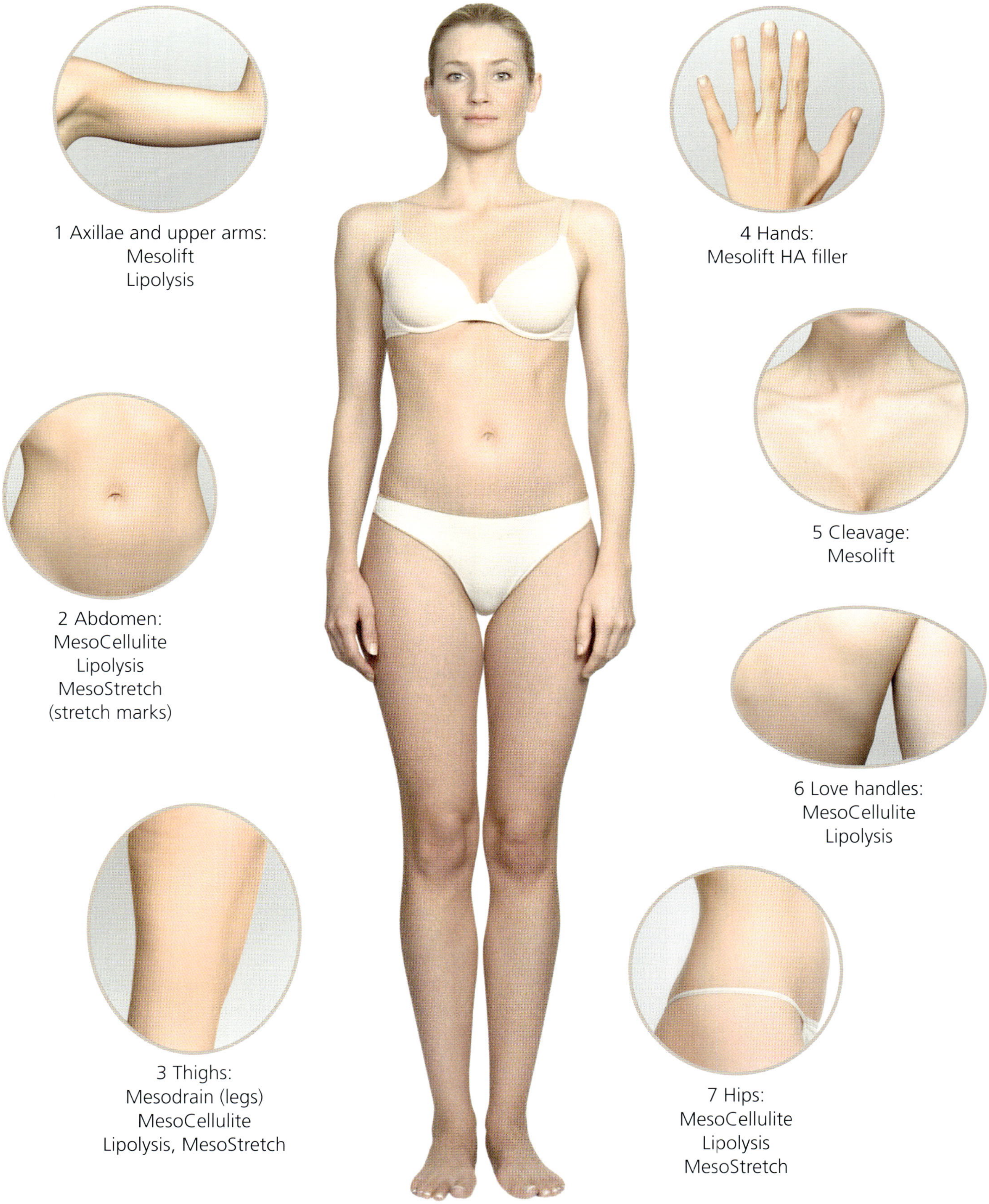

Overview: Treatment areas on the body and the possible therapy combinations.

Regional treatments

Pathological conditions and manifestations, which are often highly distressing for patients and thus need treatment, are not a major indication group for mesotherapeutic treatments. The successful treatment of skin aging manifestations, cellulite, hair loss and connective tissue weakness has helped mesotherapy make a breakthrough in many countries. Improved appearance in these areas is achieved without surgery, by stimulating the circulation of blood and lymph, and by tissue purification and regeneration. A high degree of patient satisfaction, reduced treatment time and lower cost characterize this innovative treatment method. In some cases, a *build-up* series of two to six sessions (depending on the severity of the problematic changes) may need to be followed by regular maintenance therapy.
In the latter case, the treatment intervals range from once a month to once every three to six months.

Examples of conditions needing long-term care
Prevention of skin aging, androgenetic hair loss, venous and lymphatic insufficiency.
However, a long-term effect can also be achieved in many patients, so that the treatment may only need to be resumed after several years or when required.

Examples of conditions needing short-term care
Diffuse hair loss, cellulite/lipolysis, scars, stretch marks.

The goal of the first session is to achieve tissue *repair*. This lays down the basis for sustained *regeneration*. Patients need to be informed that no great miracles can be expected after the first time, and that they are even likely to experience initial reactions.
The esthetic medicine methods described here cannot be judged using the same benchmarks as curative medicine, where any treatment must have scientific back-up. In mesotherapy, the evidence lies mostly in client satisfaction, as in the saying "Beauty is in the eye of the beholder". These subjectively perceived improvements can only be backed up by relatively few practicable and objective ways of verifying treatment success. Neither guidelines nor double-blind studies exist, and the latter would be difficult to perform for methodological and technical reasons alone. There are some histomorphological studies, together with case reports, non-interventional treatment observation studies and in-vitro trials. Biopsies, for example, are tolerated by the tiniest minority of beauty treatment clients. Very few practices produce standardized, high-quality photo documentation series for scientific purposes. The reasons for this are that independent practices have little spare time and money for the purpose, and that this therapy is currently not linked to university courses in Europe. In addition, the medical treatment methods used in mesotherapy hold no particular interest for either the pharmaceutical or the cosmetics industry.

8.1 Mesolift, Mesoglow, Mesobotox

The term *skin* aging refers to changes caused by biological senescence, and to those attributable to the environment or to behavior and lifestyle. Aging, hormonal changes and nicotine, but also the sun, wind and cold, all cause the skin to lose its tone, elasticity and shine.
Basically, the recommended way of delaying the aging process is consistent care with moisturizing creams and anti-aging products containing sunscreen, started at an early date. However, the use of creams which act only on the upper layers of the skin can prevent neither the fat redistribution that occurs with age, nor the sagging and increasing atrophy of the skin. The contours of the face change over the course of the years: the cheeks collapse inwards, "hamster cheeks" develop and the submandibular region begins to sag. The eyes and mouth appear smaller, the lip margins become more indistinct and the face appears tired. Lines turn into wrinkles and furrows.
Whereas decorative cosmetics can hide a lot on the face, the neck and hands will always betray a person's true age. A safe, long-lasting and affordable treatment method for skin rejuvenation, which can turn back the clock in the best-case scenario, is a desirable option. The consequences and causes of skin aging can be countered globally and in a natural way with Mesoglow and Mesolift. Early, even preventative treatment with Mesoglow is the best option. Promising methods in more advanced cases are repeated anti-aging Mesolift, as well as complex treatment combinations including HA fillers, laser treatments and medical peeling. If Botox is used in a combined facial treatment regimen, it should always be carried out first. Mesolift and HA fillers can then be given after two weeks, even in a single session, starting with Mesolift over an extended area, followed by targeted volume augmentation.
In practice, one tends to proceed pragmatically. The selected procedure is guided by the individual findings and by the patient's wishes. Sometimes, results can be seen after the first treatment or over the next few days; in most cases, however, the success of the treatment is enhanced by regular repeat treatments (additive effect).

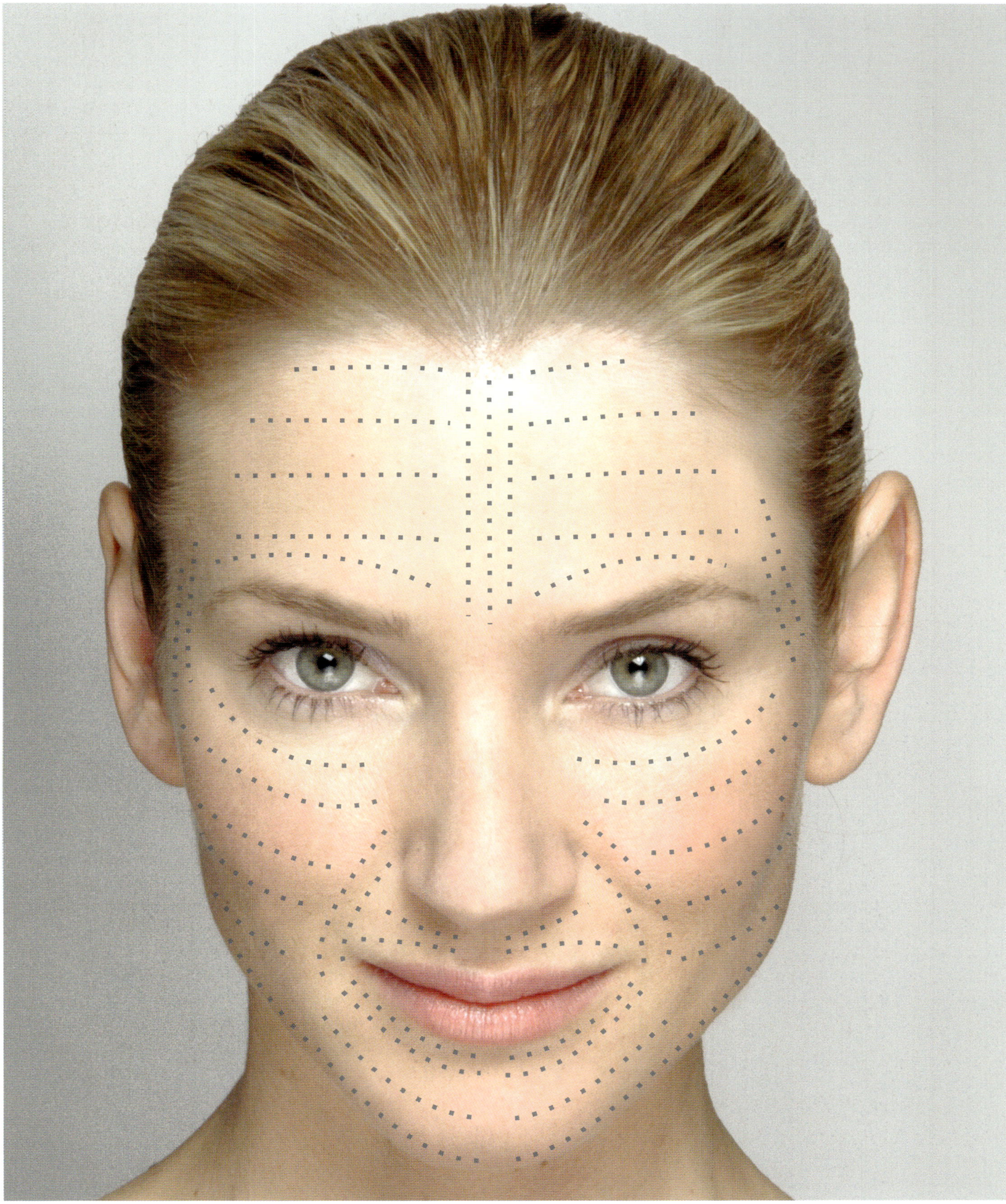

When planning a treatment for the face, it will be necessary to organize the sequence and the combination of the various measures: lipolysis, Botulinum toxin, Mesolift, filler. The figure shows the injection plan for an epidermal Mesolift treatment.

8.1.1 Studies

Both visual and palpable improvements are achieved, corresponding to the results of in-vitro studies.

1. The Pitié-Salpêtrière Hospital study
Impact of injection mode on the anti-aging effect of mixture composed of hyaluronic acid and multivitamins injected using the U225 biophymed mesotherapy gun into human skin maintained in survival. Paris 2006. The conclusion of the in-vitro study of the effectiveness of the Mesolift method was as follows:

"The experimental model presented herein, using human skin maintained in survival provided both visual and quantitative evidence that injection using the Biophymed mesotherapy gun in the rapid-pulse (high frequency) mode increases the anti-aging effect of [a] mixture of hyaluronic acid and multivitamins. The enhancement of the anti-aging effect associated with gun injection was documented in terms of a significant increase in the mitotic index in the epithelium (indicative of cell regeneration) and in collagen content (indicative of dermal reconstruction)."

2. NCTF Study
This study was sponsored by the French manufacturer of the long-established revitalization cocktail NCTF, the company Filorga. Its aim was to provide scientific evidence of the biorevitalization potential of this nutrient mixture, again by means of intensive laboratory testing.
NCTF 135® is a complex revitalization cocktail consisting of:

- 13 vitamins
- 23 amino acids
- 6 minerals
- 6 coenzymes
- 5 nucleic acids
- 2 antiradicals

+ HA (0,025 in NCTF135® or 5 mg/g in NCTF135® HA).

In-vitro tests conducted by an independent research centre specializing in cellular and molecular pharmacology, confirmed its extensive anti-aging efficacy:

Anti-aging efficacy
1 Stimulation of cell growth: + 147 % human fibroblasts in 72 h
2 Active redensification of the dermis + 256 % extracellular collagen in 72 h
3 Cell protection 90 % protection from free radicals (after 24 h of UVA and UVB radiation exposure)
4 Viscoelastic regeneration + 366 % elastase inhibitor gene expression

8.1.2 Discussion

Both studies provide impressive confirmation of the positive clinical experiences with Mesolift. Whereas the predominant purpose of the first treatment is to repair and stabilize already damaged skin structures, a marked rejuvenation effect in the form of firmer and smoother skin can be seen after the second and third sessions. The number of build-up treatments, taking place at 2-week intervals, depends on the patient's response. Fournier's experience applies when it comes to the visual effect of an increase in skin volume:

"1 mm in the face is like 1 km on the road."

The dermis consists largely of collagen and connective tissue. Collagen is a structural protein of connective tissue and gives the skin its firmness and tensile strength. The fibroblasts, the cells in the dermis which produce collagen, are stimulated by the injected mixtures, strengthening the skin's connective tissue and activating cell function.
NCTF 135® HA, TKN HA oligovit, Toskani Cocktail Anti-Aging, Toskani Cocktail Anti-Aging plus Mesolift, the Toskani Cocktail for skin firming, Reparestim-HA® or Revitacare® are specific mesotherapy products which provide the skin with an optimum supply of important vitamins, minerals, antioxidants, amino acids and other cell building blocks such as hyaluronic acid. Among other things, the active biological substances inhibit the breakdown of HA by free radicals, thus prolonging the water-binding effect of this polysaccharide. The effect of microinjecting these revitalizing active substances is to stimulate the metabolism and mitochondrial activity of skin cells and also to intensify the flow of blood and lymph, i.e. to enhance the microcirculation. The result of this is detoxification, purification and regeneration of the skin. Skin quality increases and moisture can be bound more effectively, so that the skin appears firmer and more elastic. It gets the desired radiance with a visible increase in volume. Superficial fine lines on the face, neck and cleavage are reduced for up to 18 months.
Several sessions at 2-week intervals will be needed. Their number depends on the patient's age and skin characteristics, and should include at least three build-up treatments. The patient's daily activities are not restricted after the treatment sessions. In principle, the treatment can be performed anywhere on the body, but the most commonly selected areas are the face and neck, cleavage or hands (backs of the hands and fingers). Non-interventional treatment observation studies of 120 practice cases yielded a satisfaction rating of 7.35 (on a subjective assessment scale of 1–10); there was agreement between the doctor and patient ratings. More than 1 million of these treatments have already been carried out worldwide.

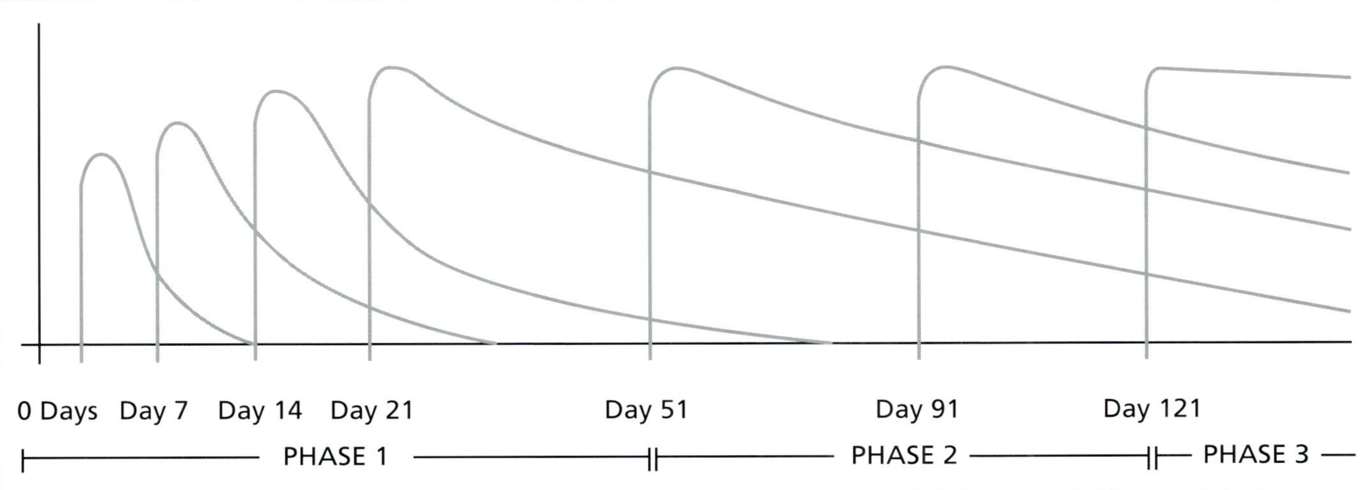

Cumulative effect of repeated Mesolift treatments on cell revitalization and thus on skin thickness and quality (theoretical model) Source: Filorga, Paris

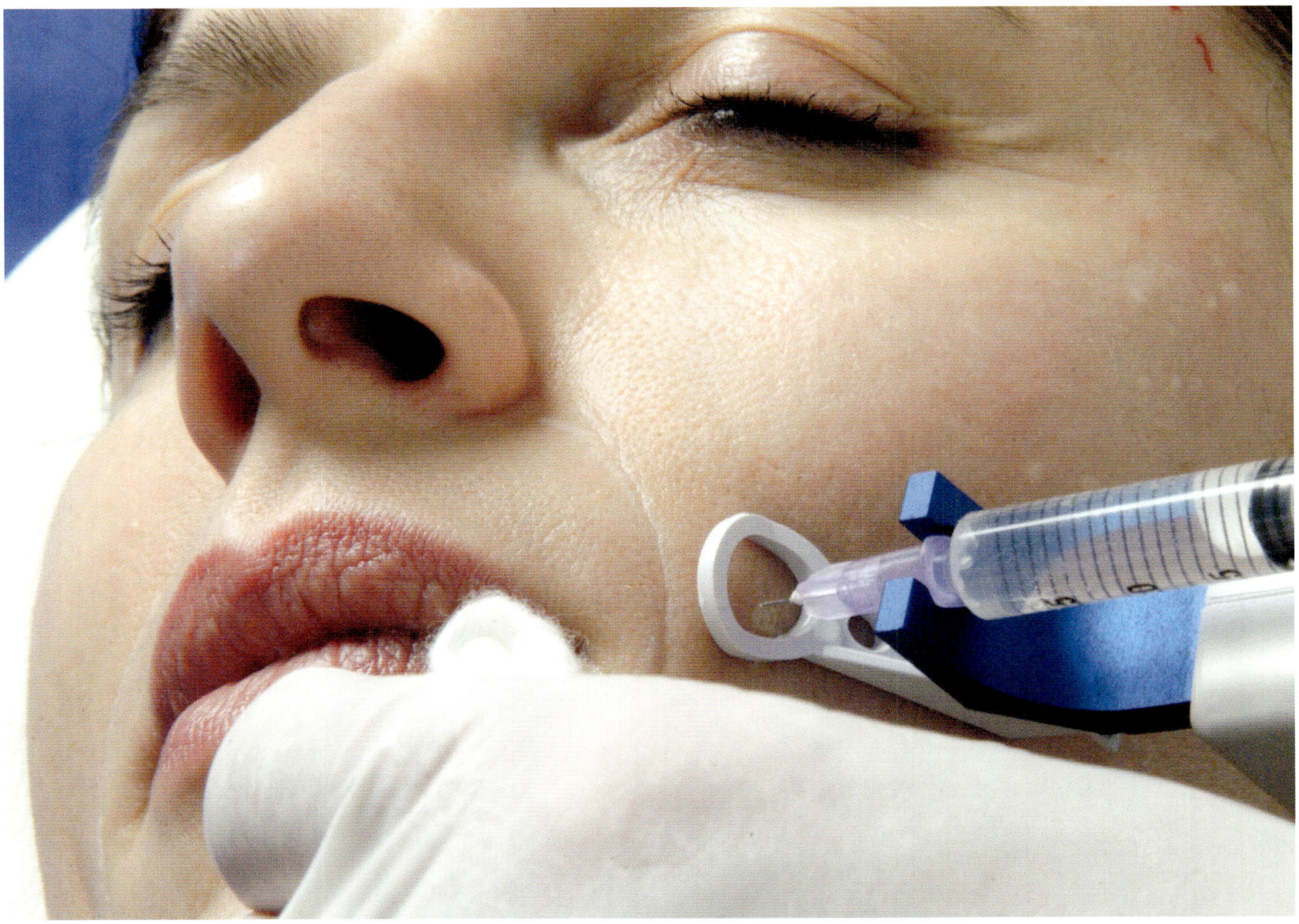

The epidermal microinjections cover a large area of the skin of the face; only the nose and eyelids are left out. A fine line of injections along the lip margin gives an attractive, natural volume.

8

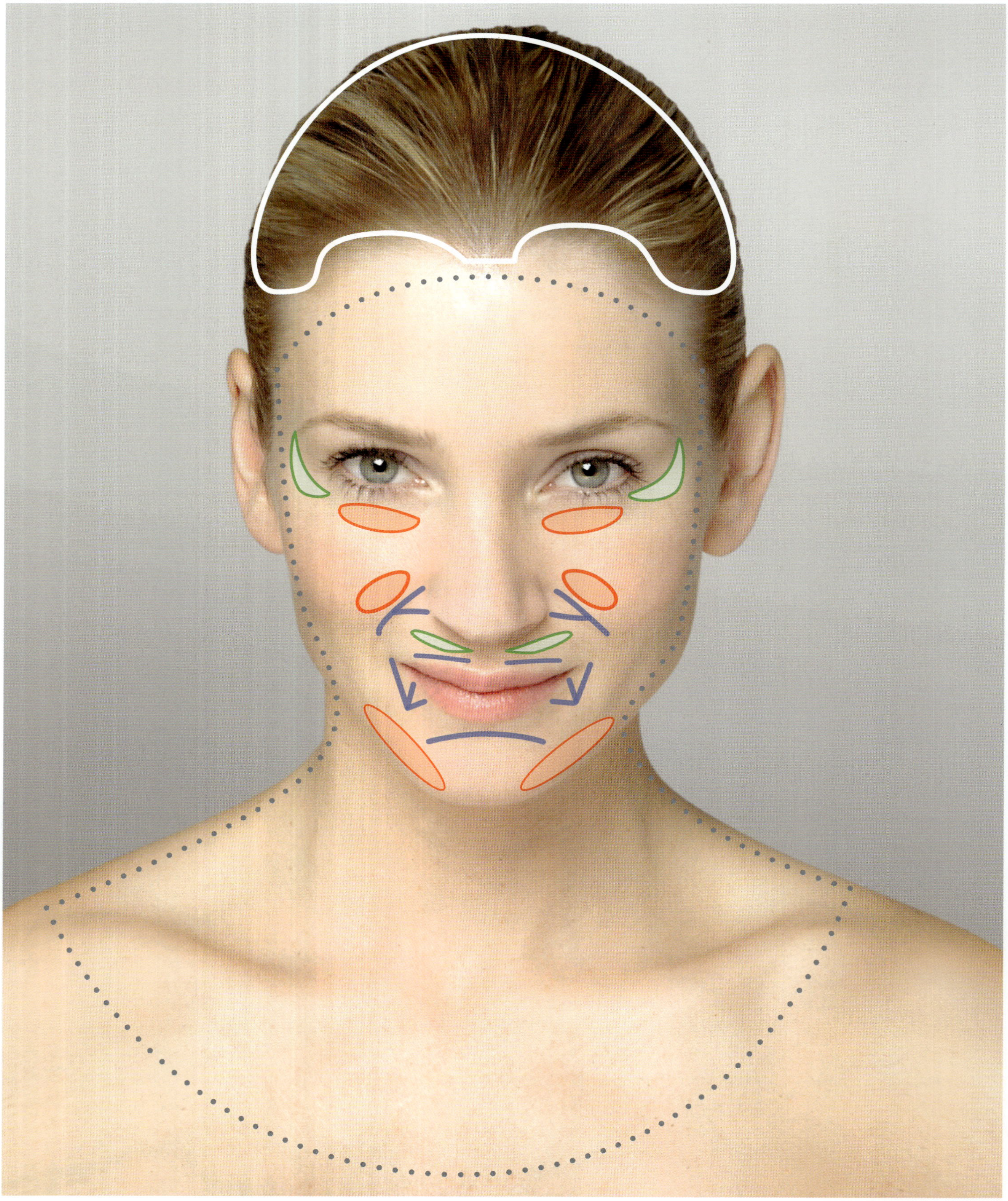

Combining various facial treatments: extensive coverage with Mesolift (• • •), adding volume with fillers (▬), reducing volume with lipolysi (⬭), musc e relaxation with Mesobotox (⬭). Treatment of hair loss with MesoHair (▭).

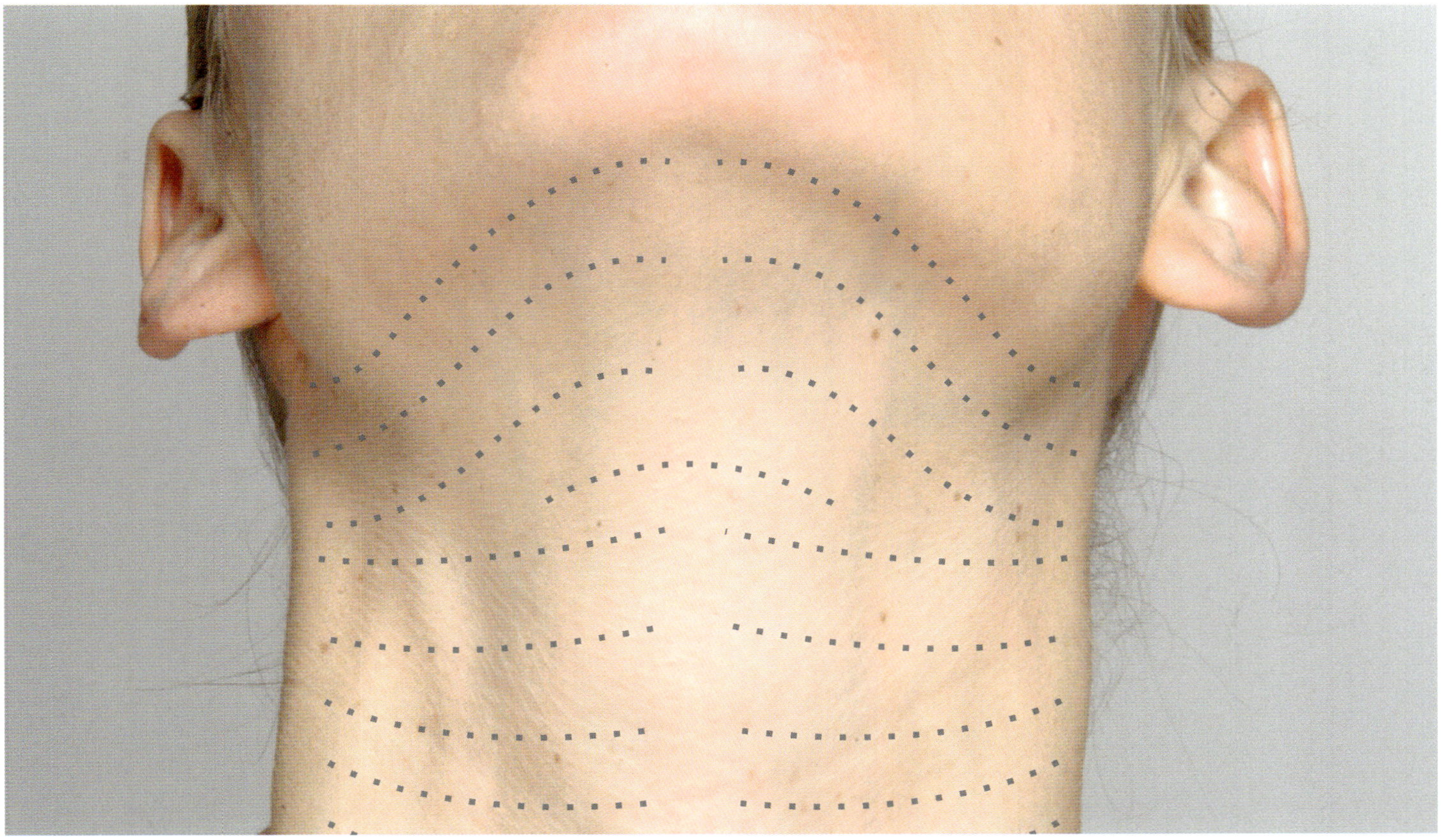

Injection diagram for epidermal firming treatment in the submandibular region.

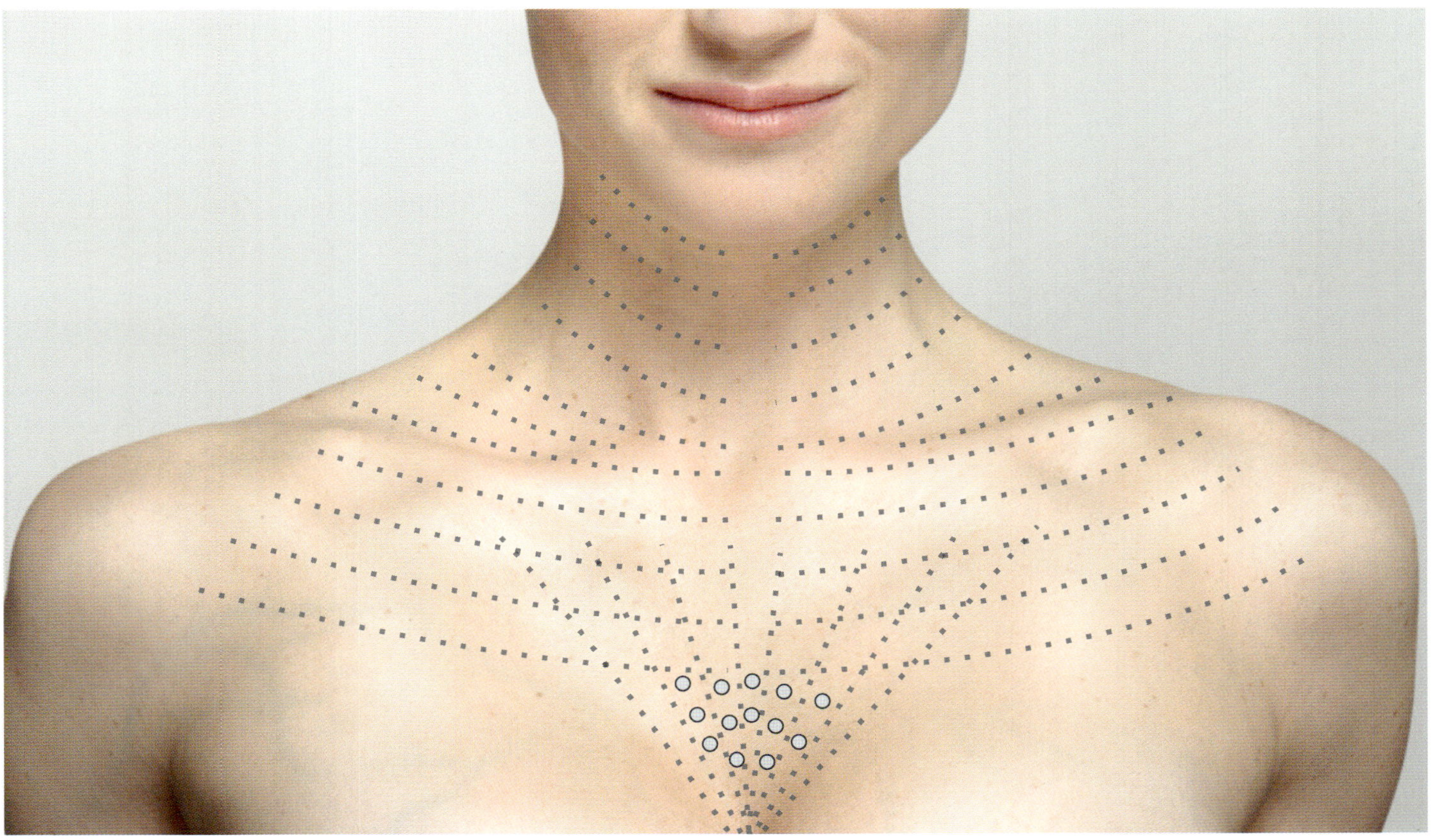

Large-area skin rejuvenation with Mesolift for neck and cleavage. Dots = serial injection technique, lines = epidermal technique.

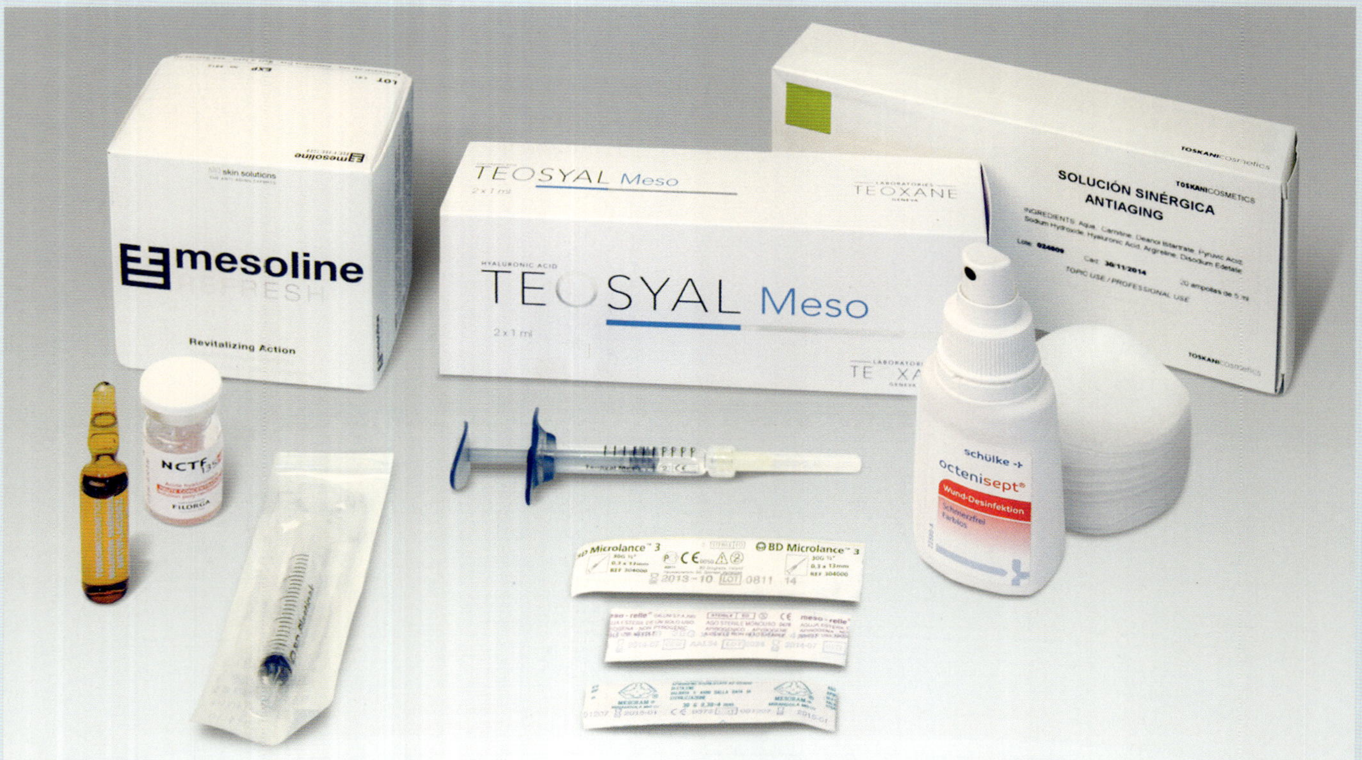

Materials needed for Mesolift.

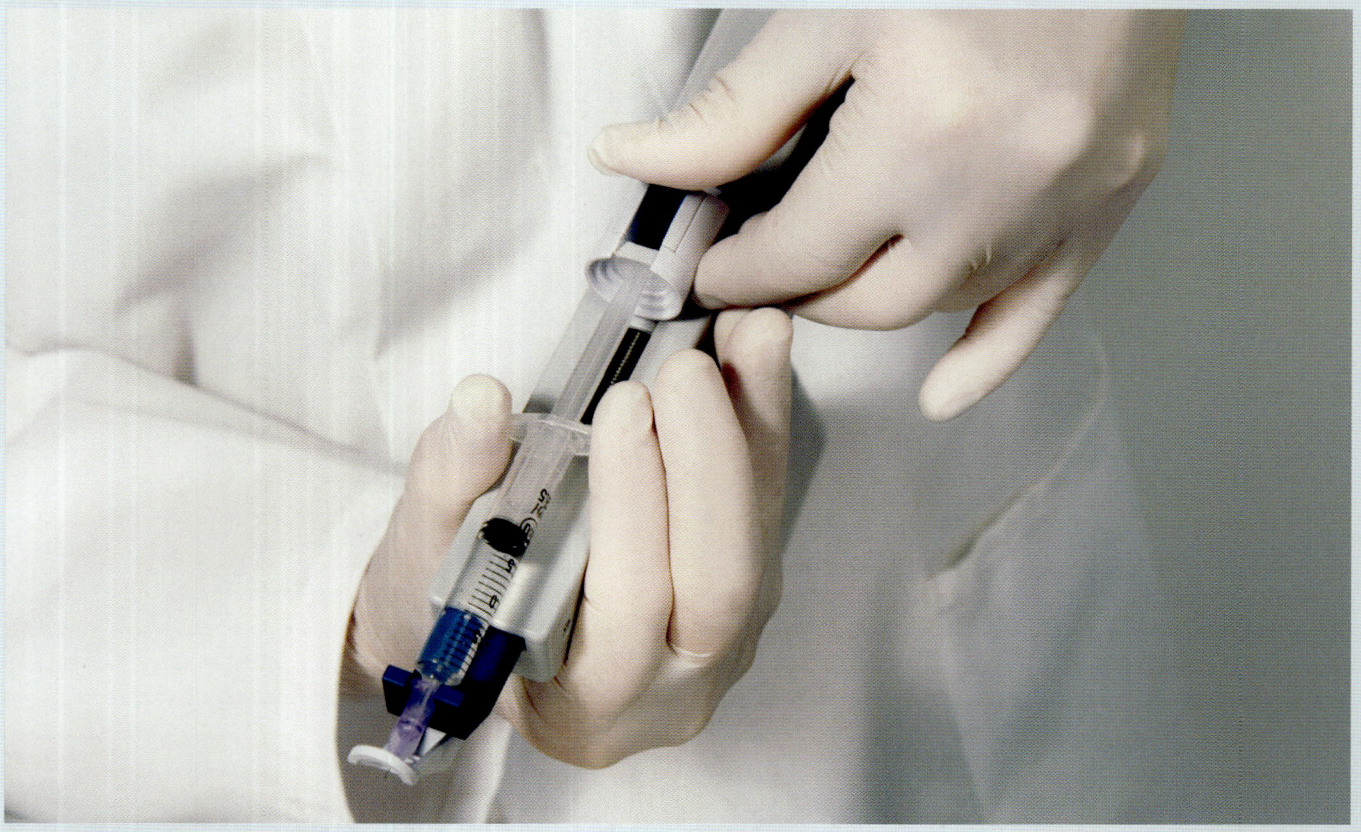

A mesogun should always be used on the face: the figure shows how to insert and lock the syringe into the injector.

Preparing a firming cocktail

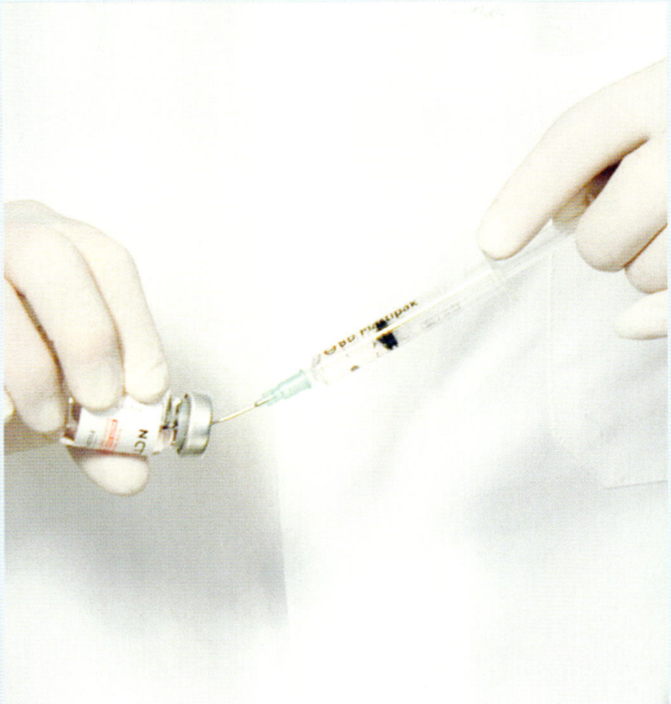

Draw up 1 ml of NCTF into a 2.5-ml syringe.

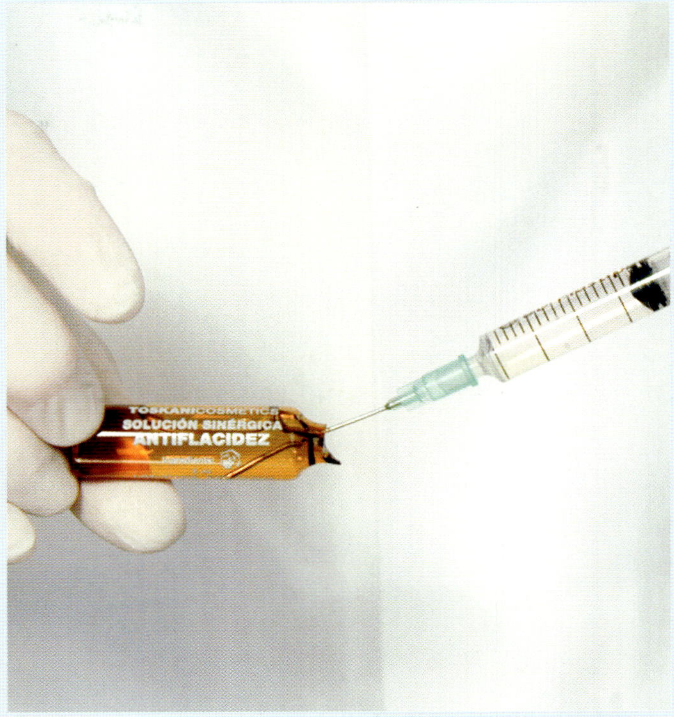

Add 1 ml of firming cocktail (ready-made product from Toskani or DM-Silk).

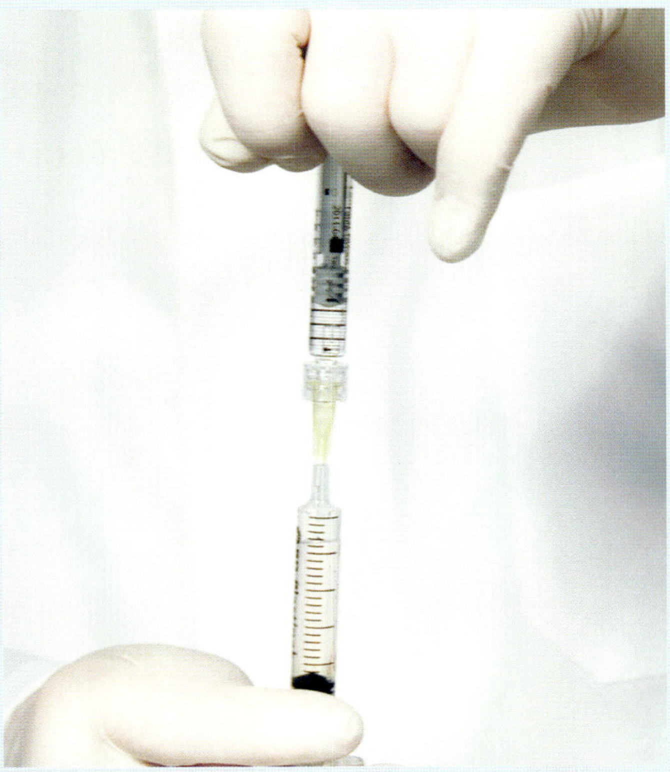

Now add 0.3 ml of non-cross-linked HA to the aqueous phase using a fine needle.

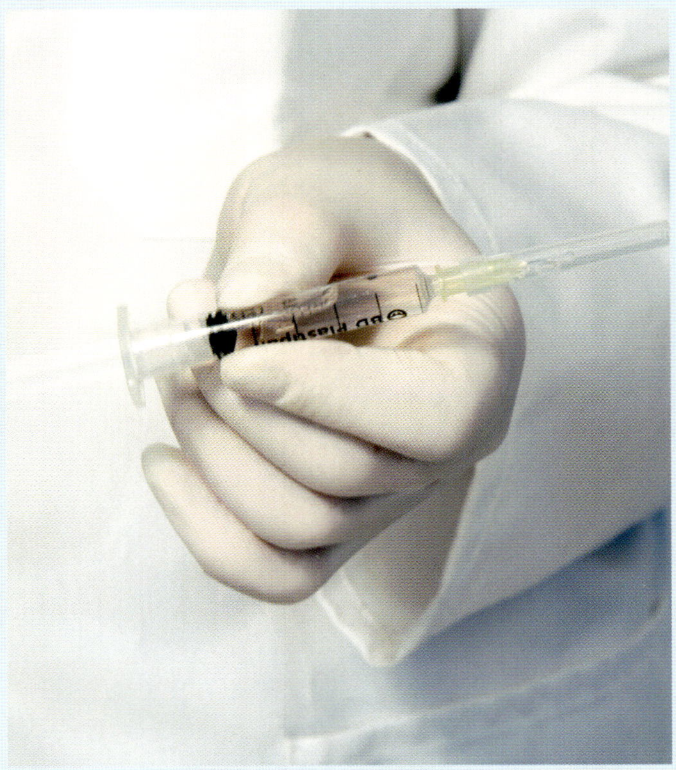

Finish by shaking gently to homogenize. Expel any air from the syringe and fit a short 4-mm needle. Check that the needle is patent, after which the syringe can be inserted into the injector.

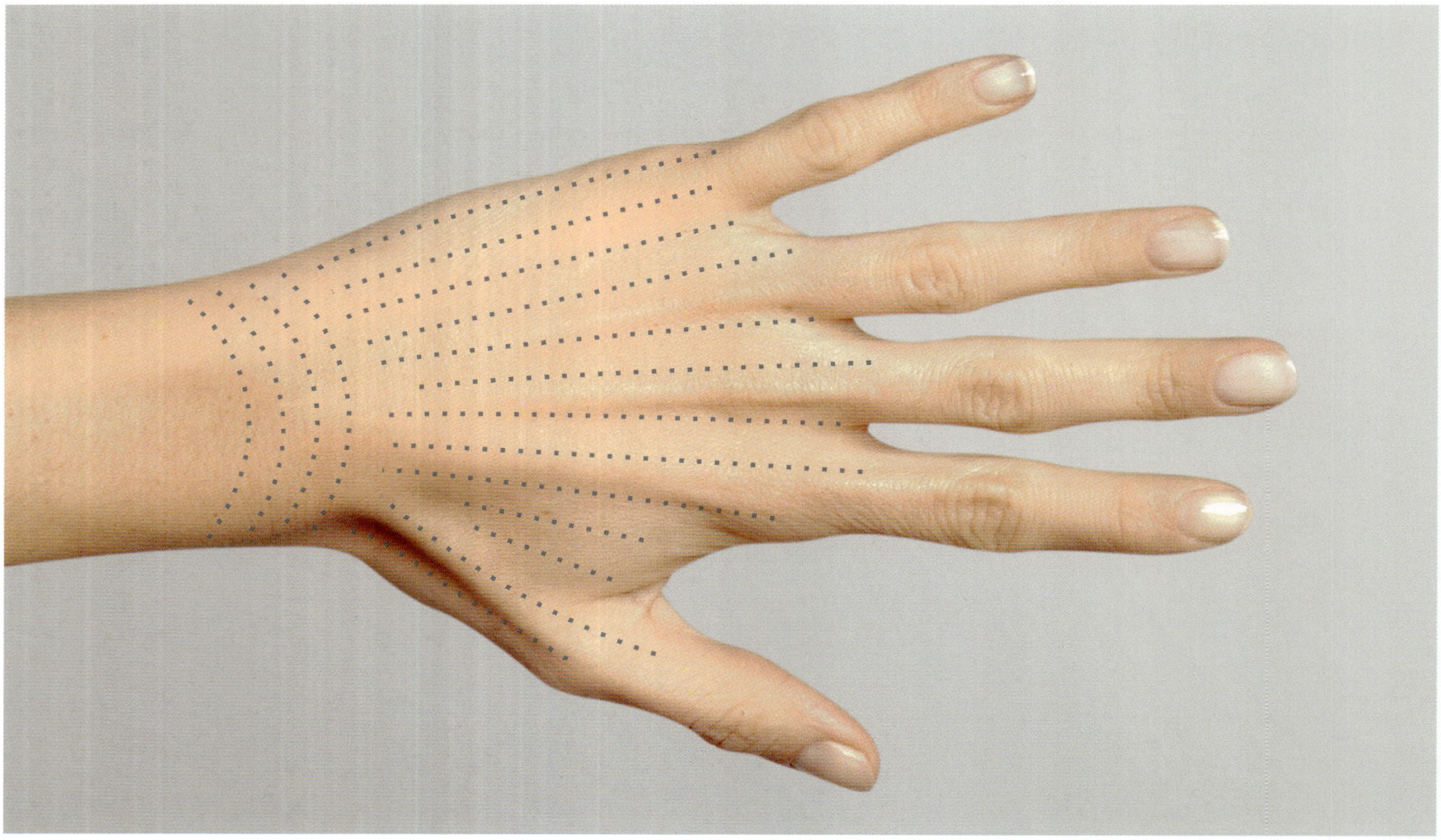

The backs of the hands and the neck betray a person's true age. Inquiries about the rejuvenation of specific areas like these are on the increase.

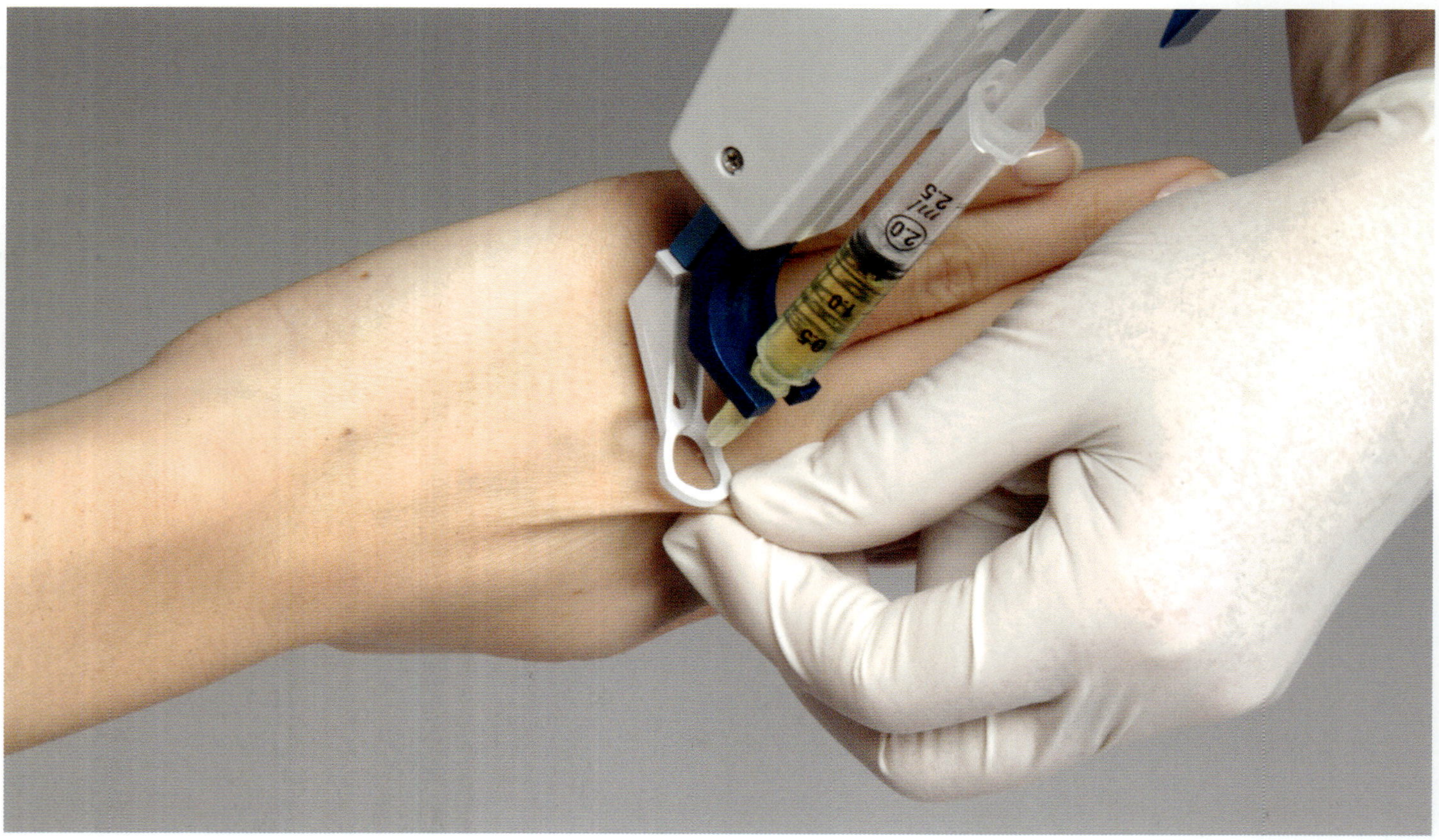

Mesolift, possibly filler and the treatment of pigment spots can be combined here.

8.1.3 The Mesolift treatment

Mesoglow (Light but long)	
Simple mixture	Lidocaine 1 % 0.5 ml + pentoxyfilline 0.5 ml + vitamin C Rotexmedica 0.5 ml + calcitonin 100 0.2 ml
Alternative	Procaine 1 % 1 ml + NCTF 135® HA 1 ml
Technique	Epidermal nappage + point-by-point injections 1–2 mm deep into the deeper lines
Location	Whole face, neck, particularly over the carotids, cleavage, backs of the hands
Needles	Mesoram or Mesojet 4 mm, 45° angle

Mesolift (Rejuvenation)	
Simple mixture	NCTF 135® 2 ml + Teosyal Meso® 0.3 ml + LA 0.2 ml
Alternative	Pur Mesoline® refresh, Toskani antiaging plus Mesolift o.a.
Technique + location	See above

Mesotight (Anti-sagging)	
Mixture	NCTF 135® 2 ml + Teosyal Meso® 0.3 ml + LA 0.2 ml
Alternative	Pure Mesoline® refresh, Toskani antiaging plus Mesolift etc.
Technique + location	See above

Mesorelax	
	Toskani Cocktail Anti-Aging with Argireline®
Technique + location	See above

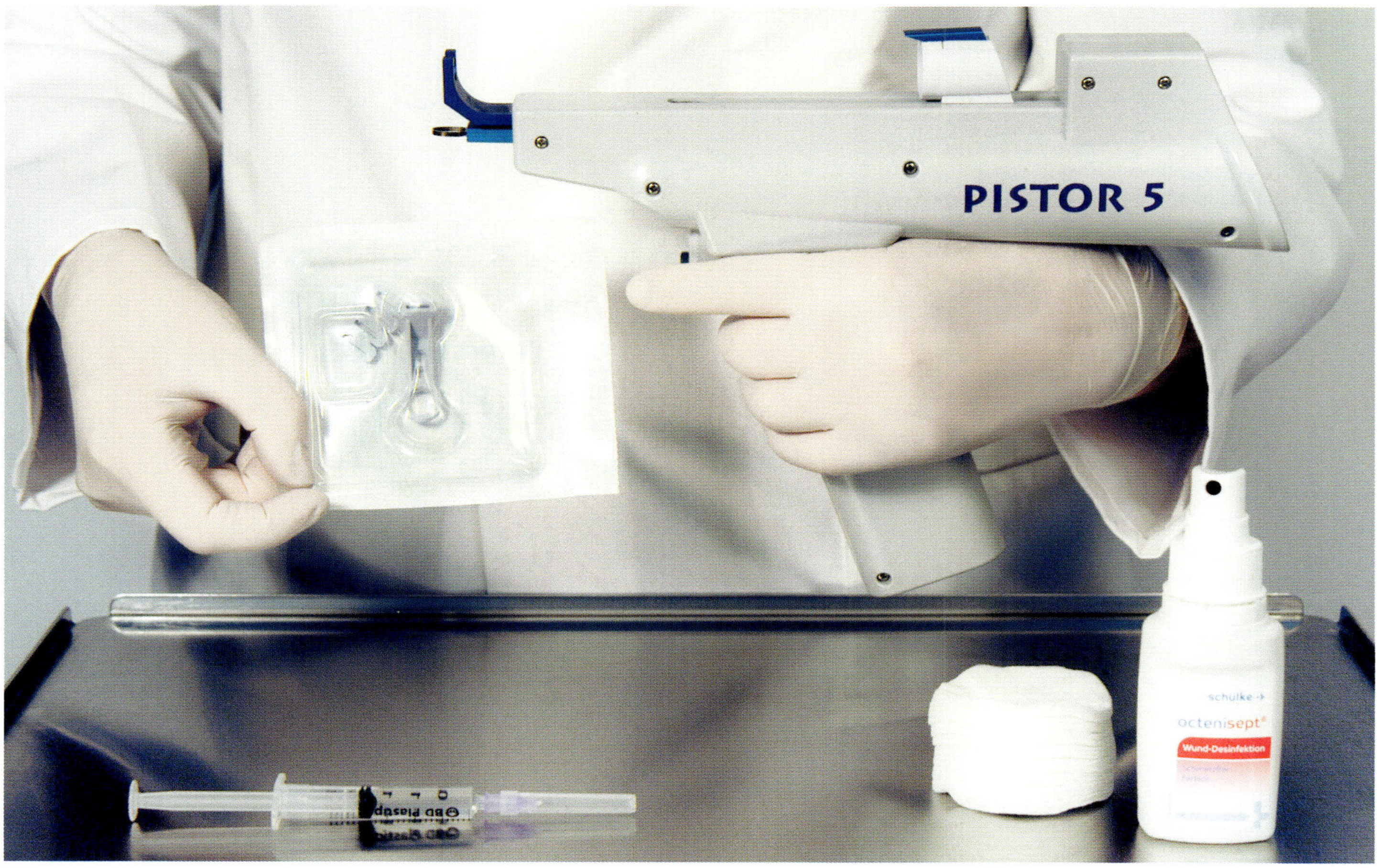

A new skin stabilizer should be fitted for each treatment.

8.1.4 Mesobotox

Mesobotox refers to the addition of small doses of Botulinum toxin to a regenerative isotonic mesotherapy mixture. This is injected not into a target muscle, but intradermally. On the one hand, this leads to direct relaxation of the small skin muscles and, on the other, to mild relaxation of the deeper muscles (as a result of diffusion). Examples of how these individually tailored cocktails are used in specific areas include, e.g. to *widen* the mouth and eye region (6 IU in 0.5 ml Anti-Aging cocktail per eye and lip, respectively), at the neck and cleavage (10 IU in 1 ml Anti-Aging cocktail each). However, it is also possible to use 20 IU in 2 ml Anti-Aging cocktail to achieve global relaxation of the face. When working around the eye, do not inject past the boundary represented by the eyebrow ridges. Side-effects are not likely. In practice, considering the low Botox doses involved, a product strength of 50 IU (Bocouture® or Vistabel®) tends to be used instead of 100 IU. The effect persists for at least six months, and initially skeptical Botox "refusers" often find that this starts them off on classical Botox treatment.
Anatomical studies demonstrate the considerable complexity of the anatomical relationships of the highly differentiated facial musculature, with its frequent overlaps and asymmetries, making precise intramuscular injection difficult. There are thus many factors which favor this gentler variant of Botulinum treatment. Former concerns that Botox could not be mixed with other ingredients without losing its effect have long since been thrown out by the clinical evidence of its efficacy. It is important for the mixture to be isotonic and for it to be used immediately after it is prepared.

8.1.5 The "tension column" technique

A new technique from Spain potentiates the effect of Mesolift by producing traction vectors. It is used to give greater firmness and padding to zones of more severe tissue sagging. Using a targeted infiltration technique, 0.5–1 ml each of the Mesolift mixture is injected intradermally into defined points and then massaged in with a circular motion against the underlying bone. This forced tissue expansion then leads to a mild, local fill-and-lift effect. The "tension columns" are constructed at strategic points, such as the temples to firm and lift the lateral part of the eye and the mid-face region, periorally to firm and lift the area around the mouth, or in the angle between lower jaw and neck to firm and lift and neck.

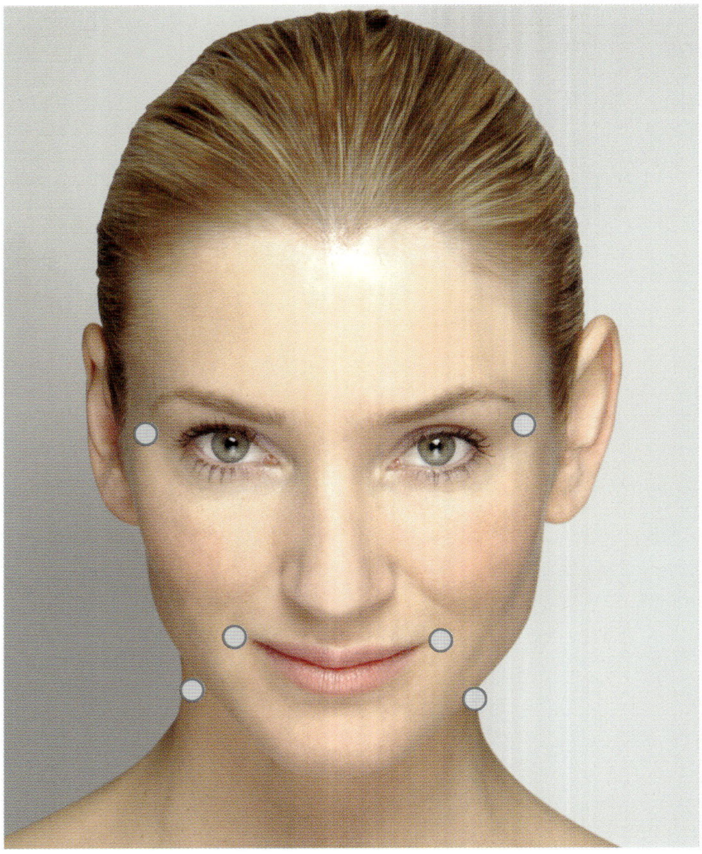

Anatomical positions of the "tension column" injection points, front view.

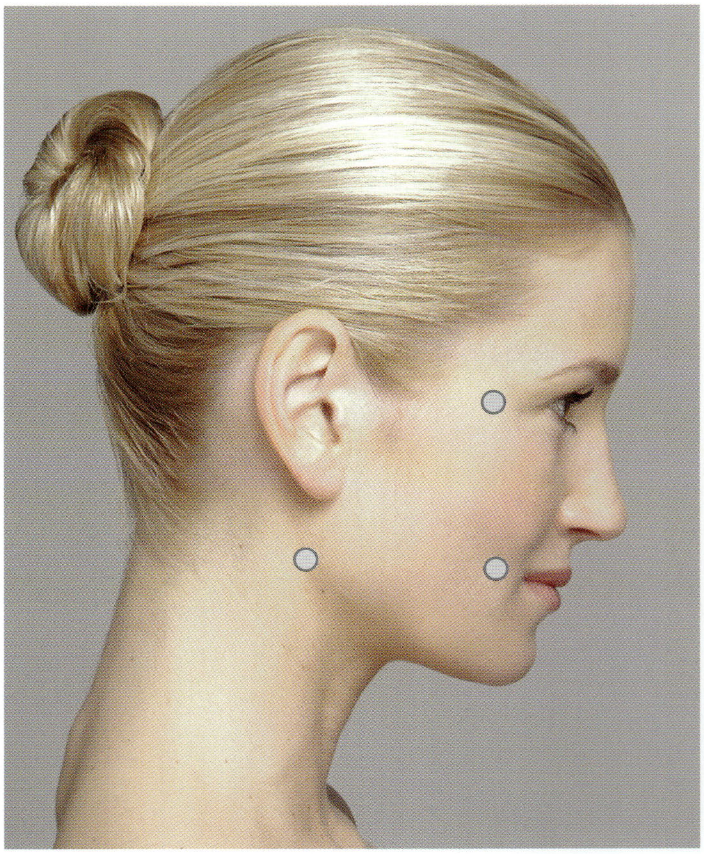

Anatomical positions of the "tension column" injection points, side view.

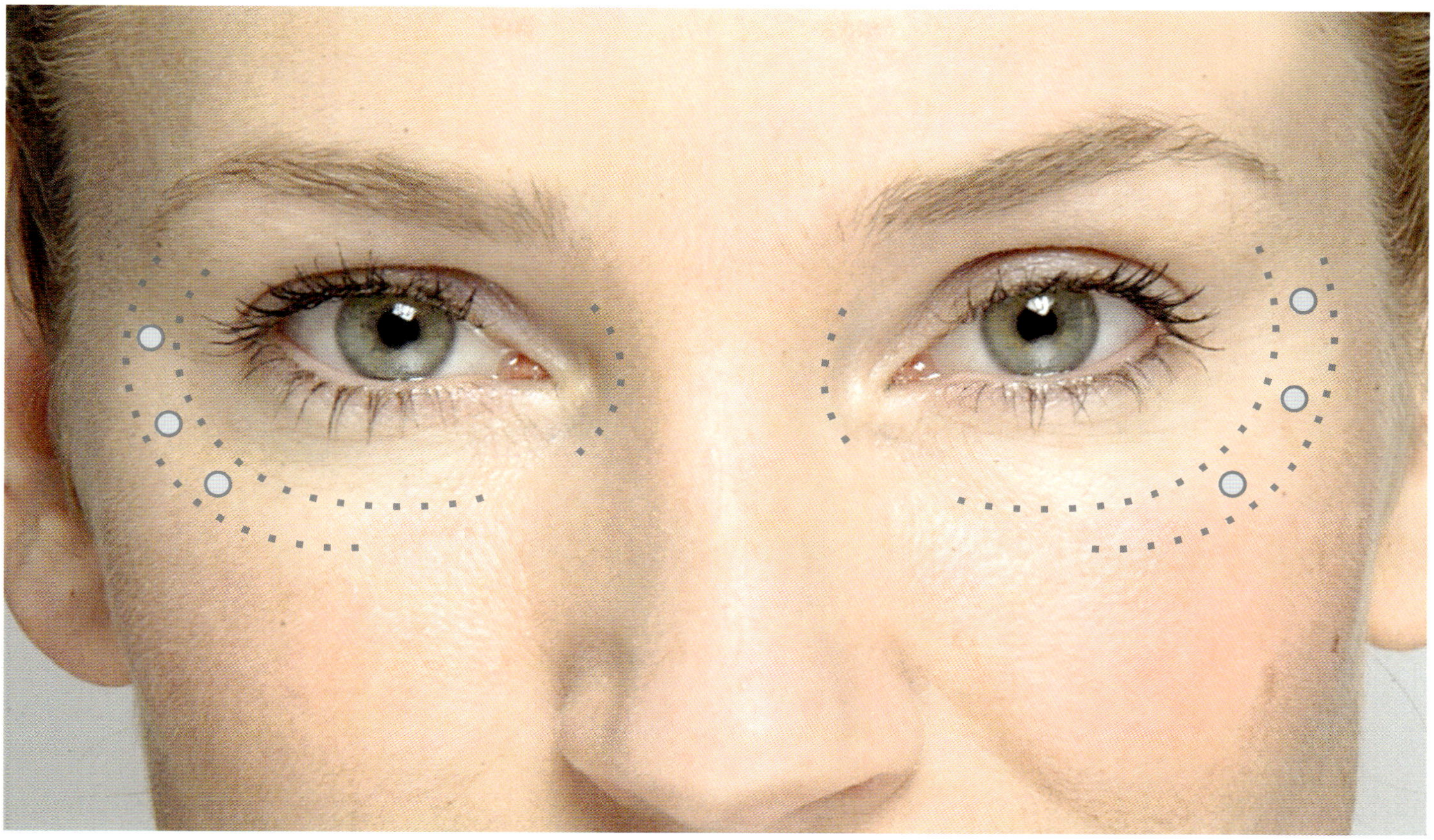

Injection technique for Mesobotox: intradermal nappage and serial injections to smooth fine lines and widen the eye openings.

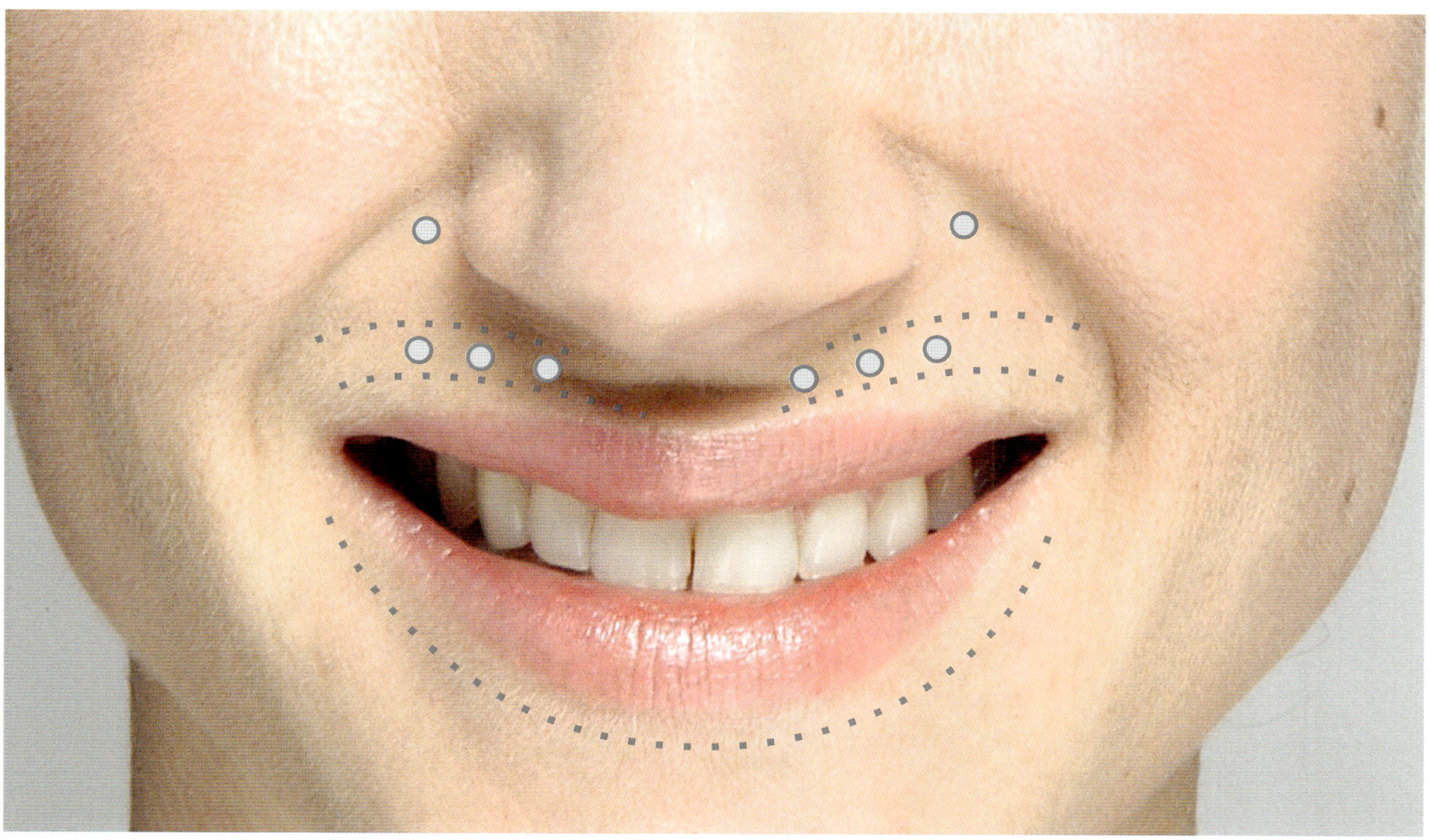

Injection technique for Mesobotox: intradermal nappage and serial injections to smooth stubborn lines around the mouth and to open up the mouth region.

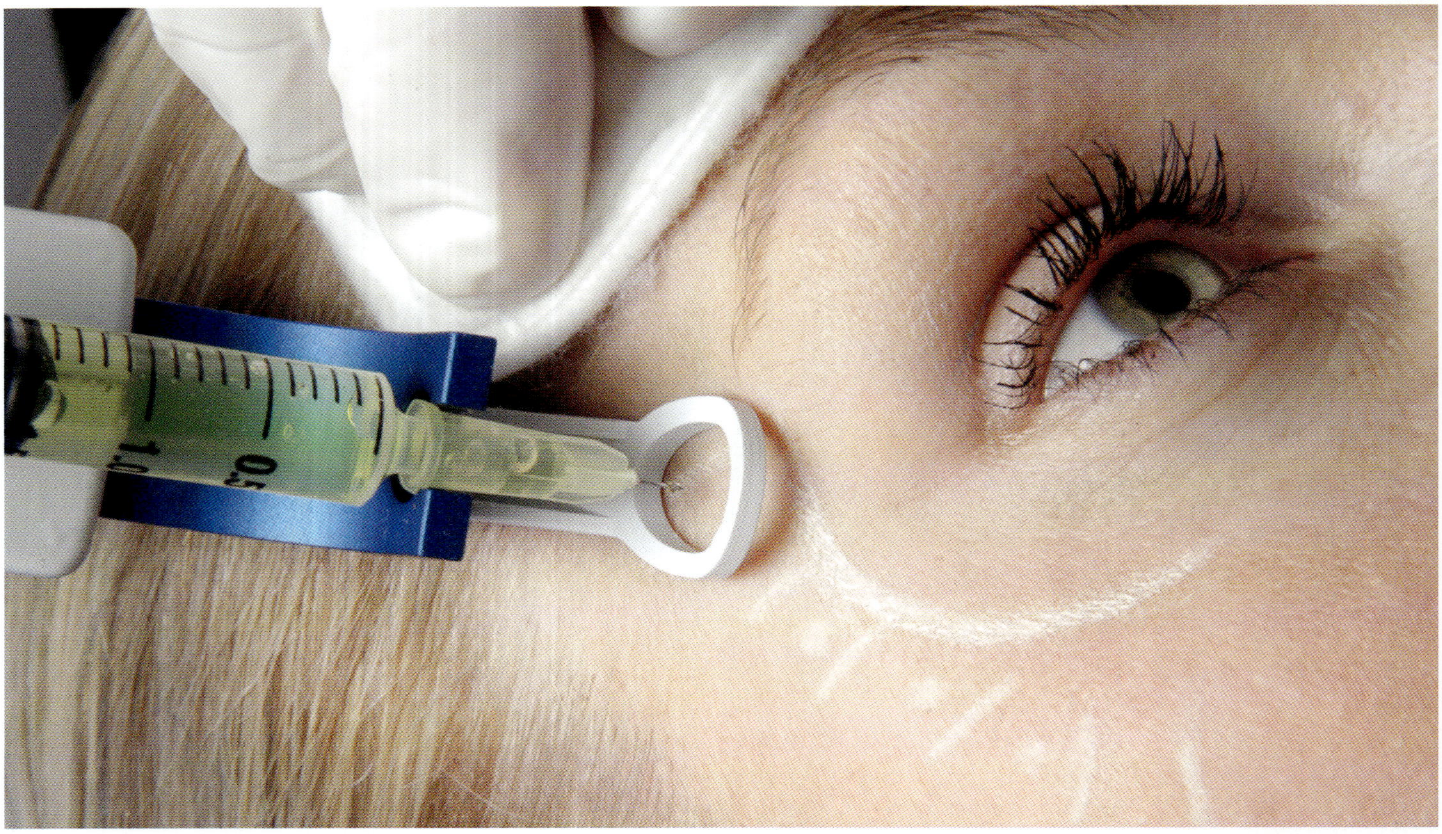

In Mesobotox, a combined technique is used to achieve both relaxation of the small superficial skin muscles …

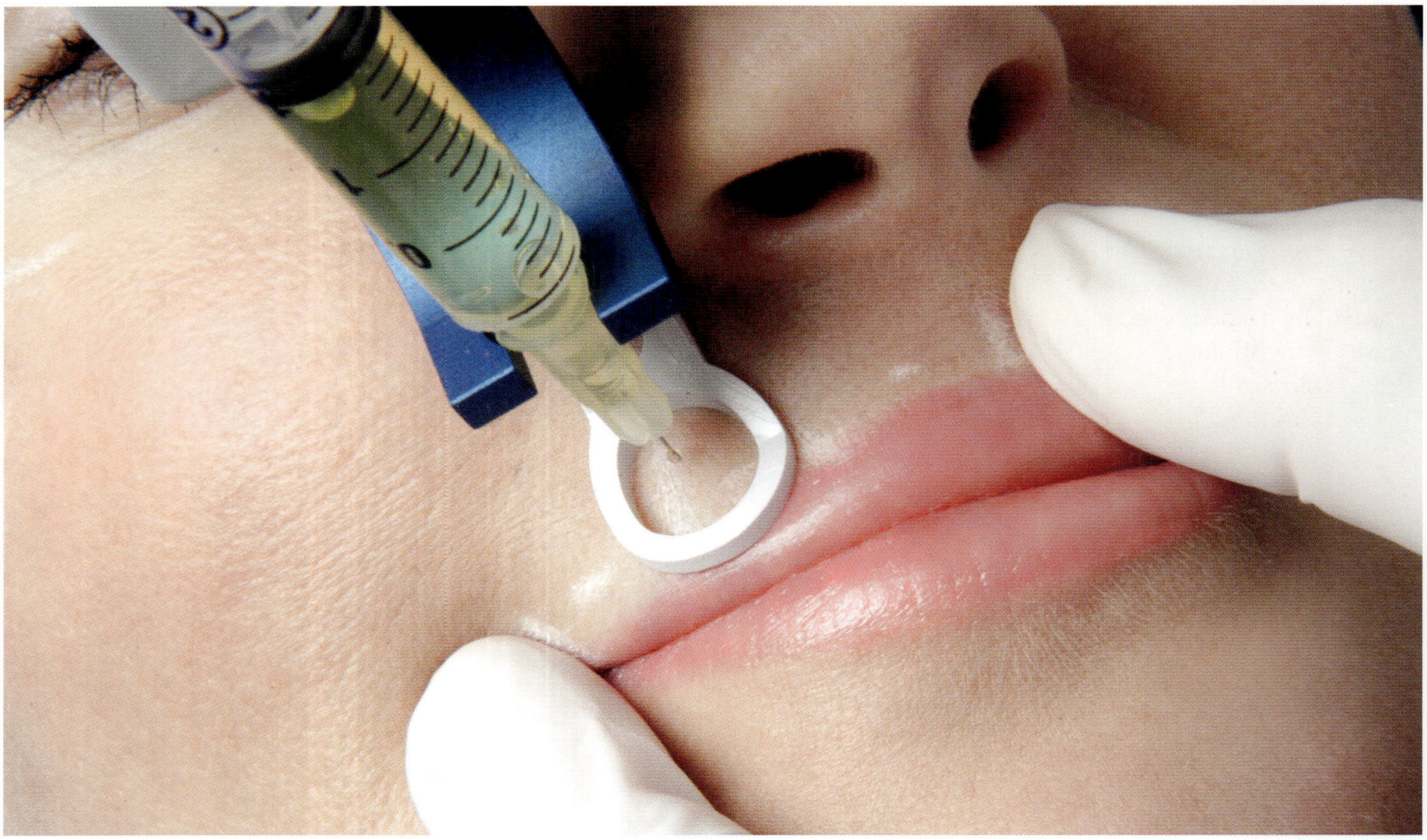

… and a diffuse and thus discrete effect on the deeper musculature.

8.2 MesoHair

Thick, luxuriant hair is a sign of youthful dynamism. A full head of hair communicates a positive impression to our fellow humans. Consequently, both men and women suffer greatly from another typical sign of aging: hair loss.
The daily loss of up to 100 individual hairs is normal. During washing, the only hairs that are lost are those already in the resting phase, that would have fallen out in any case. The most common type of hair loss in men, so-called androgenetic alopecia, has a genetic cause. It develops due to an inherited hypersensitivity of the hair roots to dihydrotestosterone (DHT), formed in the body from the male hormone testosterone. It is typical to see either a *receding hairline* at the front, or thinning of the hair at the back of the head in a *tonsure* pattern.
A certain degree of androgen-related hair loss is also normal in women over 50, particularly in the parietal region, caused by the hormonal changes during the menopause. This also includes a loss of hair volume due to a progressive decrease in hair thickness. However, this type of hair loss is also increasingly found in younger women, for unknown reasons. A periodic increase in hair loss may occur in spring and autumn. This rise in hair turnover is a normal, self-regulating physiological process. Post-partum alopecia, this time caused by hormonal changes following childbirth, is another form of physiological hair loss.
Acute hair loss can be experienced as totally traumatic from the psychological point of view, and rapid and effective intervention is often needed. When the history is taken, the patient will need to be asked about the duration and severity of the hair loss, previous treatments and any medication (taken orally, including food supplements; ask about DHEA and topical treatment, e.g. with minoxidil), exposure to toxins (thallium, arsenic, mercury, chemotherapy), concurrent disorders, e.g. of the thyroid, or iron deficiency (lab tests will be needed).
Mesotherapy should not be recommended in patients with high autoimmune activity, e.g. in (sub)total alopecia areata, in FFA (=frontal fibrosing alopecia with folliculitis and destruction of the hair follicles by scarring) or in patients with long-standing baldness, because of the poor chances of success. If definitive destruction of the hair follicles has taken place, the only remaining option is the *classical* method of autologous hair transplantation, in which so-called micrografts (individual hair follicles or small groups of two to three hairs) are transplanted. However, in all other forms of non-pathological hair loss, there is a very good chance of achieving successful and safe treatment with MesoHair. Prompt intervention is ideal, to prevent atrophy of the hair follicles and excessive apoptosis of the keratinocytes. The aim is to increase the anagen and reduce the telogen phase. This can be demonstrated using a trichogram (see Figure, page 89). The Trichoscan® is another diagnostic method. Most patients refuse a traction test or a skin biopsy. In contrast, photographic documentation of the treatment course, which is also shown to the patient, is desirable and considerably increases compliance.

8.2.1 The hair phases

1 Anagen phase
Duration c. three to seven years, active pigment production, growth c. 1 cm/month, > 80% of all hair on the head.

2 Catagen phase
Duration two to four weeks. The hair shaft detaches itself from its blood supply, hair color is lost; two to three percent of hairs are in this phase at any point in time.

3 Telogen phase
The most severe hair loss, up to 15% of hairs are in this phase. It can last three months.

The revitalization cocktail injected into the scalp in MesoHair leads to stimulation and regeneration of the hair roots. Hair loss of any sort is arrested in most cases. Provided that the hair roots are still vital, it results in renewed and often continuing hair growth, together with improved hair quality. Six sessions at one-week intervals will be needed. This is followed by three treatments every two weeks with subsequent monthly maintenance treatments, if required.
Hair growth in unwanted places or shedding (increased hair loss caused when the telogen hair falls out) is not generally likely. New hair becomes apparent after about two to three months. Patients should wash their hair before the treatment and must not dye their hair or have a perm for the first 24 hours. Incidentally, the scalp is not particularly sensitive to pain, although stimulation of the many acupuncture points is often perceived as unpleasant.
Any other problems, such as dandruff or seborrhea, can also be treated during the MesoHair therapy. In these cases, a homeopathic adjuvant is added to the mesotherapy mixture, in the form of Ferrum Sulfur comp. from Wala or Wiedemann Homöokomplex BH. Contrary to public opinion, the scalp is very well perfused, which is why the antifibrotic agent pentoxyfilline tends to be used as a vasoactive agent.
Buflomedil can lead to severe hyperemia of the scalp even at doses of just over 0.2 ml. The purpose of the active substances used in MesoHair is to energize the keratinocytes in the matrix, i.e. to improve the terminal microcirculation, thus improving micronutrition of the hair follicle.

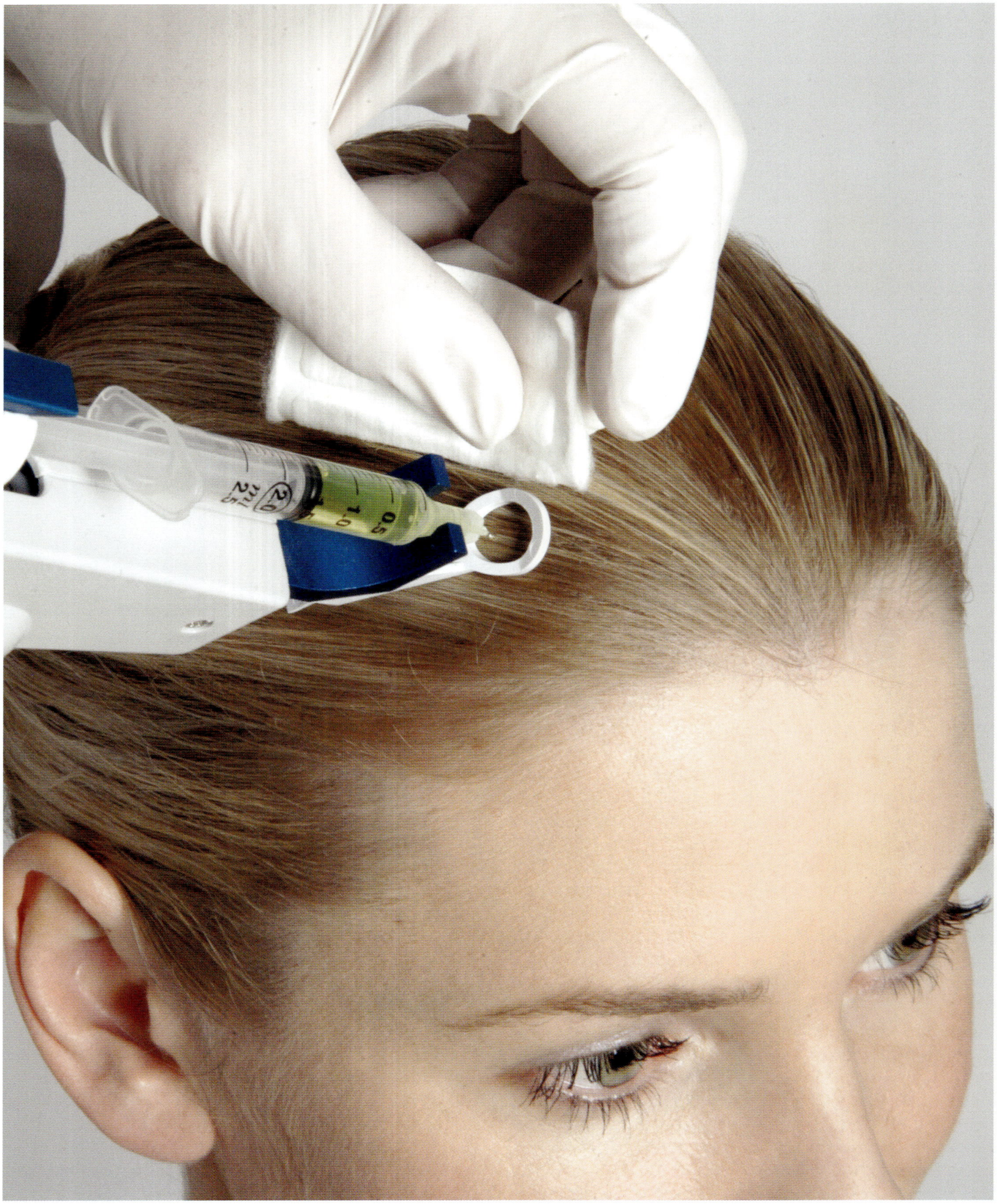

The hair loss treatment may be administered manually or using the mesotherapy injector. Needle length 4–6 mm (Mesojet is best).

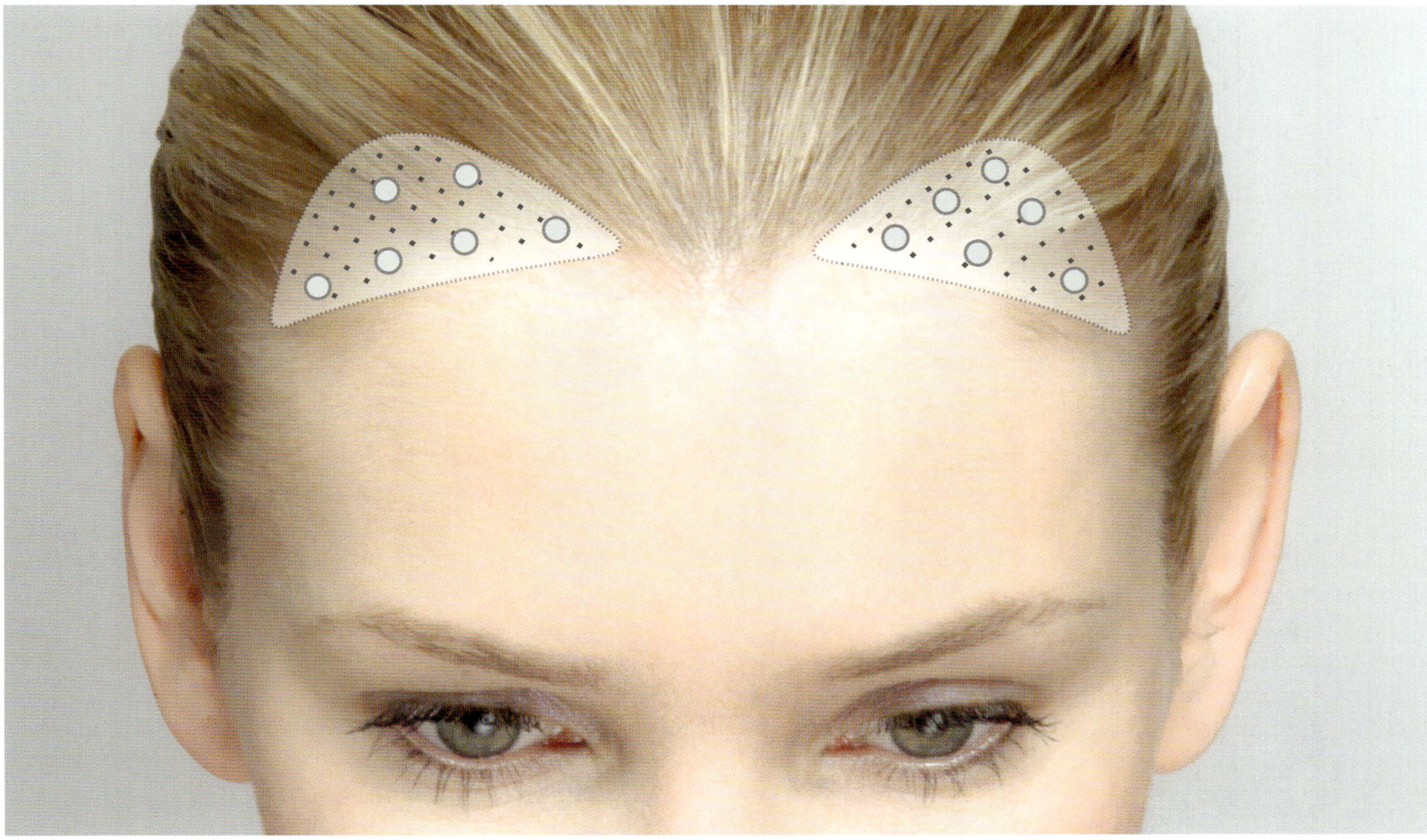

Treatment zones and injection technique in frontal hair loss. Tonsure pattern or circular hair loss (alopecia areata) is treated analogously.

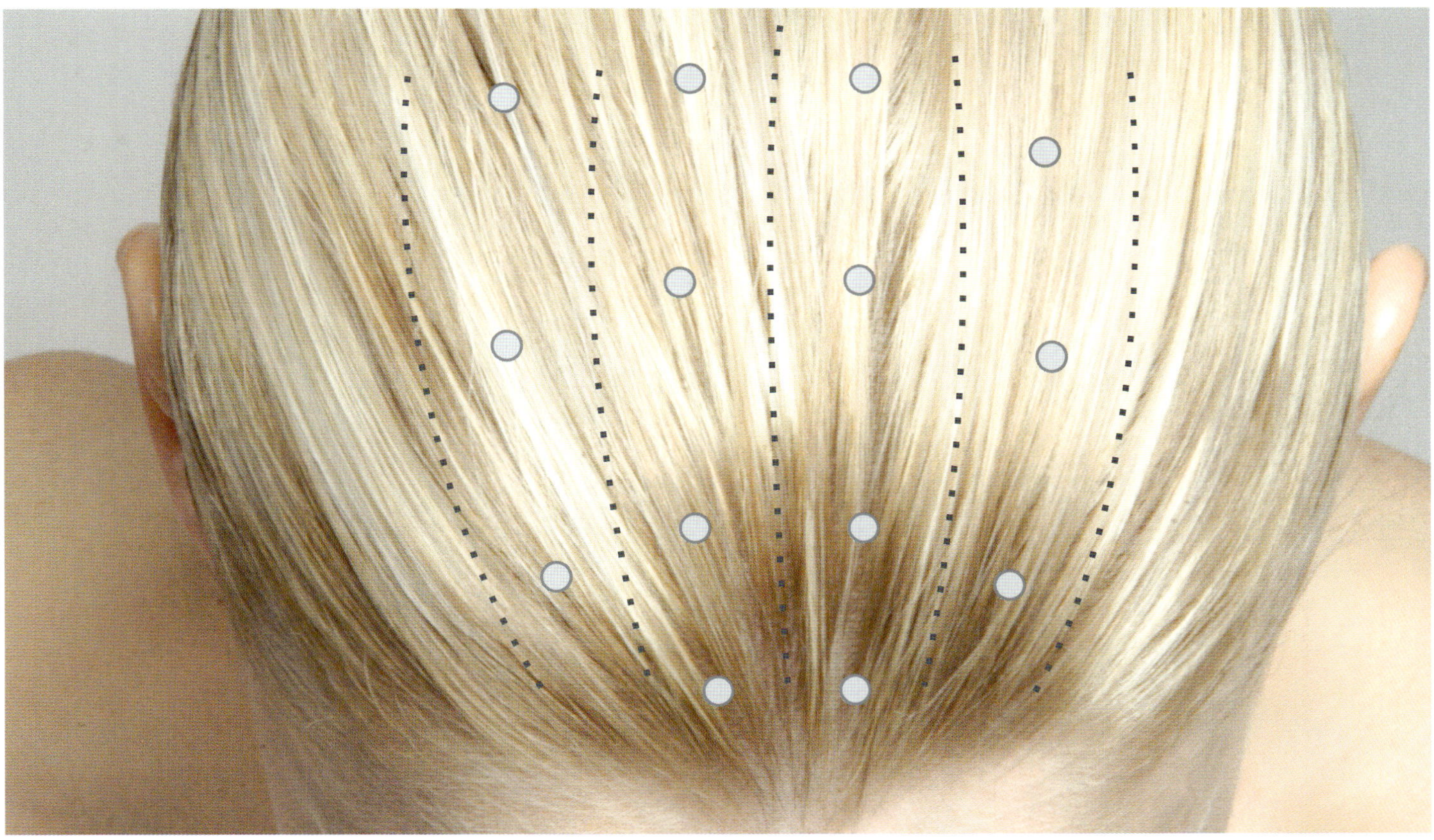

Treatment zones and injection technique in hair loss in the parietal region. Epidermal lines are an option only in cases of severe thinning or where a bald spot has formed.

The non-interventional treatment observation studies carried out to date, particularly in diffuse and often also stress-induced hair loss, confirm the excellent efficacy and tolerability of mesotherapy. No other hair-specific medication was permitted in these studies. The global success rates show a doctor and patient satisfaction rate of about 80%. Cessation of hair loss was achieved after four sessions in 90% of cases, with new hair growth on the bare patches in 50–70% after three months. The younger the patient, the better the result (Petit 1983–1992, 150 cases; van der Niepen 1992, 150 cases, DGM 2009–2010).

8.2.2 MesoHair treatment

MesoHair is not indicated with highly active autoimmune processes, such as extensive alopecia areata, alopecia totalis or frontal fibrosing folliculitis. Definitive destruction of the hair follicles may also be assumed if the head has been bald for a long time.
Mesobotox is a new treatment variant for hair loss. It relaxes the muscle fibers of the scalp and could thus dilate the blood vessels indirectly, ensuring a better supply of nutrients for the follicles.
Gradual or sudden hair loss can affect anyone. Women aged between 50 and 70 years alone generally lose 20% of their head hair. In men, a receding headline or tonsure pattern hair loss are often genetically pre-programmed, even at a young age. Stress or a deficiency in vital nutrients can also play a role. However, shampoos and tinctures are totally incapable of reaching the hair root, embedded 4 mm deep into the scalp, and often produce little success. The increasingly available food supplements (cosmecueticals) have a similar problem: the active substances are distributed throughout the body, and reach the target area with difficulty. Anti-androgen tablets need to be taken for life if their effect is to be maintained. Minoxidil, a frequently prescribed agent, needs to be applied locally twice a day, which is an unacceptable inconvenience for a lot of patients. Many patients who consult a physician or alternative practitioner specializing in this method have already been through a long odyssey of unsuccessful treatments. Relative to its global success rate of 80% after about 3 months (cessation of hair loss, new growth, increased volume) and also the likelihood of a long-lasting result, the time investment of mesotherapy is quite negligible: 6 treatments at weekly intervals, followed by monthly maintenance therapy if required. Risks and side-effects, apart from the mild injection pain, are virtually unknown. In alopecia areata and androgenetic hair loss in women, treatment costs may be recovered under private insurance schemes, because both forms are regarded as pathological.

8

Examples of active substance mixtures in MesoHair treatments	
1. Dexpanthenol 0.5 ml + biotin 0.5 ml (or Cocktail Hair Toskani 1 ml) + procaine 1 % 1 ml 2. Procaine 1 % 0.5 ml + Thymus extract 0.5 ml + NCTF 135® HA 0.5 ml 3. Cocktail Hair 0,5 ml + Cocktail FCE 0,5 ml + Tauricol 0,5 ml + Rutinel 0,5 ml 4. Cocktail Hair + Cocktail Anti-Aging Toskani 0.5 ml each + procaine 1 % 1 ml	
The following may be added if required: 1. Buflomedil or pentoxyfilline, Silicor, taurine, caffeine 10 % or carnitine, 0.2 ml in each case 2. Finasteride or futasteride, 0.2–0.5 ml in each case	
Technique	Epidermal nappage in hairless areas, point-by-point infiltrations 2–4 mm deep and 1 cm apart in the affected area. Disinfection is often difficult; however, the risk of infection on the head is very low.
Needles	Microlance 13 mm at a 45° angle or Mesojet/Mesoram 4 mm at a 90° angle. In sensitive patients, one can also work with the Mesorelle needle and with the aid of an injector in C mode.
Location	The whole region of hair loss, particularly the parietal area, tonsure, receding hairline, patches of circular hair loss. Intensive diffusion processes ensure distribution of the active substances throughout the scalp.

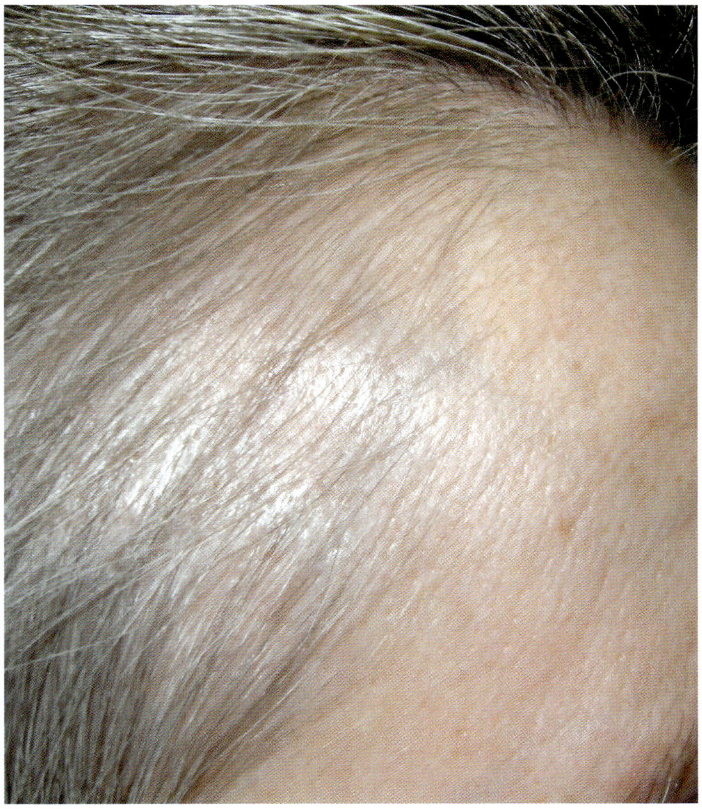

Baseline status at the first MesoHair treatment.

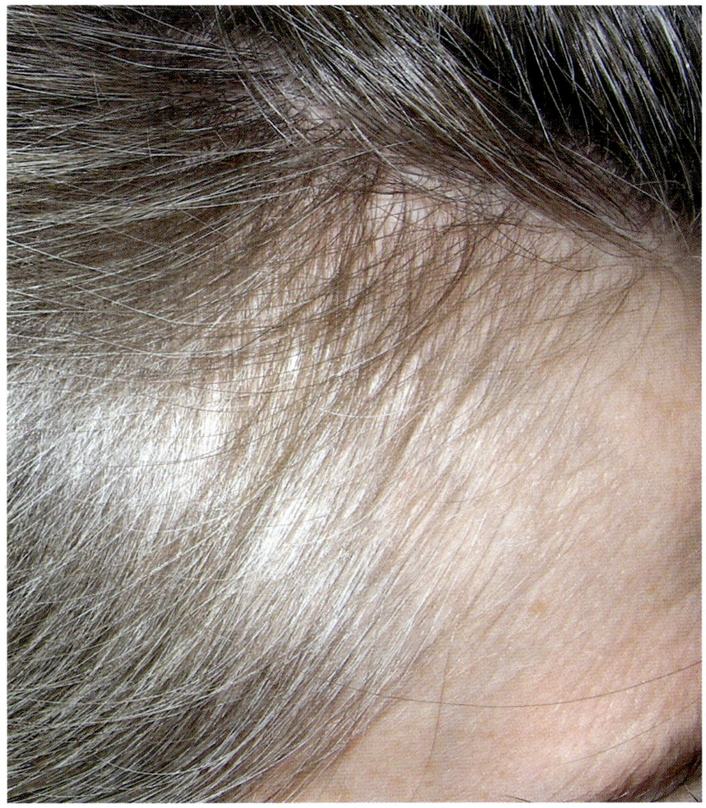

Treatment result after 10 sessions, corresponding with the same female patient's trichograms as shown below.

1) Trichogram – before

FINDINGS: hair root type (%)

Site of hair removal	Anagen Root sheath with	without	Total	Catagen	Telogen	Dystrophic	Broken
Frontal	40	20	60	–	60	–	–
Parietal/Vertex	50	35	85		15		
Margins of a lesion/patch	80	5	85		15		
Occipital							
NORMAL (%)			> 80	< 5	< 20	< 5	

EVALUATION

Normal findings
Findings correlate with clinical diagnosis
Please note the following

Date of treatment 30 09 08

i. A. B.

2) Trichogram – after

FINDINGS: hair root type (%)

Site of hair removal	Anagen Root sheath with	without	Total	Catagen	Telogen	Dystrophic	Broken
Frontal	60	30	90	–	10	–	–
Parietal/Vertex							
Occipital							
NORMAL (%)			> 80	< 5	< 20	< 5	

EVALUATION

Normal findings
Findings correlate with clinical diagnosis
Please note the following

Date of treatment 09 03 09 (Day Month Year)

i. A. B.
Assessed by

The before-and-after trichograms of the MesoHair treatment, provided by the University of Munich, impressively document the clinical results after 10 sessions: more hair in the growth phase, less hair in the resting phase.

8

8.3 Treatment of cellulite and localized fat deposits

"I have only one line, and I'm sitting on it" was the mischievous comment made by the venerable Frenchwoman Jeanne Calment. She died in 1997 at the Biblical age of 122 years, and still holds the record as the longest-lived person in the world. Those lucky individuals who can make that sort of claim nowadays are either totally lacking in vanity, full of self-confidence or heavy on the scales.

Overweight is a subject that (quite literally) moves the world, or that should move it. It has taken on epidemic qualities. Practices of esthetic medicine will also need to tackle it, as the success of any *body styling* mission will depend to a key extent on the choice of individual treatment strategies. At the first contact with the patient, the practitioner will already need to decide if the following are present:

- pathological overweight requiring treatment, with a BMI > 30 (gross obesity)
- general overweight (obesity) with a BMI > 25
- localized fat deposits, abnormal fat distribution (also referred to as lipodystrophy)
- local structural changes in the adipose tissue (cellulite) in an individual of otherwise normal weight.

The aim is to develop an individually tailored concept for each case, accompanied by procedures which you yourself may not offer, but which you feel are advisable and which you wish to recommend, or which you would like to inform the patient about.

The options for outpatient injection methods are explained in this section; these may be performed immediately after the appropriate practical training has been completed. As is so often the case, lifestyle counseling and personal coaching are essential accompanying measures in this area of treatment, if permanent results are to be achieved.

The visual arts in particular readily demonstrate that ideals of beauty have changed considerably over the centuries. Whereas balanced proportions of face and body have been the ideal that we have aspired to since antiquity, the individuals depicted in those times tended to look somewhat stocky; it was only in Renaissance and Baroque art that their proportions became considerably more ample. Pale was regarded as beautiful, and the skin was smoothed with special "biological" preparations, as a book from the year 1689 reveals: "Place a mouse in olive oil until it has broken down almost completely, press it through a cloth and dab the skin with the liquor…". Biochemically speaking, this is not as perverse as it sounds (the liquor would contain amino acids, hyaluronic acid, carnitine, antioxidants, unsaturated fatty acids, etc.), and the same applies to the traditional vinegar and lemons diet (vitamin C, base formers, detoxification, purification, tissue firming).

The slim silhouette has only been regarded as ideal since the Romantic period; since the 20th century, it has all gone further downhill in terms of weight, at least when it comes to style-setting fashion models. However, just having a perfect WHR (waist to hip ratio) of 0.7 is a classic, totally achievable and desirable goal for the great majority of women. Another sensible for the figure is a waistline of ≤80 cm for women and ≤94 cm for men, the figures associated with the lowest cardiovascular risk.

8.3.1 Practical procedure in body styling

Carry out the inspection with the patient standing, preferably in front of a full-length mirror. The patient, undressed down to underclothing, points out his or her "problem zones" and the treatment goals are worked out jointly. Unrealistic ideas and requirements need to be cast aside and the patient guided towards an appropriate solution. Motivation and plenty of patience are needed.

Mark the target areas, taking into account any asymmetry. Take photographs in one or two views, measure circumferences and document the results, then ensure that the patient's informed consent and treatment cost forms are signed. Disinfect the skin, if the first treatment session is scheduled to take place. Treatment should start with the milder protocols. These must be documented in detail with respect to the active substances and injection volumes. If these are well tolerated, the therapy may be more aggressive next time. The treated regions should be marked on a body diagram and the technique used (mesotherapy and/or lipolysis) documented.

The number of sessions may vary between one (small, circumscribed regions of low severity, e.g. mild cellulite, small jowls or slight bags under the eyes) and more than ten. The interval between sessions should range between two (mesotherapy) and six weeks (lipolysis).

At each session, treat no more than one large zone (abdomen, thigh, buttocks, hips) or two small ones (e.g. upper arms and axillary fat). Effective protective medication against hematomas after the treatment consists of five globuli of Arnica D4 given orally or the addition of the homeopathic preparation Wiedemann Homöokomplex-BH to the injection. The use of Mesojet needles can also prevent hematomas. Diphenhydramine (Sedativum Hevert Ampoules, 0.5 ml in 10 ml) may be added to the mixture for lipolysis or for patients with an allergic predisposition. Some therapists even give a pulse of oral prednisone if severe reactions are likely (e.g. lipolysis in the area around the eyes). In most cases, however, the topical application of some Retterspitz® äußerlich or medical taping are sufficient to relieve any inflammatory reactions on the body.

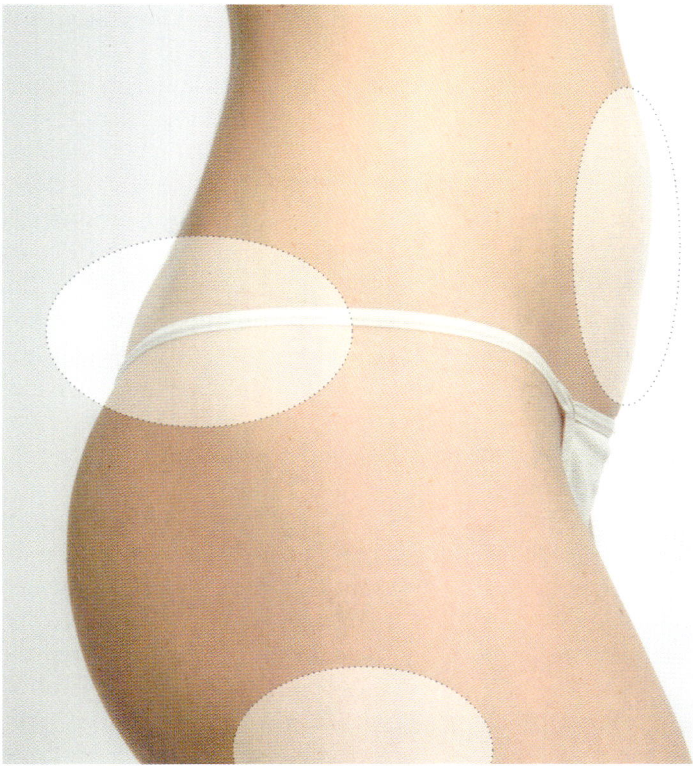

Fat deposits and treatment zones: hip, abdomen, thigh.

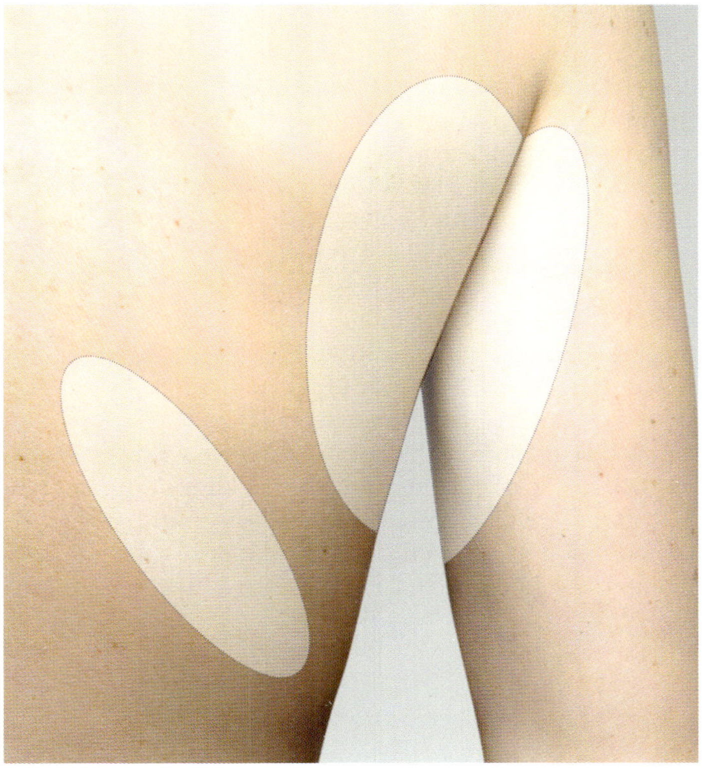

Fat deposits and treatment zones: upper arm, axilla, love handles.

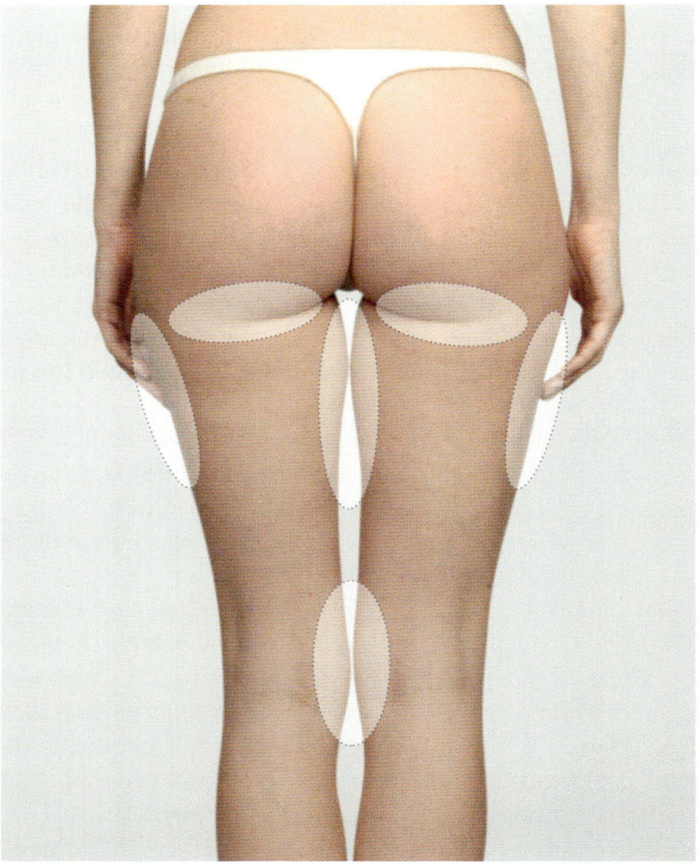

Fat deposits and treatment zones: inner thighs and knees, saddle bags (outer thighs), banana rolls (buttocks).

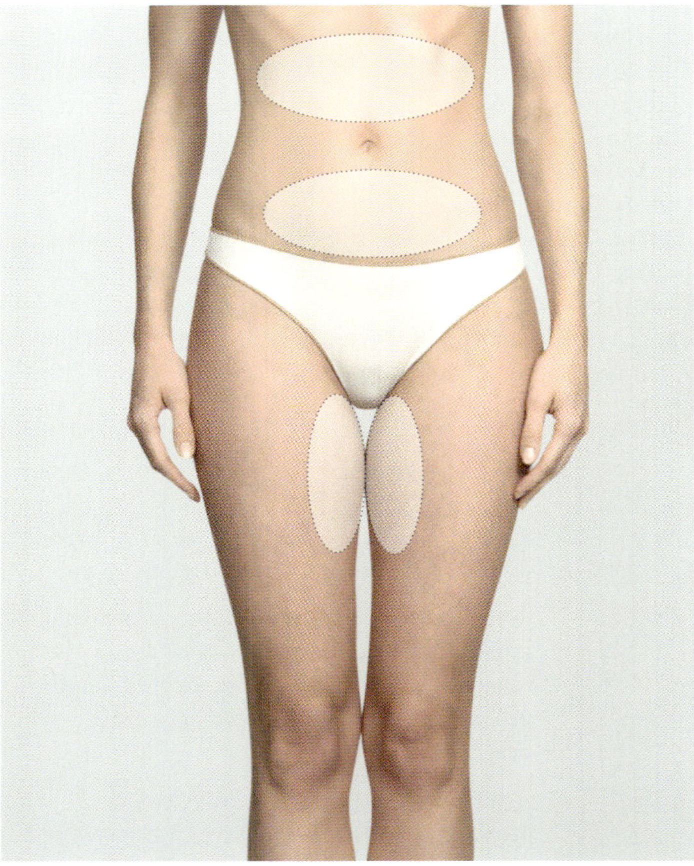

Fat deposits and treatment zones: upper and lower abdomen, thighs.

Contraindications to deep (subcutaneous) lipolysis injections include a prolonged prothrombin time value on anticoagulant therapy , together with allergy or intolerance to the medication (caution: soy allergy; test for this by creating a welt with dilute active substance). Furthermore, pronounced obesity or a lot of loose skin following weight loss are not indications for lipolytic injection methods. However, they are very suitable as follow-up treatment of any uneven skin areas after liposuction or to boost the skin's reaction to that therapy.
As a general rule, local treatment alone will not suffice if the BMI is > 30, and will only lead to patient dissatisfaction. However, it is perfectly possible to offer medical support for targeted reduction at the critical sites, to aid the patient's motivation to adopt lifestyle changes (diet, exercise). For many women, it is a problem to lose weight from the face or breasts, but not around the abdomen or thighs. Mesotherapy and lipolysis can be an effective aid in this situation.

8.3.2 Definition of cellulite

Cellulite is a segmented lipodystrophy of the subcutaneous adipose connective tissue, often associated with venolymphatic stasis. Thus, the crux and focus of local treatment is to improve the disrupted microcirculation. 80–90% of the female population is affected by this problem. Its severity is determined by many factors: apart from genetic, hormonal and complex biochemical factors, a key role is also played by the mind (stress as a trigger and aggravator) and by lifestyle (diet and exercise).
Apart from the clinical staging of the condition, other potential diagnostic methods include ultrasound measurement, thermography, total body densitometry or xeroradiography.
A lab test is also advisable (metabolism, thyroid function).

Histology of cellulite	
Phase 1	Panniculitis, deformed adipocytes, incipient lymphatic stasis, fibroblast proliferation, microhemorrhages
Phase 2	Increased fibroblast activity, collagen neogenesis, capillary sprouting. The increase in the density of the connective tissue fibers produces so-called orange peel skin, i.e. incipient edematous fibrosclerotic panniculopathy
Phase 3	Aggravation of the symptoms in the form of dermopanniculopathy with collagen hyperplasia and pronounced sclerosis of the deep dermis and subcutaneous tissue

Photo documentation and circumference measurements are a helpful part of the evaluation process.

8.3.3 Physiology of cellulite

The number of adipocytes in the body is already determined at birth. Generalized adipocyte hypertrophy is referred to as obesity, while the regional form may be described as cellulite or a fat deposit (lipodystrophy). A key physiological difference between these forms lies in the ability of fat to mobilize when a person is dieting: this happens easily in obesity, but with difficulty in localized lipodystrophy. The discovery of two specific adipocyte receptors explains this phenomenon:

- ß-adrenergic receptors 1,2,3: activate adenyl cyclase and have a lipolytic effect
- α-2-receptors: inhibit adenyl cyclase and have an antilipolytic effect. They occur in very large numbers in the lipodystrophic zones.

A further role is played by intracellular c-AMP and phosphodiesterase which, in turn, regulate lipase activity. Any drug which acts on these regulation mechanisms either accelerates or slows lipolysis.

8.3.4 When it's more than just cellulite

At your esthetic practice, you will also be confronted by the epidemic phenomenon of obesity. The success of the "body styling" mission will depend to a crucial extent on the advice you give and on the choice of individual treatment strategies.
Even at the first contact with the patient, you will already need to decide which of the following is involved:

- pathological overweight requiring treatment (BMI more than 30)
- general overweight (obesity, overeater)
- localized fat deposits, abnormal fat distribution (also referred to as lipodystrophy) or
- local structural changes in the adipose tissue (cellulite) in a woman of otherwise normal weight.

If you take holistic medicine seriously, you will try to develop an individually tailored concept in each case, and will also recommend or inform patients about procedures which you yourself may not offer, but which you feel are advisable. The injection methods that can be performed on an outpatient basis are explained in greater detail in the following section

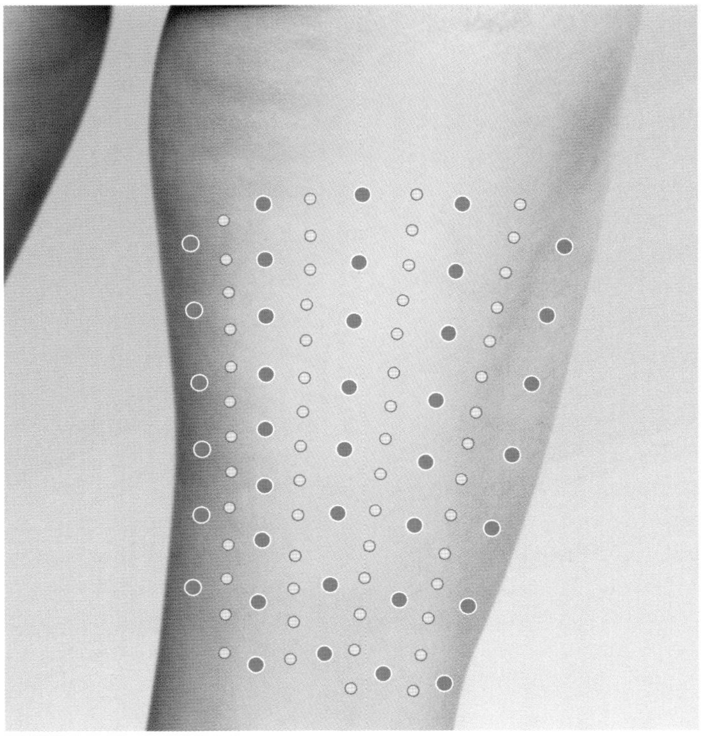

Treatment of cellulite on the back of the thigh with mesotherapy and lipolysis: using the serial technique, inject 0.2 ml doses of the mesotherapy cocktail to a depth of 6 mm, with individual infiltrations of 0.5 ml each of lipolysis cocktail at 1.5 cm intervals to a maximum depth of 1.5 cm. The depths of the injections depend on the thickness of the fat pad. Total volume: mesotherapy 10 ml per side + lipolysis 25 ml per side. Mesotherapy alone is sufficient for milder forms, at 20 ml per side.

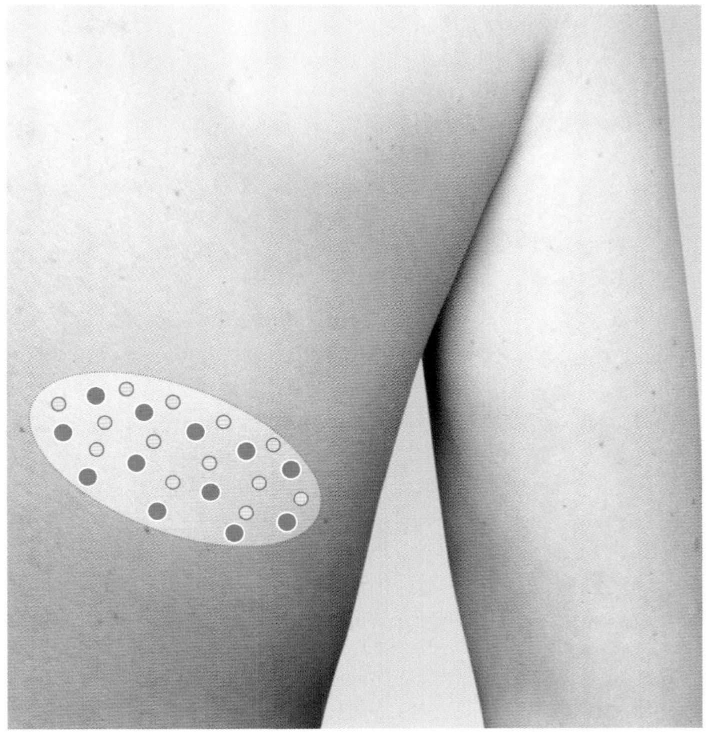

Treatment of the back of the upper arm, axillary fat and love handles with mesotherapy and lipolysis: using the serial technique, inject 0.2 ml doses of the mesotherapy cocktail to a depth of 4–6 mm with individual infiltrations of 0.5 ml each of lipolysis cocktail at 1.5 cm intervals to a maximum depth of 1.5 cm. The depths of the injections depend on the thickness of the fat pad. Total volume: mesotherapy 10 ml per region + lipolysis 10 ml per region. Mesotherapy alone is sufficient for milder forms, at 10 ml per region.

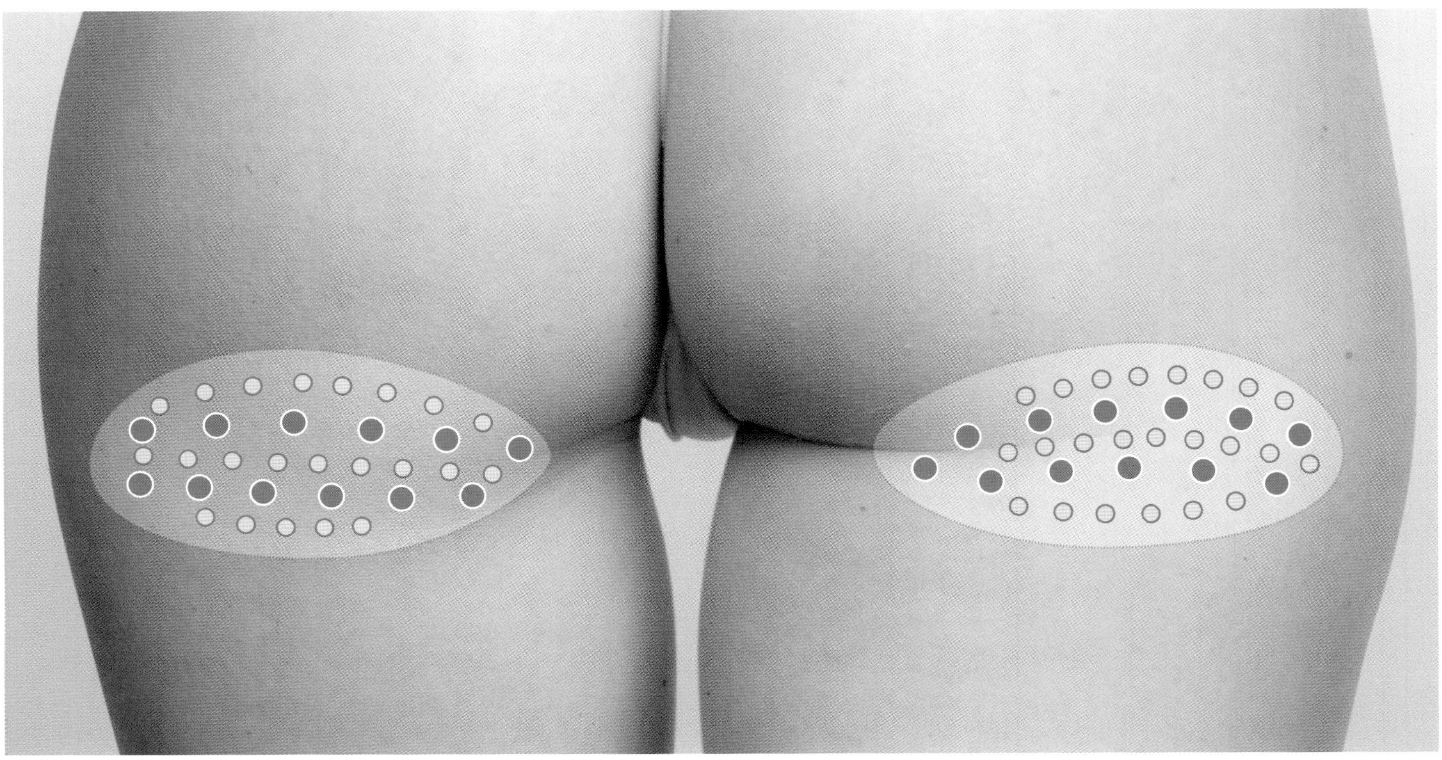

Treatment of banana rolls with mesotherapy and lipolysis: using the serial technique, inject 0.2 ml doses of the mesotherapy cocktail to a depth of 4–6 mm with individual infiltrations of 0.5 ml each of lipolysis cocktail at 1.5 cm intervals to a maximum depth of 1.5 cm. The depths of the injections depend on the thickness of the fat pad. Total volume: mesotherapy 10 ml per side + lipolysis 10 ml per side. Mesotherapy alone is sufficient for milder forms, at 10 ml per side.

8.3.5 Injection methods

After surgical intervention (liposuction, lipo-aspiration), mesotherapy is the most effective medical cellulite treatment method for local accumulations of fat and disruptions in adipose tissue structure. In most cases, repeated treatments lead to targeted reduction in the problem area. Xeroradiography and MRI scans show a marked reduction in adipocyte size and a finer cell structure. If thicker fat stores are present in addition to the superficial cellulite, the most effective method is a combination with so-called injection lipolysis. With these methods, care is needed with the various drug mixtures, injection techniques and depths. The total amount used depends on the extent of the changes. Systemic effects due to absorption are likely if more than 20 ml is used. The treatment is administered directly into the area showing the changes. The active substance quantities depend on the extent of the changes and on the individual constitution of the patient.

8.4 Mesotherapy in cellulite

Examples of drug mixtures
Mesotherapy, superficial administration 1–6 mm, mixed technique

M1: Procaine 1% 2 ml + L-carnitine 2 ml + caffeine 10% 2 ml + Buflomedil 2 ml + BH 2 ml
M2: NaCl 2 ml + PPC/DC 2 ml + Asiacen 2 ml + pentoxyfilline 2 ml + Cynomax 2 ml
M3: Procaine 1% 2 ml + PPC/DC 2 ml + Buflomedil 2 ml + Silicor 2 ml + Rutinel 2 ml

Ready-made products: Cocktail anticellulite (large areas) + Cocktail anticellulite spot (node infiltrations) from Toskani, 5 ml each + vasoactive agent 1 ml + LA 1 ml.

Injection technique M1–3: serial injections and nappage, depth 2 mm (face) – 6 mm (body), treatment interval at least 2 weeks.

8.5 Lipolysis for local fat pads

Lipolysis syringe, subcutaneous infiltrations, depth 4–6 mm (face), 6–15 mm (body)

Lipolysis injections are in particular demand for small fat pads, e.g. on the abdomen, legs (saddle bags), knees, upper arms, hips, and for small lipomas. This method is also an esthetic aid for the face (nasolabial fat, double chin, hamster cheeks, "moon face", bags under the eyes).

The lipolysis syringe is suitable for penetrating and dissolving small fat deposits. The active substance combination contains Lipostabil N, which is introduced into the affected regions with fine needles, allowing it to exert the desired effect. The result becomes fully apparent after a few weeks. To achieve optimum results, these injections are repeated some three times at intervals of six to ten weeks. A reduction in the thickness of the fat layers of about 1 cm may be expected per session. The treatment costs and risks of injection lipolysis are a great deal lower compared to surgical liposuction.
The patient needs to be informed extensively and in detail about the universal side-effects: pain and itching, swellings, reddening and hematomas are caused by the active substances and are simply part of the process, even with the best injection technique. The main symptoms subside gradually after three days, while the main effect sets in after the fourth week. The patient must not take part in any sports/ physical activity on the day of the therapy and should drink plenty of water or, even better, apple spritzer, to avoid circulatory reactions or dehydration. Vegetable stock or bitter preparations (artichoke, chicory, Bitterstern® drops, Urbitter® Bio Granulate) are recommended and can help boost any additional weight loss that may be desired. A heparin gel or Retterspitz® compresses are recommended for local cooling and against the hematomas.
The active substances are distributed across and into the depth of the subcutaneous tissue by diffusion; they may be either metabolized in situ or transported away by the blood. They leave the body naturally together with the mobilized fat.
Experience has shown that the best results are achieved with special needles (Thiebaud 6 mm with 5-sided bevel or BD Hypoint 0.4 x 13 mm). This ensures that the multiple injections cause little pain and that the formation of hematomas is minimized.
The frequency of the sessions is one every 6 weeks (in winter is best), with a total of 3–10 sessions depending on severity and extent. This is not a treatment for systemic obesity, but for localized fat deposits with and without connective tissue weakness. The greatest advantage of lipolysis lies in the additional firming effect on the skin. The patient needs to be warned that there is a long waiting time of at least 6 weeks before a visible result is achieved. This waiting time may last up to 3 months for those notorious fat pads around the eyes.
If venous and lymphatic insufficiency is also present, then concomitant classical mesotherapy for drainage and toning of the veins is also recommended. The same applies to the commonly seen "stress factor", which can be treated with the mesotherapeutic anti-stress protocol.

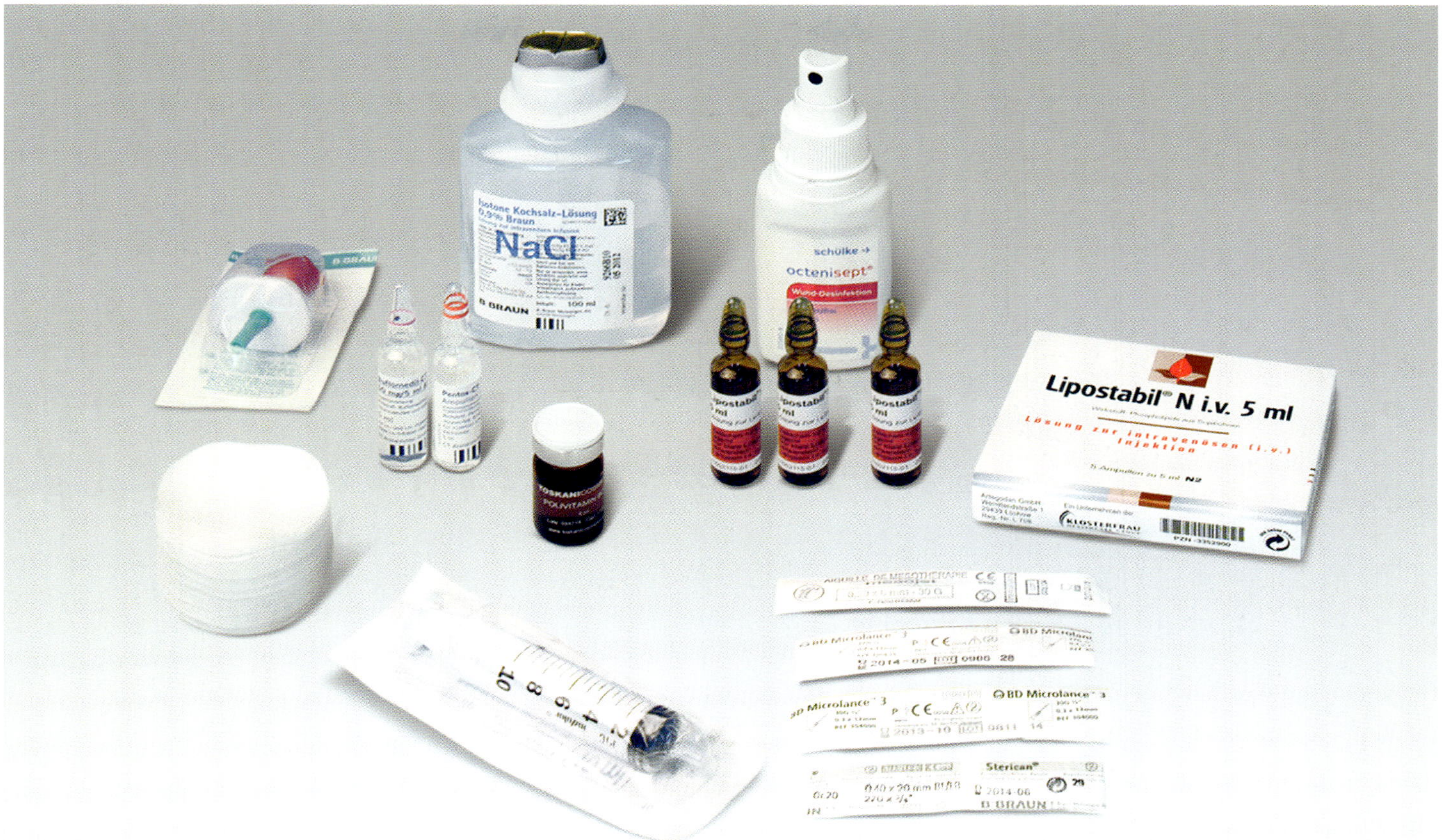

Materials required for lipolysis.

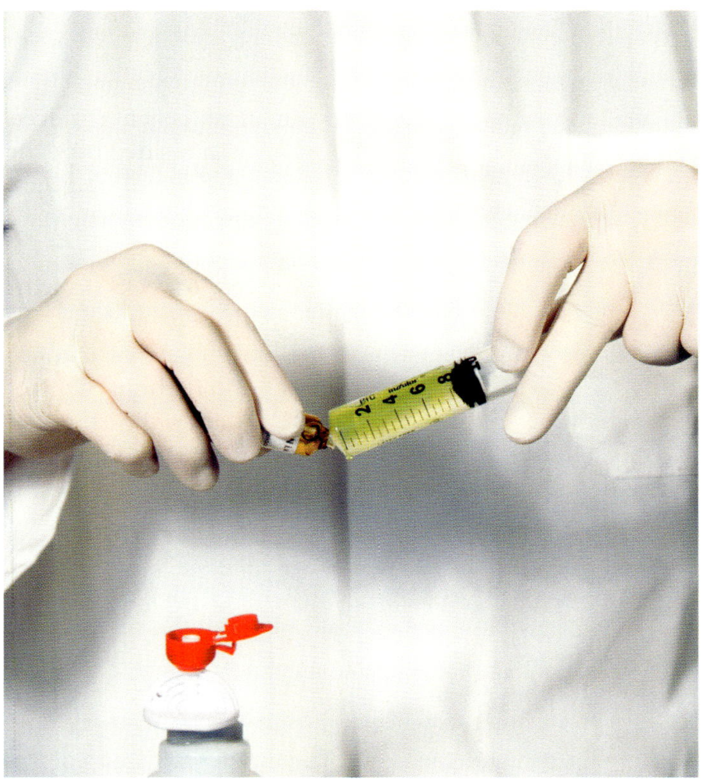

Mixing the two components for lipolysis (aqueous phase 5 ml + PPC/DC 5 ml).

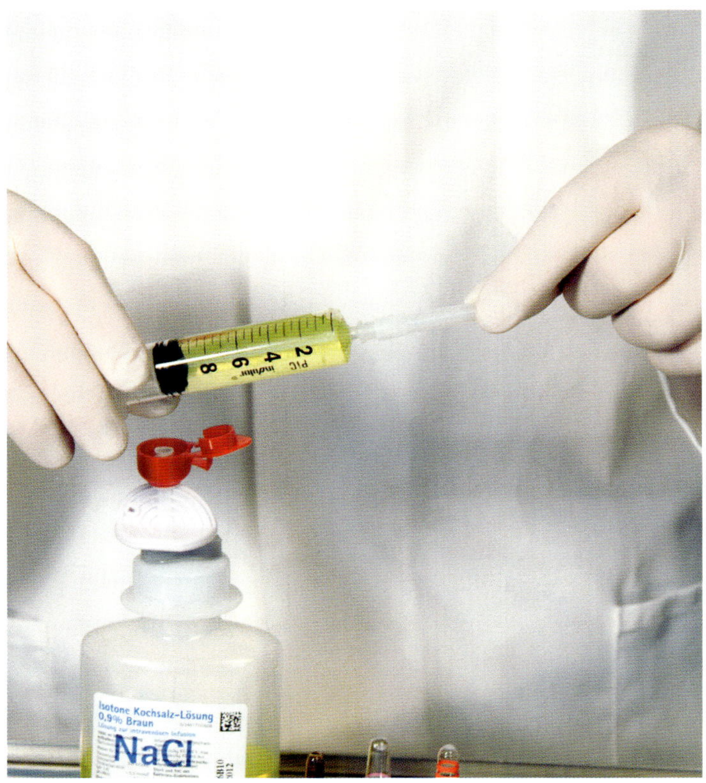

The cocktail is ready to use once the appropriate needle is fitted. It should be used immediately after preparation.

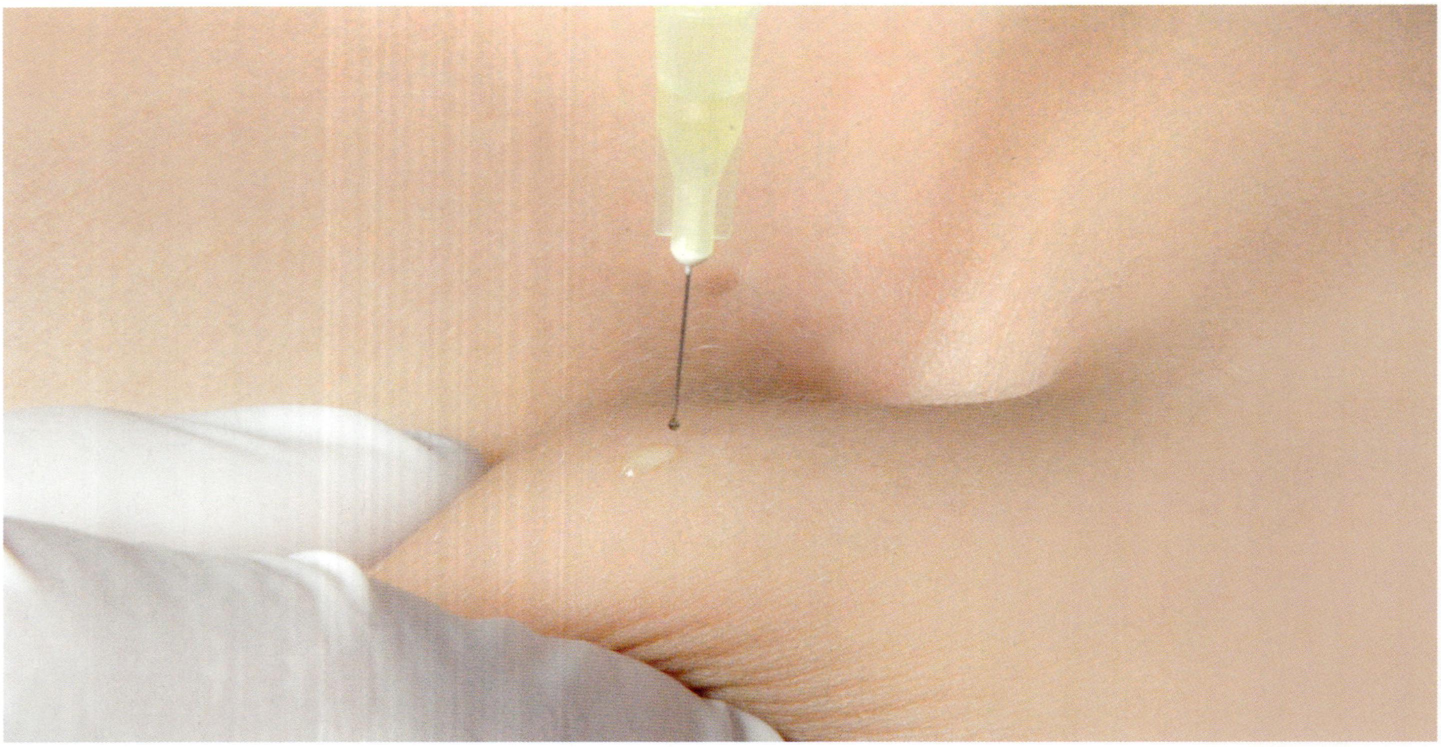

While lipolysis injections to the body are not particularly painful, side-effects are to be expected.

8.5.1 Lipolysis protocol

Use an infusion vial containing 100 ml 0.9 % NaCl + 1 ampoule (5 ml) Polyvitamin BCAE Toskani + 2 ampoules (10 ml) Buflomedil. The solution may be prepared in advance and keeps in the refrigerator for several days with a sterile venting spike.

- Label the vial.
- Mix with equal parts of Lipostabil (5 ml + 5 ml) and use immediately!
- Maximum dose per patient: 100 ml of the mixture. At the start of treatment or if the patient's constitution is delicate, do not exceed 50 ml (= 5 times 10-ml syringes).
- Massive side-effects are possible if these dose limits are not observed: circulatory problems, diarrhea, dehydration.
- When treating the body, it is best to inject with the BD Hypoint™ 0.4 x 13 mm needle, only into the adipose tissue.
- Never inject into muscle (this is very painful)!
- The distance between the injections is generally 1.5 cm. Distribution of the active substances through the adipose connective tissue takes place by diffusion. The maximum depth of injection is 1.5 cm on the body and 6 mm on the face.
- Exert maximum pressure on the plunger, maximum volume per injection 0.5 ml.
- Never inject into existing hematomas!
- Ensure a long treatment interval of c. 6 weeks.

8

8.5.2 Doses

Inject pure Lipostabil only into small lipomas (quantity equivalent to volume) and nasolabial fat pads (0.2 ml per point, 3 injections per side).

Face: dilute Lipostabil
On the face, inject 0.5 ml per point, always maintaining a distance of 1.5 cm. Insert 6-mm needle vertically, pinch the skin into a roll with the fingers if necessary, to protect underlying structures.

- Cheeks: up to 2 ml per side.
- Hamster cheeks: maximum 2.5 ml per side.
- Double chin: 3–5 ml.
- Bags under the eyes – lower lid (into fat only, not into any edematous swelling!): 0.3 ml (3 x 0.1 ml) per side, divided into 2–3 tangential injections into the three fat compartments using a 1-ml syringe and (important!) the Mesorelle 4-mm needle, always working manually. Depth of injection 2–3 mm.

Caution: Hemorrhage risk, retrobulbar hematoma in the worst-case scenario; this may lead to blindness and must be incised. The eye must not be injured, no pressure, no ice. Severe swellings around the eyes are normal; the patient needs to be informed beforehand about the likely restrictions (down-time up to 3 days). The best results are achieved in younger individuals without excess sagging skin. Number of sessions: 1 to 5, according to severity.

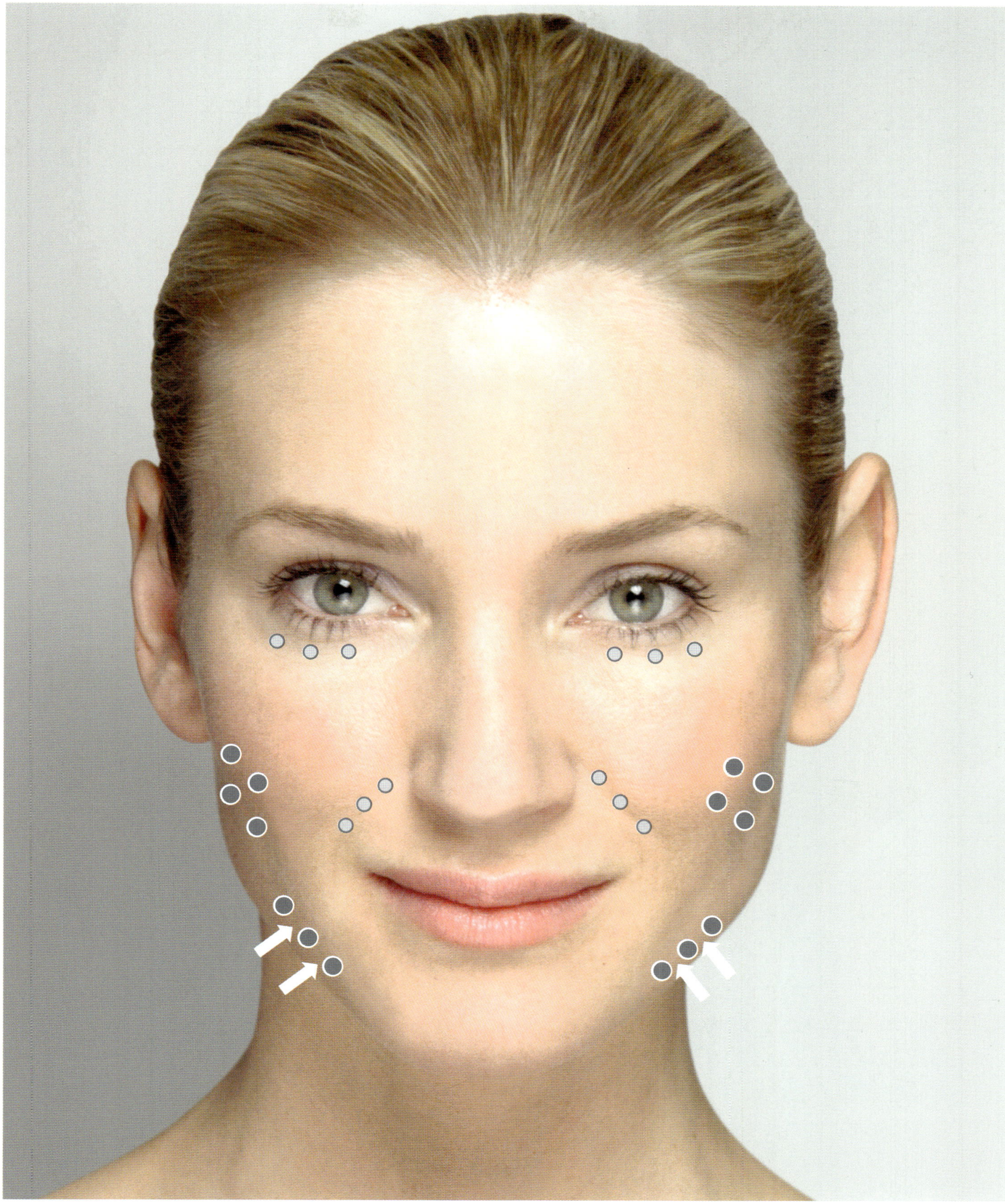

Lipolysis options on the face. The treatment of prolapsed fat around the eyes is associated with increased risk.
Dark gray dots = infiltration, Light gray dots = serial injection technique.

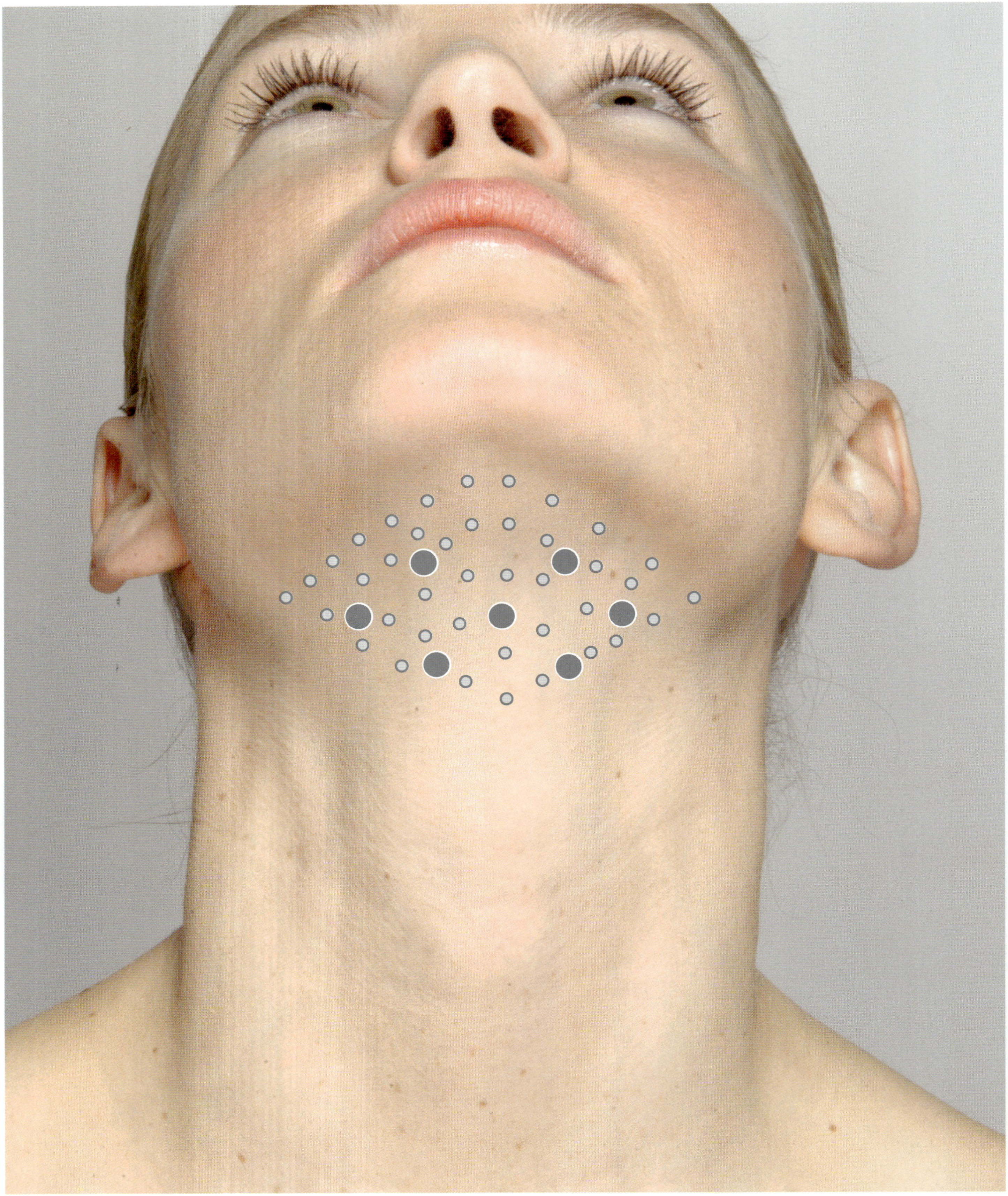

Treatment of double chin and sagging in the mandibular region.
Mesotherapy with cellulite cocktails (0.2 ml/point by serial injection) and/or lipolysis (0.5 ml/Infiltration).

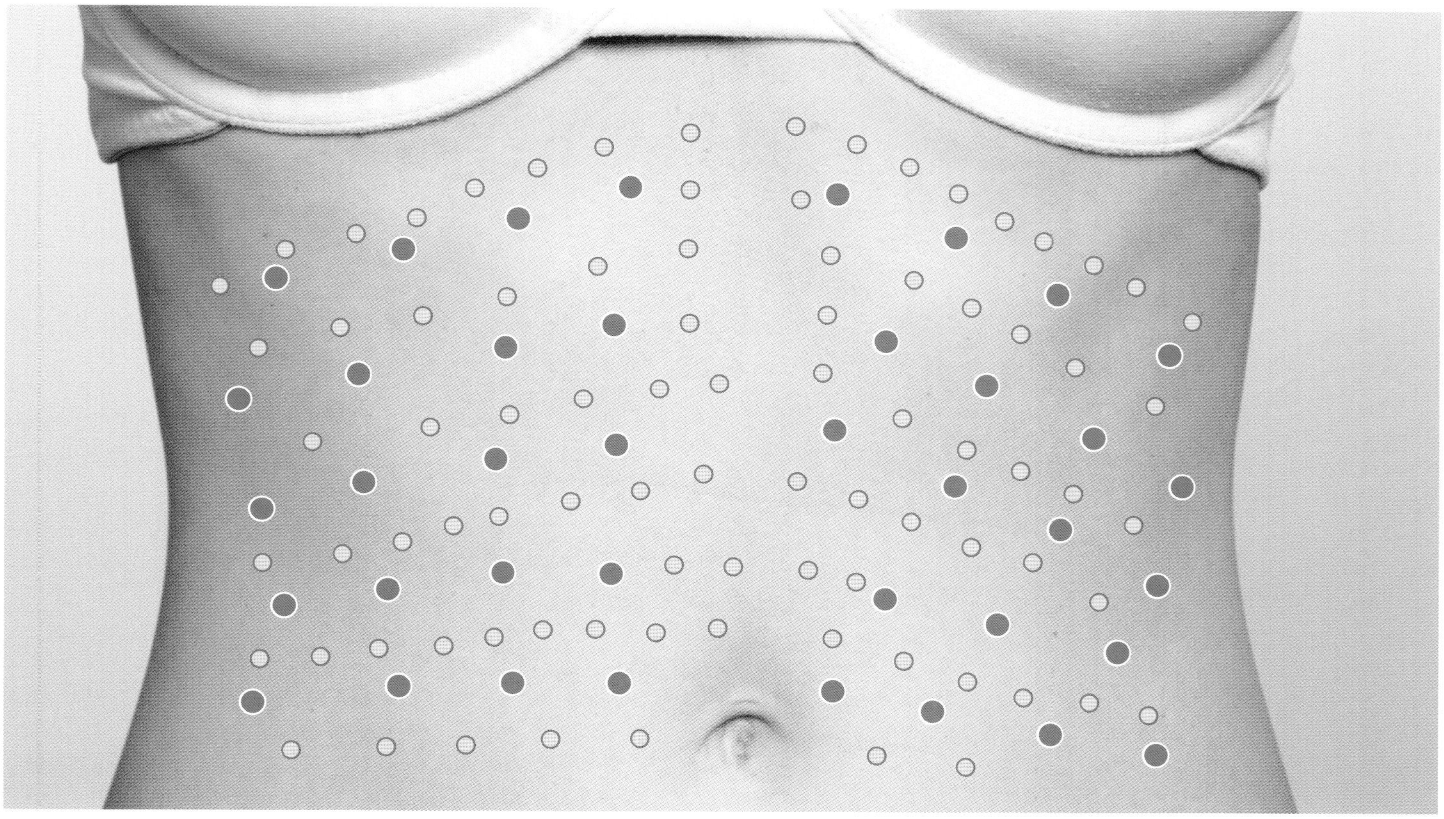

Combined treatment of fat deposits on the upper abdomen with 1. lipolysis (infiltrations) and 2. mesotherapy (serial injections). A treatment interval of 2 weeks should be cbserved in sensitive individuals.

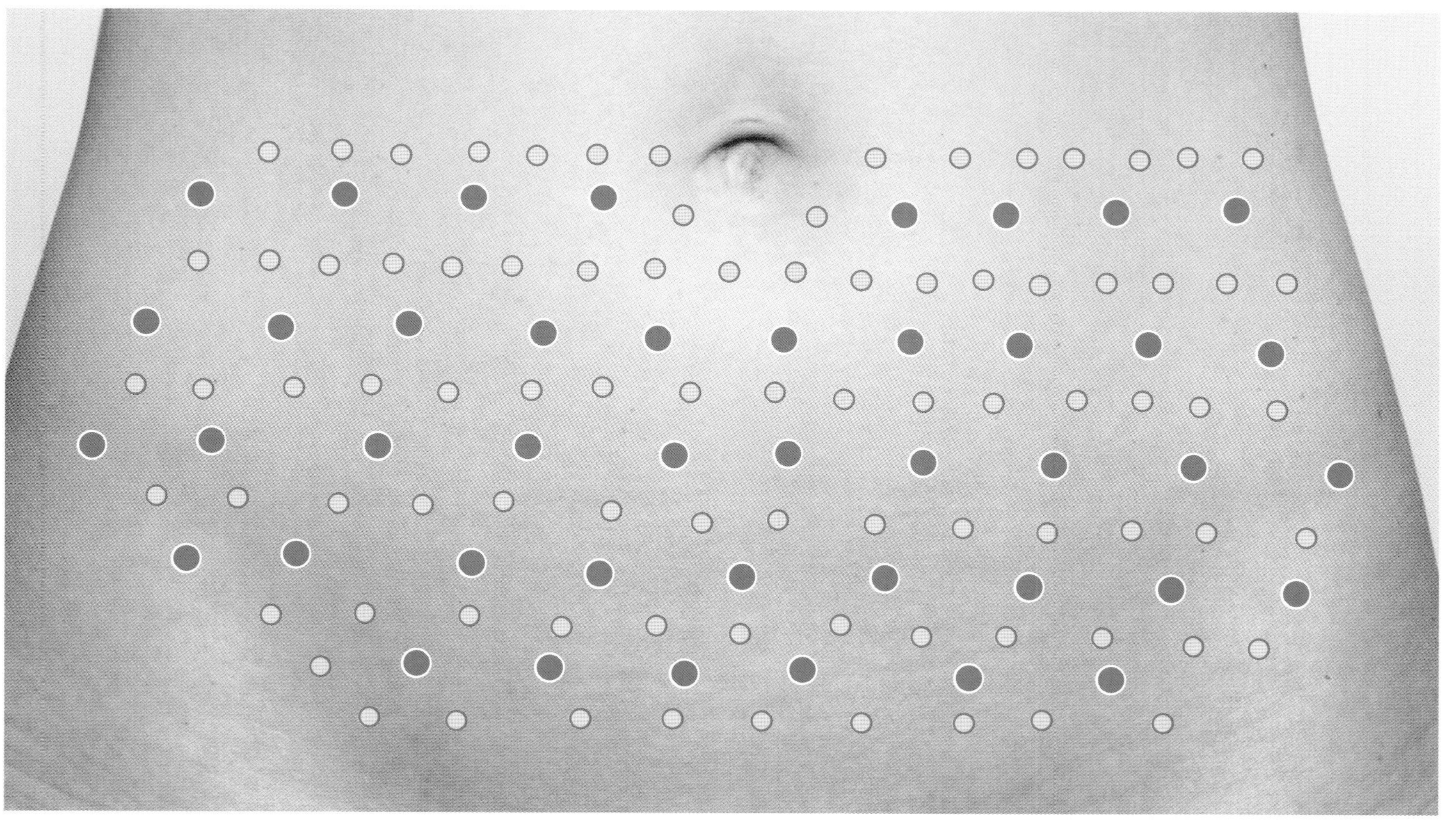

Combined treatment of fat deposits on the lower abdomen with lipolysis and mesotherapy. Due to the volume limits for the active substance, it is not possible to treat more than 1–2 regions per session.

Body: dilute Lipostabil

Maximum 50 (–100) ml on the body.

- Axillary fat: anterior 6–10 ml per site, posterior 10 ml.
- Upper arms: posterior 15–20 ml per site.
- Love handles: 5–15 ml per side.
- Hips: 10–20 ml per side.
- Upper abdomen: 40 ml.
- Lower abdomen: up to 80 ml.
- Banana rolls: 10 ml per side.
- Saddle bags: up to 50 ml per side.
- Knee: cranial side 10–20 ml per side, medial side 10 ml (caution: there is a higher risk of thrombosis here).
- Thigh, extensive: up to 50 ml per side.
- Gynecomastia in men (caution: differential diagnoses need to be considered): 10–20 ml per side.

Side-effects: swellings, itching, pain and reddening starting immediately after the injection and persisting up to about three days. All side effects occurring after doses of up to 50 ml are harmless and should have disappeared after three days. In contrast, the lipolytic effect persists for up to six weeks. Caution is needed on the inner sides of the knees, where more serious complications have been reported. Connective tissue sclerosis (retractions or necrosis) may occur. In some cases, this may be due to poor perfusion, e.g. where there are large lipomas.

Cellulite and fat deposits

The two techniques are combined. The addition of hyaluronidase + collagenase, 2 ml each, is recommended in severe cases, e.g. the fibroslerotic form (solid adipose connective tissue, more common in men than women, and also more common on the upper than the lower abdomen and in bull neck).

8

8.5.3 Mechanism of action of Lipostabil

- The release of stored fat from the adipocyte.
- The lysis of adipocytes by causing the local accumulation of lymphocytes, plasma cells and macrophages, and by increased collagen formation (as indicated by histology results after one week).

The active substance phosphatidylcholine used in lipolysis treatment has no genotoxic or teratogenic effects in the human body (Deutsches Bundesinstitut für Arzneimittel und Medizinprodukte, the German Federal Institute for Drugs and Medical Devices, 2004). A new in-vitro study from the University of Regensburg has confirmed that destruction of the adipocyte cell membrane is achieved through lipolysis, with resultant effective and persistent local breakdown of fat. This involves cell apoptosis and not cell necrosis. The released fat is emulsified and transported away from the site of action.

Breakdown of fat by PPC – the Hasengschwandtner hypothesis

- Dephosphorylation of phosphatidylcholine by phospholipase
- Release of enzymes from the mitochondria in the adipocyte nucleus
- Initiation of an enzyme cascade which remains active for about 8 weeks: hormone-sensitive lipase, triglyceride lipase, diglyceride lipase, monoglyceride lipase
- Transport to the liver mediated by lipoproteins
- Metabolization by beta-oxidation (citric acid cycle)

The treatment itself is almost painless, as the substance is injected directly into the adipose connective tissue using fine needles. Nevertheless, the patient needs to be informed about certain type of discomfort, which occur regularly with varying severity.

Side-effects: swelling of the treated region: the substance induces an artificial inflammation, which causes the area to swell considerably at first. Most of the swelling tends to subside after two to three days. The shrinkage process now begins. It generally lasts about six weeks. It is also normal for the treated area to redden and to start itching. Pain resembling aching muscles may also develop after the treatment, although analgesics do not generally need to be administered. Because of the depth of the injections, it is possible for minor vessels to be damaged and for small hematomas to develop; these are broken down within a few days. The formation of transient nodules in the tissue is observed in rare cases. Permanent dents or asymmetries may develop if the injected fluid is not uniformly distributed, e.g. if double the recommended volume is injected into one point.

The treatment is not suitable for impatient clients who want to see an immediate result.

Normally, at least two sessions per region will be needed, with an interval of six to eight weeks between them; even three or four sessions may be necessary in some cases. The body's contours change slowly and imperceptibly. The treatment result is long-lasting, provided that there is no weight gain. A 4 cm reduction in the circumference of the abdomen and a 1 cm reduction in the thickness of the fat layer per treatment are quite common.

The first changes occur after ten days, and the breakdown process is at its most active in the fourth to sixth weeks. The lipolysis produces little or no actual weight loss. For this reason, in slightly overweight individuals, the treatment should be accompanied by appropriate changes in diet.

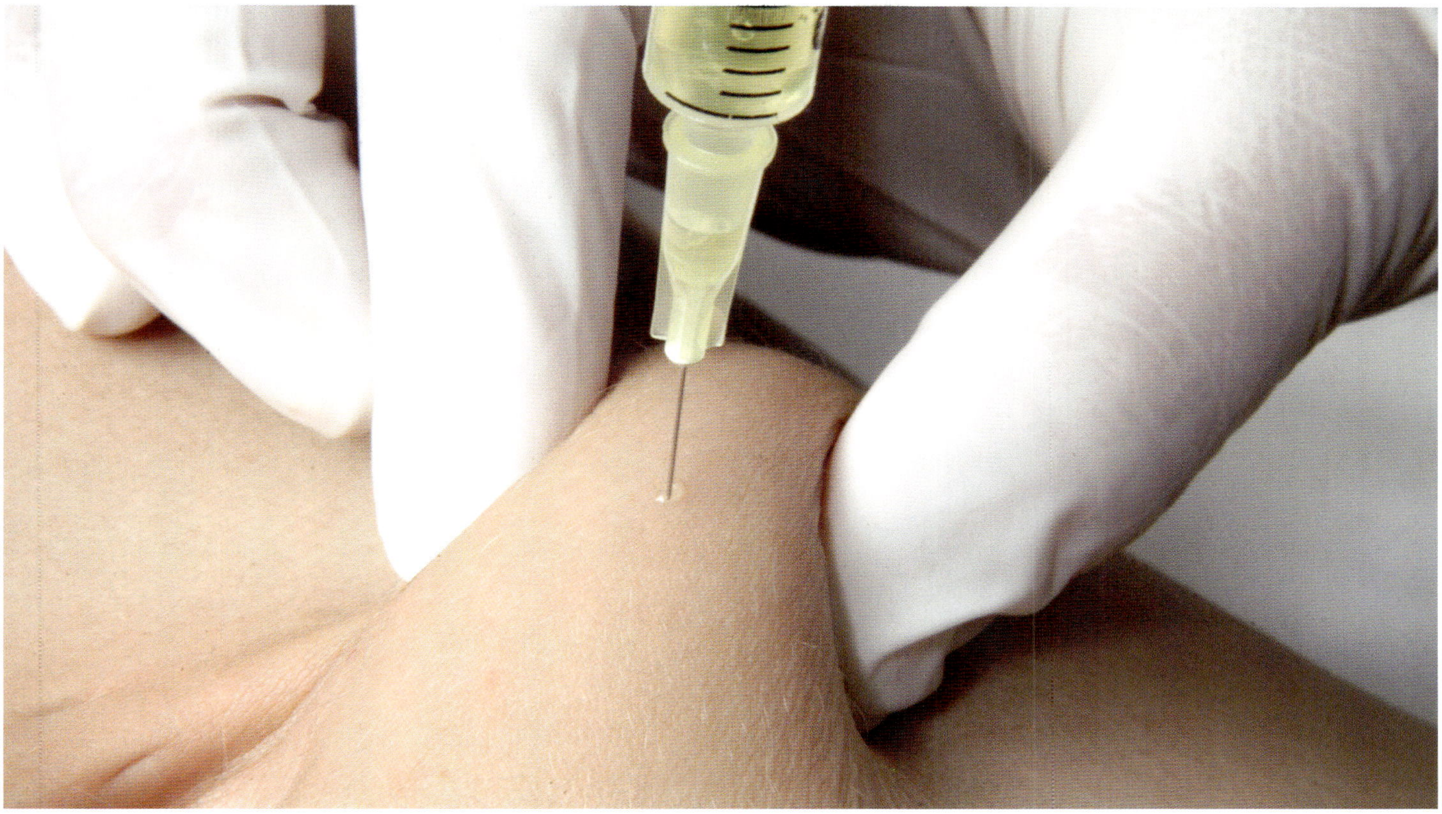

Injection technique in lipolysis: inject 0.5 ml of dilute PPC/DC per injection point directly into the adipose connective tissue to a depth of 13 mm, exerting as much pressure as possible.

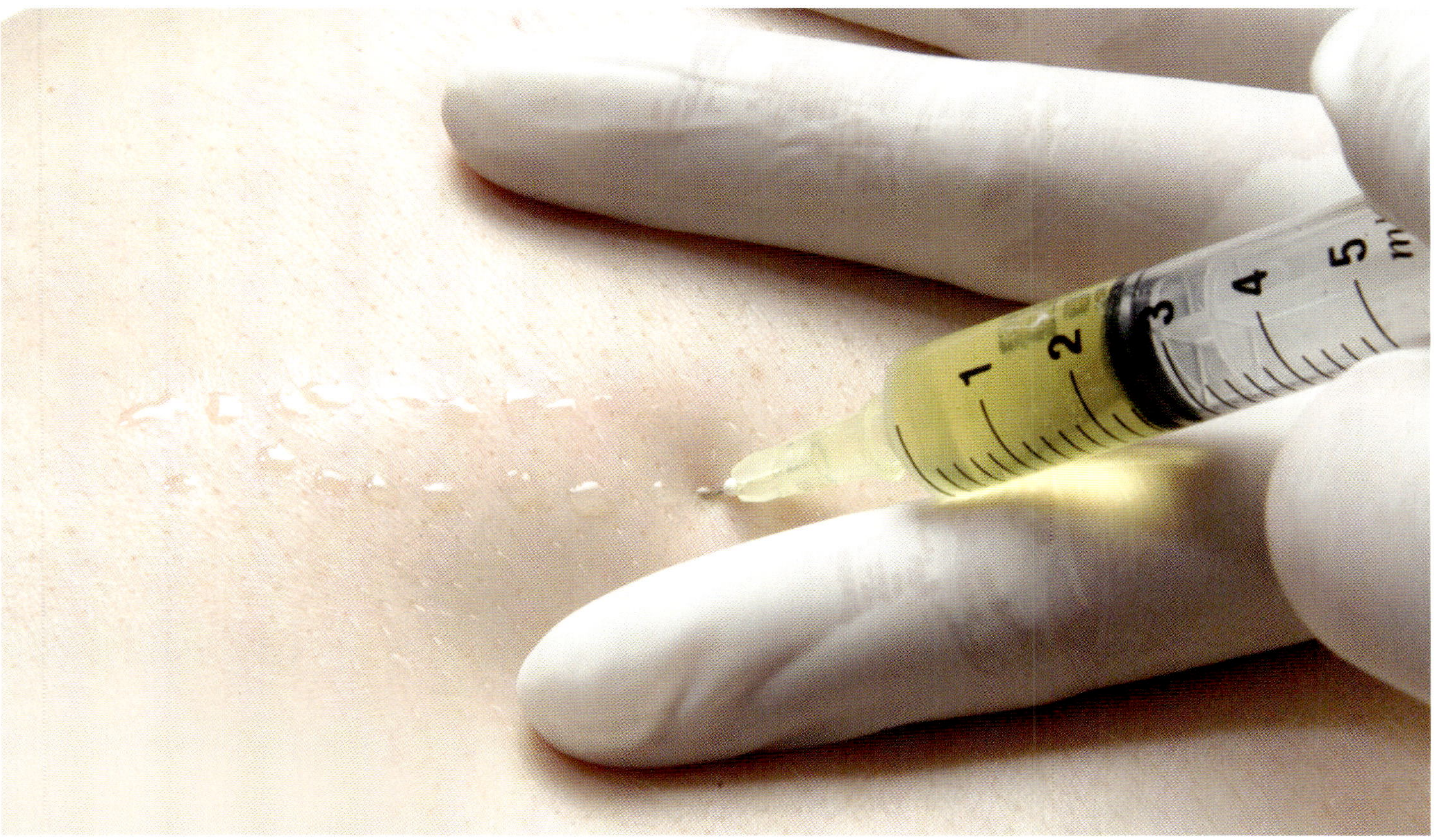

Serial and nappage technique in mesotherapy: inject 0.1–0.2 ml of cellulite cocktail per injection point to a depth of 4–6 mm.

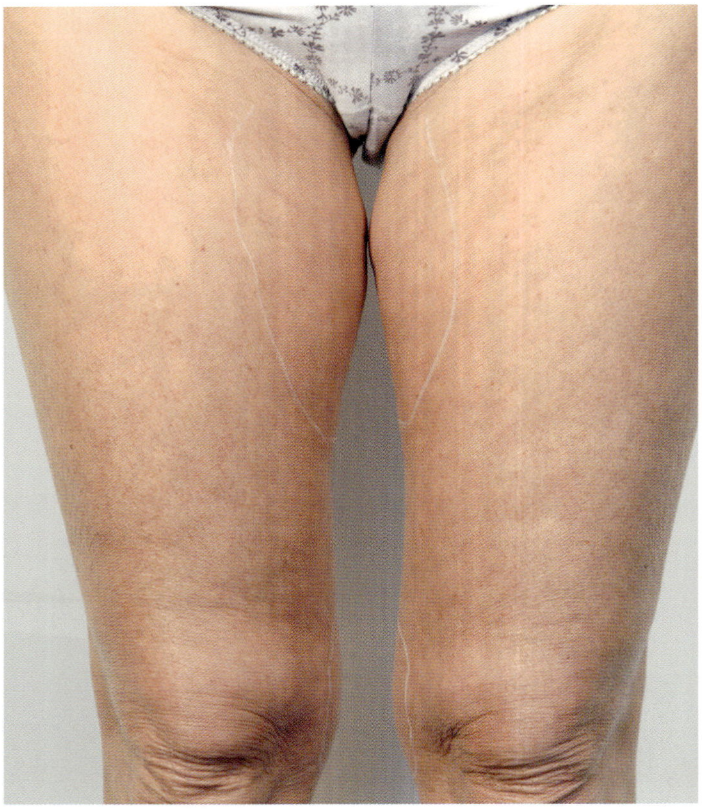

Marked treatment site, viewed from the front …

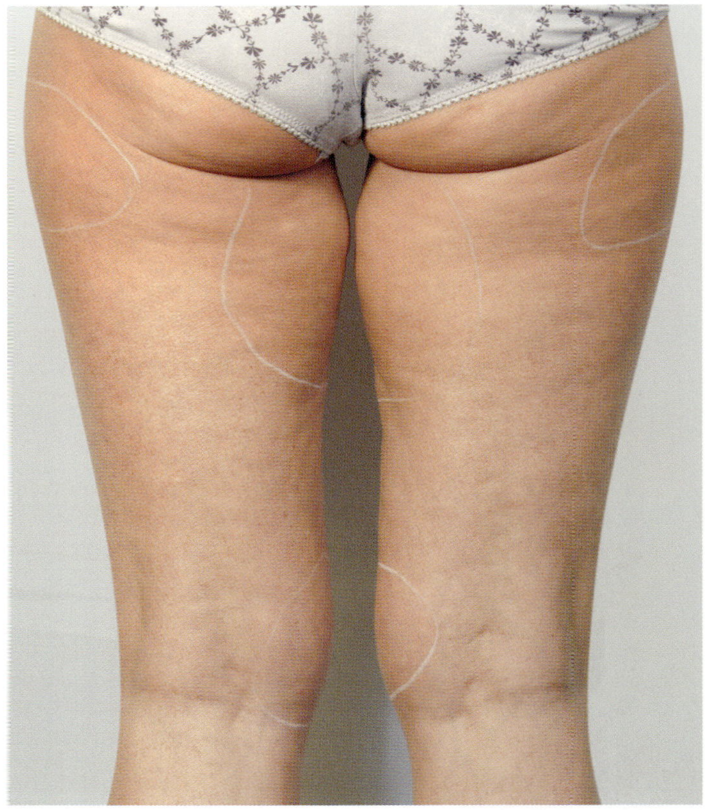

… from behind

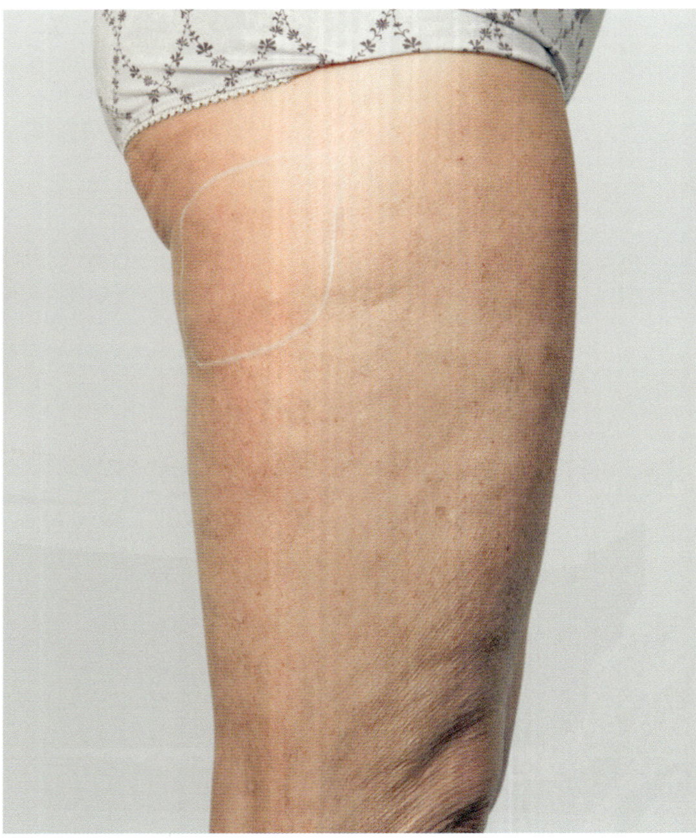

… from the side

The treatment is promising for patients with smaller fat pads and cellulite, patients who absolutely refuse to have surgery/liposuction and those who want to change their contours slowly and unobtrusively. Other well-established indications include lipomas, gynecomastia or correction following liposuction.
The best results are achieved on the face, with double chin, in the (female) abdominal and hip region, in axillary fat pads, with rolls on the back and on the thighs.

8.6 Mesotherapy for dermatological indications

The dermatological indications mark the transition from purely esthetic to curative medicine, and include venous insufficiency, precancerous skin changes, wound healing disorders and viral warts. Careful diagnostic investigations are essential here. Mesotherapy also has some interesting uses in this area, some of which are presented in this section.

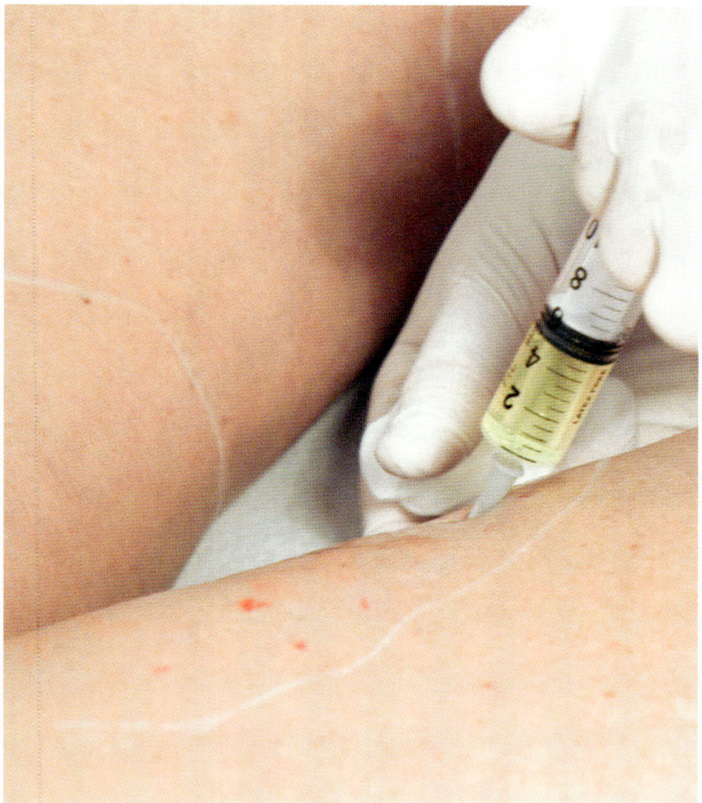

10-ml syringes are used in lipolysis.

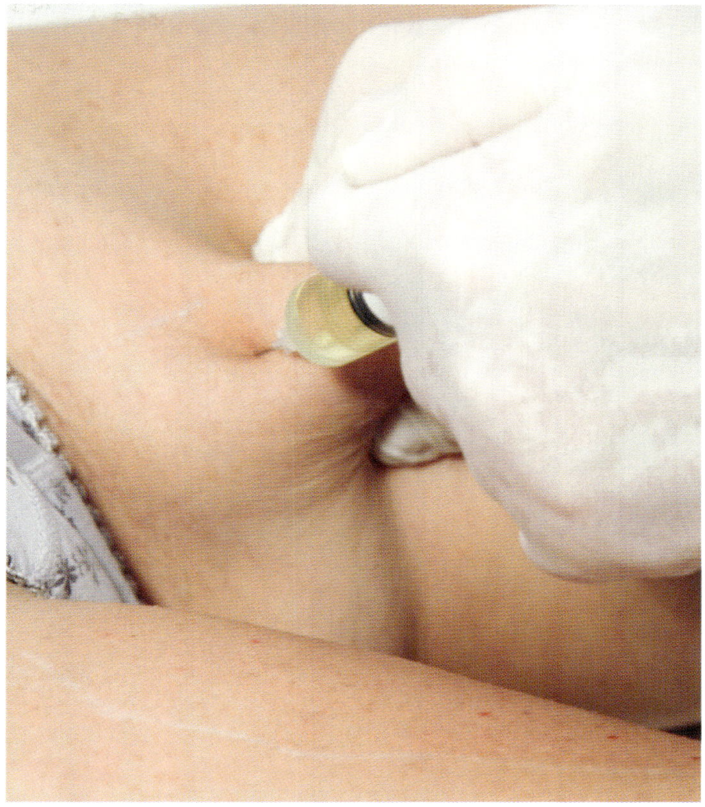

In sensitive zones, pinching the skin and inserting the needle firmly and confidently makes the pain bearable. The injection of the mixture itself is not painful.

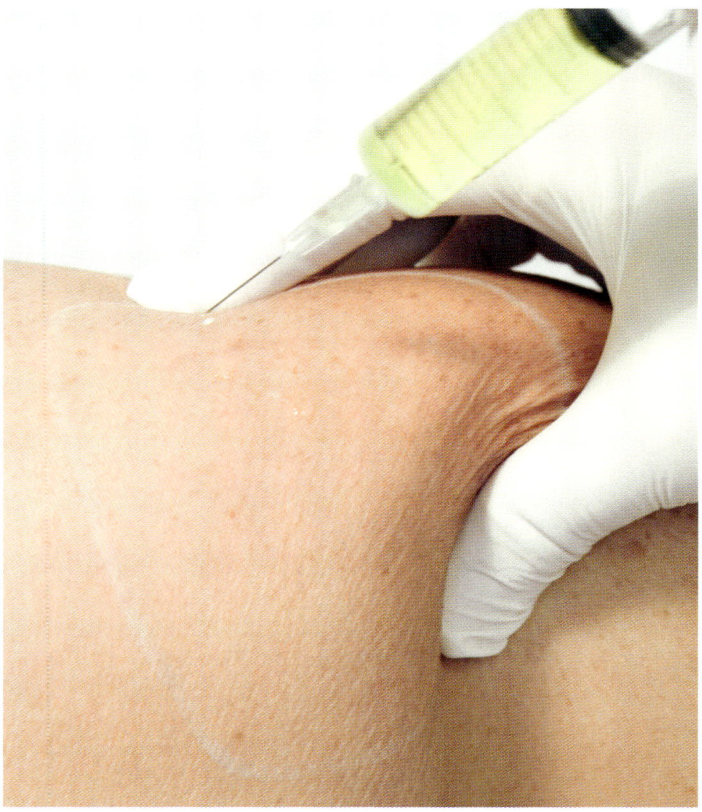

When injecting on the body, it is best to use the Hypoint™ 0.4 x 13 mm needle.

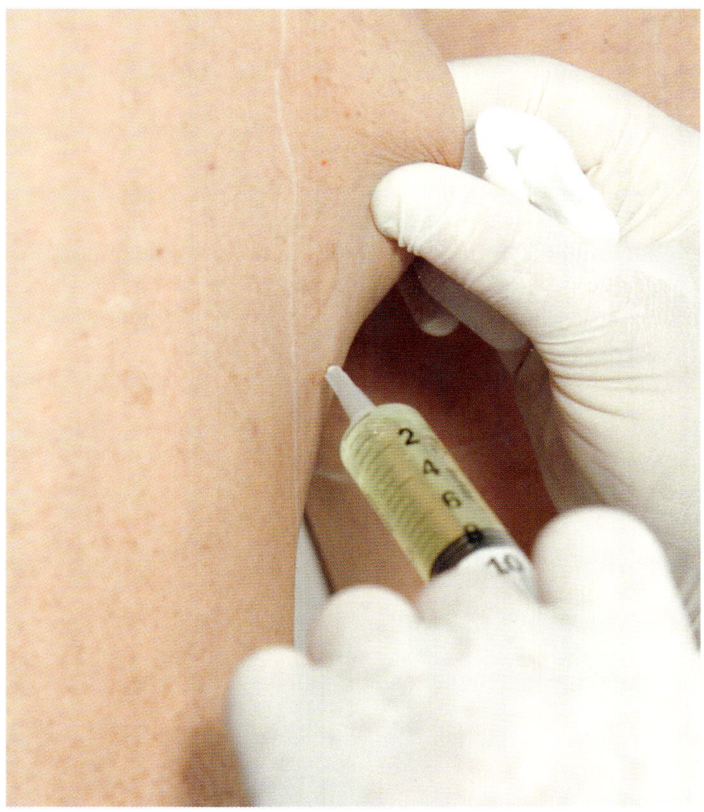

If the fat pad is small, the needle is not inserted vertically, but at a 45° angle.

8

8.6.1 Treatment of stretch marks

Stretch marks (striae) are clearly demarcated lines of skin atrophy, caused by overstretching and tearing of the connective tissue. Their causes lie in rapid growth, pregnancy, weight gain, medication, hormonal imbalances or a genetic predisposition.

Course

- Fresh stretch marks are pink to purple, 1–15 mm wide; they fade in 3–6 months.
- The older and more faded they are, the more difficult they are to treat.

Treatment

- Mesotherapy + tretinoin cream (0.05%) during the treatment interval.
- Mesotherapy, also during pregnancy, but not into the abdomen. Exposure to sunlight must be avoided!

Mesotherapy protocol

Pull the skin tight, administer intradermal nappage at 2-mm intervals along the course of the mark, including its margins.

Drug mixture for *fresh stretch marks*

Alternate the following:

- Procaine 1% 0.5 ml + Wiedemann BH 0.5 ml + Aethoxysklerol (polidocanol) 0.5% (diluted 1:10) 0.5 ml.
- Procaine 1% 0.5 ml + Calcitonin 50 0.5 ml + silorgamine 0.5 ml.

Frequency of the sessions

- Every 7 to 14 days.

Drug mixture for *older stretch marks*

- Procaine 1% 0.5 ml + NCTF 1 ml + non-cross-linked HA 0.2 ml + Buflomedil 0.5 ml (for better elasticity and trophicity).
- Procaine 1% 0.5 ml + Centella asiatica (e.g. Cefabene-Cistus Complex) 0.5 + Silicor 0.5 + Calcitonin 50 0.5 ml + Vitamin C 0.5 ml (for repigmentation and regeneration).
- Toskani Cocktails Antistriae + Skin Firming, alternating, both used in the pure state (firming, regeneration, hydration).

Frequency of the sessions

- Every 14 days.

Caution: do not treat the abdomen during pregnancy. The available time window is generally sufficient to produce good results when treating stretch marks, even after the delivery. In the latter case, the mesotherapy also aids retraction of the overstretched skin structures.

It is not only young women who develop these connective tissue tears; fast-growing male adolescents are also sometimes affected.

8.6.2 Treatment of venous insufficiency

Spider-burst veins are acquired pathological dilatations of small, superficial, peripheral veins. The causes may be hereditary, hormonal, mechanical or related to venous dysfunction. All forms can be drained temporarily by pressing down with the fingers. There are two distinct clinical forms:

- Blue spider-burst veins, which are deeper and thicker.
- Red spider-burst veins, which are more superficial and finer.

Treatment

- Surgical removal or foam sclerotherapy when associated with varicose veins, particularly insufficiency of the perforating veins (30%).
- Isolated forms can be treated by direct sclerotherapy.
- Forms associated with the menstrual cycle: mesotherapy with vein toning agents and compression.
- Diffuse, spreading, fine forms: mesotherapeutic microsclerotherapy.

Sclerotherapy

Blue spider-burst veins:

- To begin with, always use a maximum of 3 ml of pure Aethoxysklerol (0.5–1%).

Red spider-burst veins:

- Maximum 1.5 ml pure Aethoxysklerol (0.5–1%).
- Hold the skin tight, tangential injection, directly into the vessel, no aspiration.
- Interval 3 to 4 weeks.

Microsclerotherapy

For diffuse venules, as well as couperose and small skin hemangioma.

Mixture:

- Aethoxysklerol 0.5% 0.5 ml + DHE 0.5 ml.
- Epidermal nappage technique, best administered with an injector. Broad coverage of the affected area. It can and should bleed.

Frequency: Once a year.

Contraindications include pregnancy, allergy to the sclerotherapy agent, florid thrombophlebitis or thrombosis, local or systemic infections, immobilization or severe systemic disorders, hyperthyroidism, stage III or IV arterial occlusive disease.

Mesodrain

- Preventative and therapeutic.
- To clear the area, improve microcirculation and for decongestion of the legs.
- Procaine 1% 1 ml + Asiacen 2 ml + Rutinel 2 ml + pentoxyfilline 2 ml.
- Epidermal technique, the quickest way being by injecting manually across the three vascular axes of both legs.

Frequency: Every two to three months.

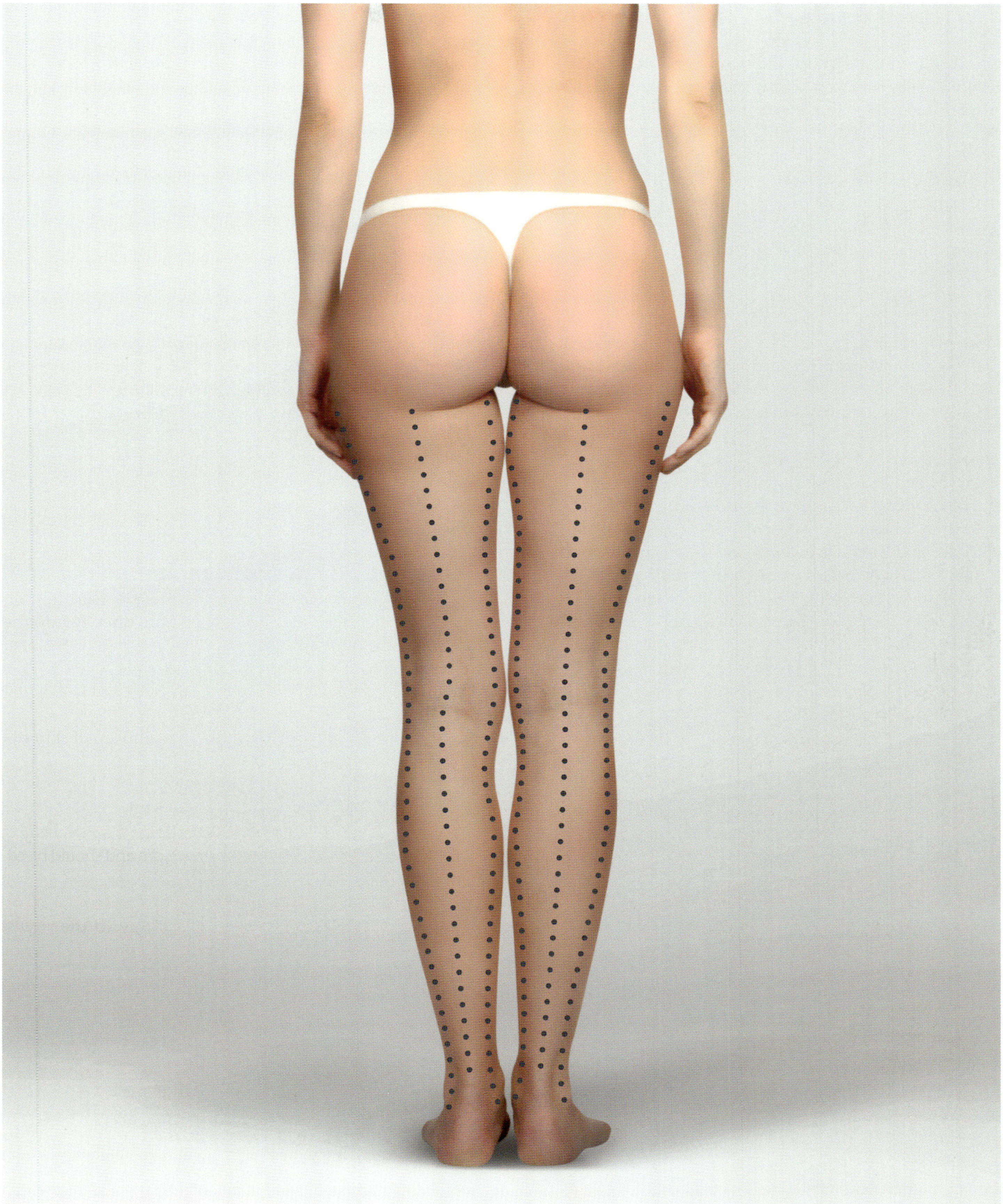

Mesodrain produces global decongestion and improved perfusion of the legs.

8.6.3 Treatment of scars

Scars are the final result of the skin's repair process following injuries. Possible causes include mechanical, chemical or physical traumas with injury to the stratum papillare, skin infections, tumors, autoimmune disorders or vascular disorders.

Wound healing phases

- Cleansing (two hours).
- Repair (up to one month).
- Granulation (up to three months).
- Maturation (up to one year).

Wounds can heal by primary or secondary intention.

Complications

Dehiscence, adhesion, pain, foreign body inclusions, keloids (this is an exceptional indication for corticosteroids, i.e. crystalline triamcinolone suspension).

Drug mixture for keloids

- Procaine 1% 5 ml + triamcinolone 0.5–1 ml.
- The sooner it is done, the more effective it will be.
- Superficial papules exclusively in the keloid region.
- Treatment intervals every three weeks. Five to six treatments, depending on extent and severity.
- Intermittent use of 0.05% tretinoin cream (Airol cream or Cordes VAS cream) and the wearing of silicon plasters is an option.
- Caution: a two-day interval must be maintained between this treatment and mesotherapy.

General drug mixture for scars

- Procaine 1% 1 ml + pentoxyfilline 1 ml + Cocktail antistriae 1 ml + Wiedemann BH 1 ml + Calcitonin 100 0.1 ml.

8.6.4 Treatment of warts (verrucae vulgares)

In many cases, it is also possible to administer allopathic active substances locally rather than systemically. In dermatological wart treatment, mesotherapy may be used for severe or treatment-resistant cases, with the following mixtures:

- Equal parts of cimetidine + lidocaine 1% + vitamin C, administered near, into and below the lesion, using a Mesorelle needle, in three to four once-weekly sessions.
- Bleomycin 1 mg per ml in 0.9% NaCl, administered into the lesion with a Mesorelle needle, 0.1 ml/injection; anesthetic cream may also be applied beforehand.

Repeat until visible results are achieved. Do not use in pregnant women or children.

Treatment of age spots, melasma, pigment disruptions

Epidermal mesotherapy with:
Glutathione 5 ml + vitamin C 1 ml + glycolic acid 1 ml (e.g. Glutamax, Ascormax, Glycomax).

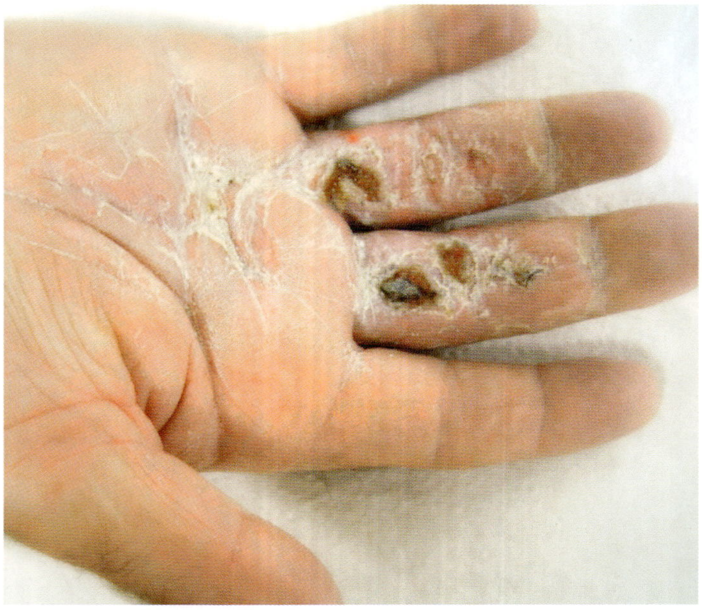

Wound healing problem with functional impairment 3 weeks after hand surgery (for Dupuytren's contracture).

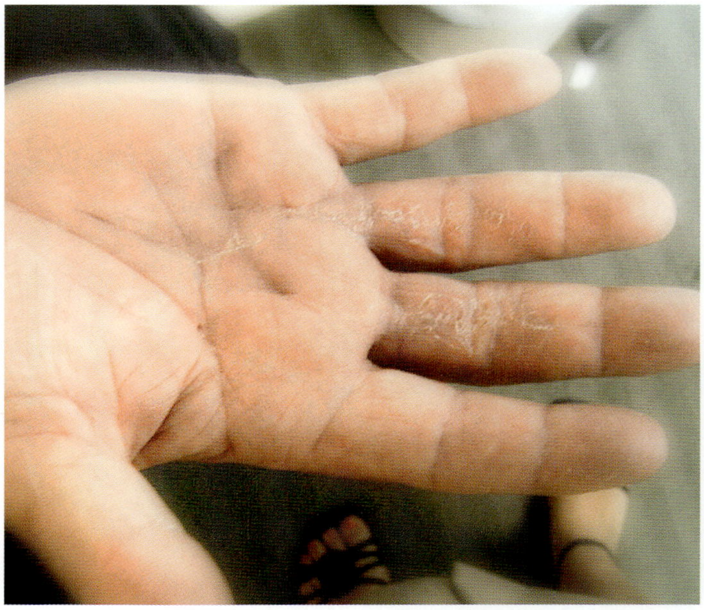

Result after a single mesotherapy session (epidermal only): full visible and functional restitution has been achieved.

9 Case histories

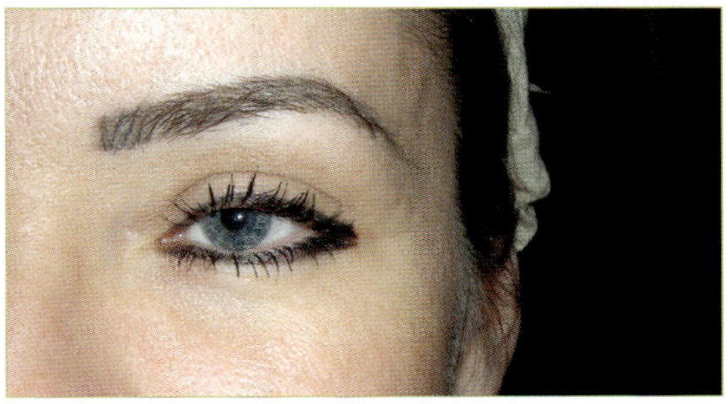

40-year-old woman having preventative treatment.

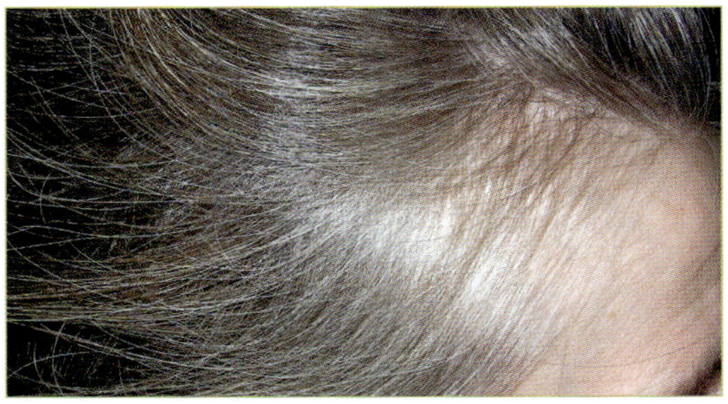

Hair regrowth in a woman's receding hairline.

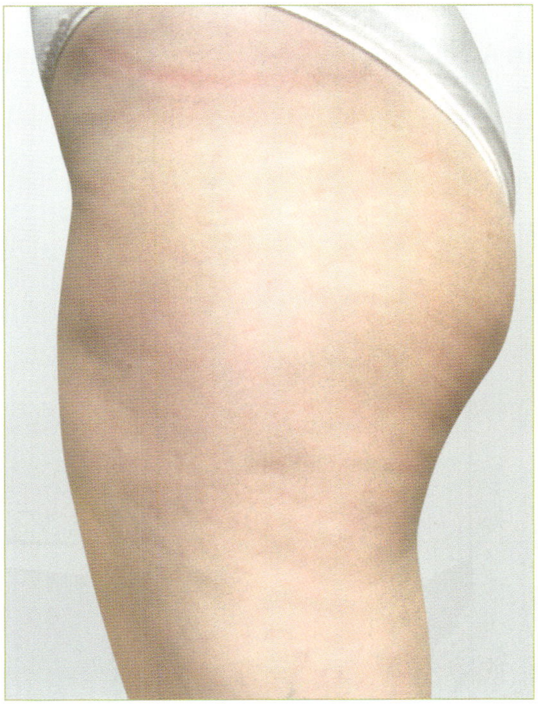

Discrete cellulite in a slim female patient.

9.1 Mesolift

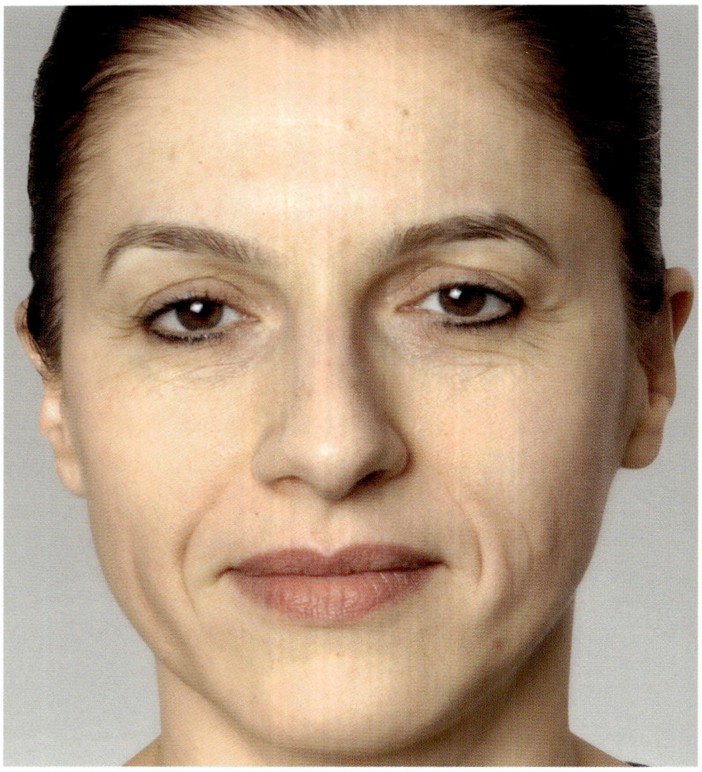

Case 1: 45-year-old woman (untreated, does not want Botox).

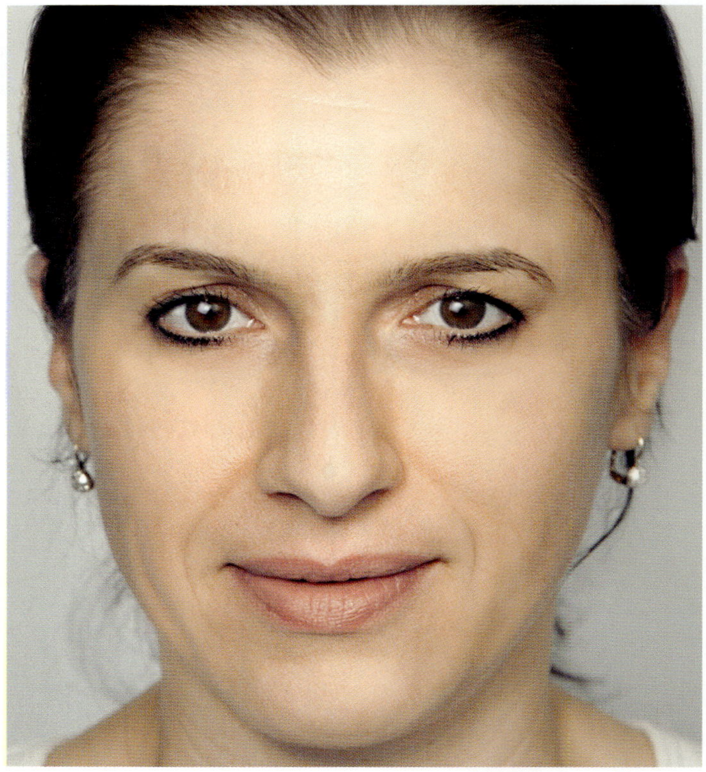

Case 1: Findings directly after the second Mesolift: marked improvement in skin structure and tone, a brightening glow effect.

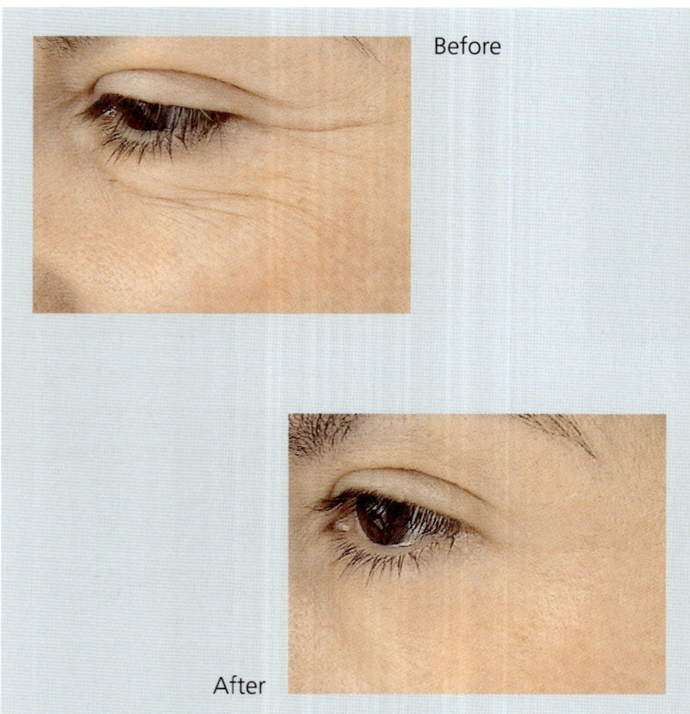

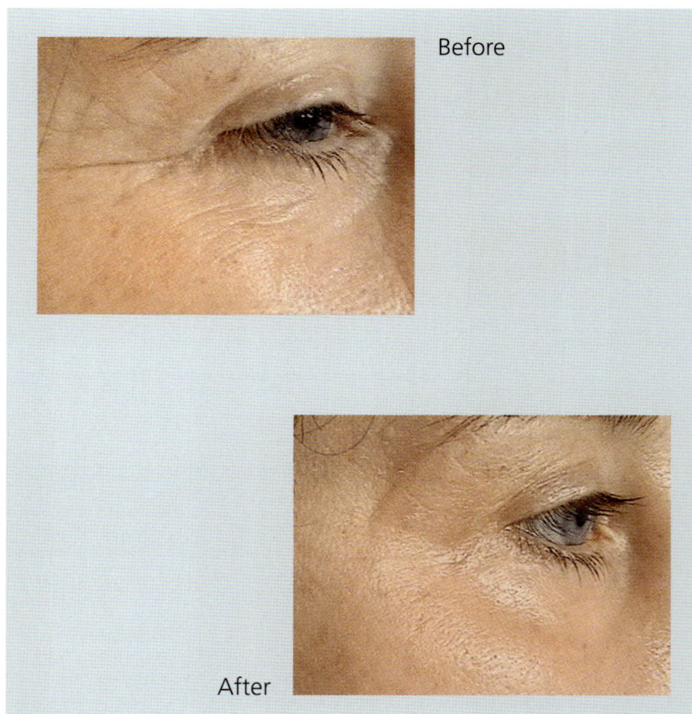

Cases 2 and 3: The results of injecting pure (non-cross-linked) hyaluronic acid was to smooth the fine structural lines (crow's feet) around the eyes. Less than 0.1 ml was injected per point, producing a small welt. Even if the substance is massaged in afterward, it can still take time for it to be integrated into the skin.

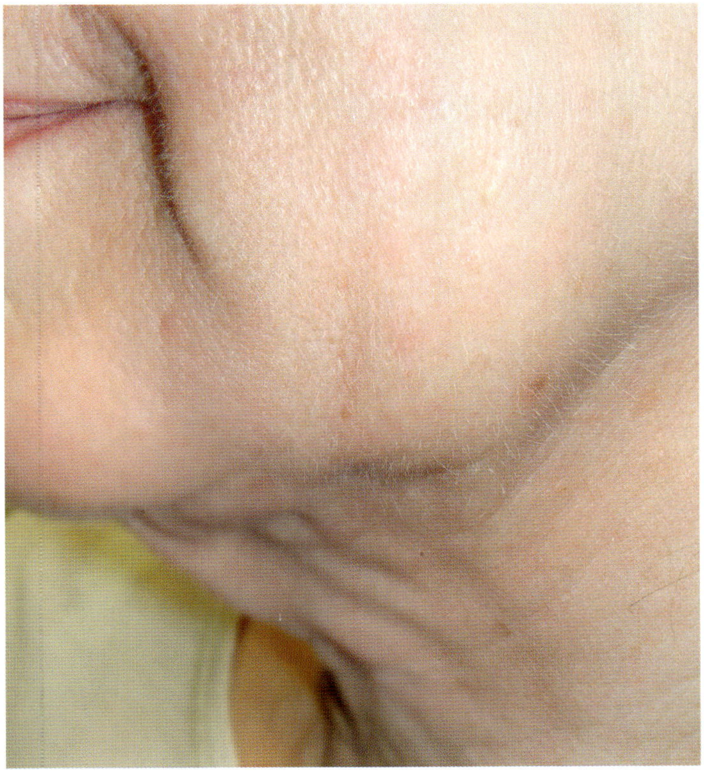

Case 4: Sagging of the cheeks, chin and neck.

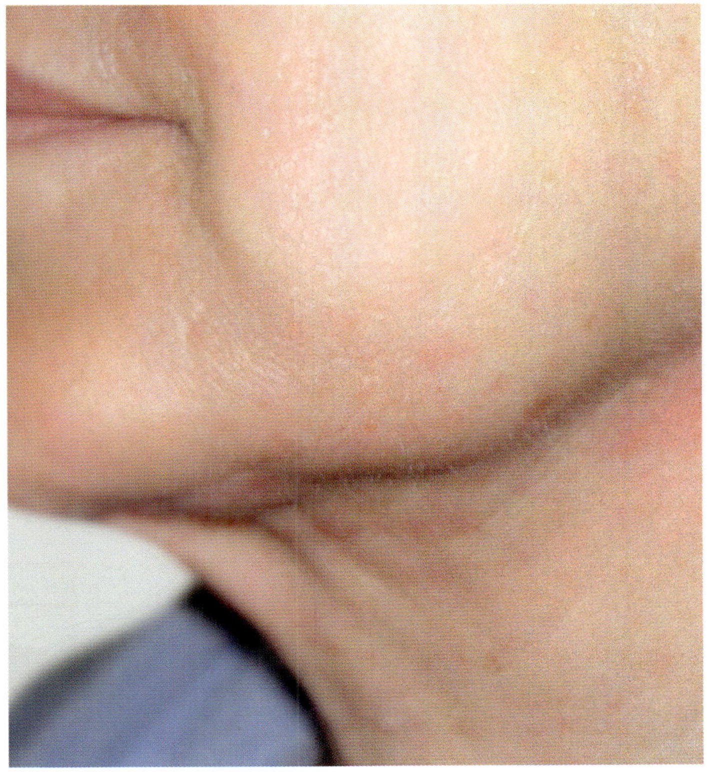

Case 4: Change immediately after the first Mesolift. Repeat treatments can enhance this improvement further.

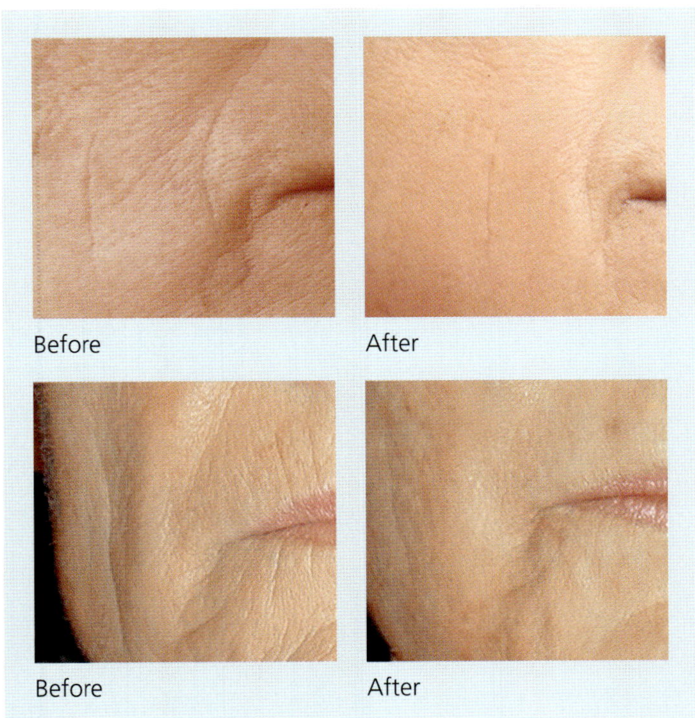

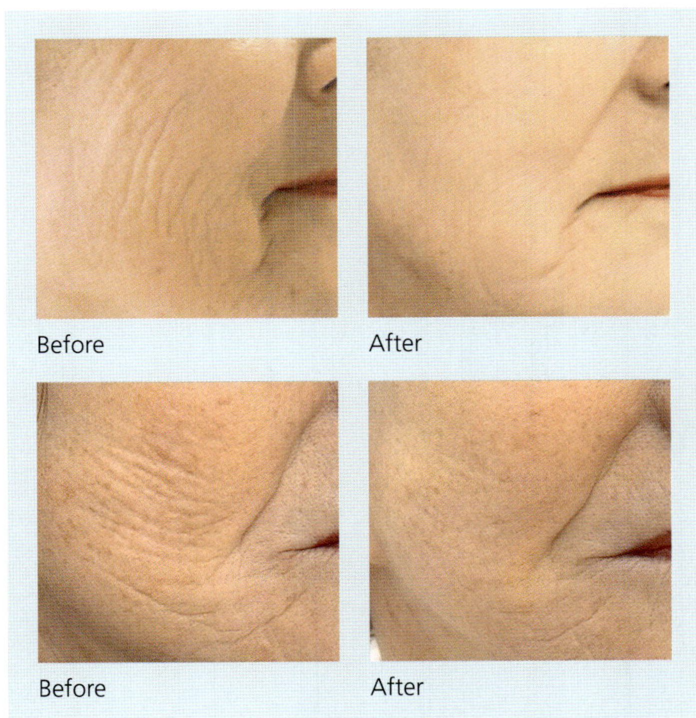

Cases 5–8: Cheek areas with large skin pores and/or creased skin.

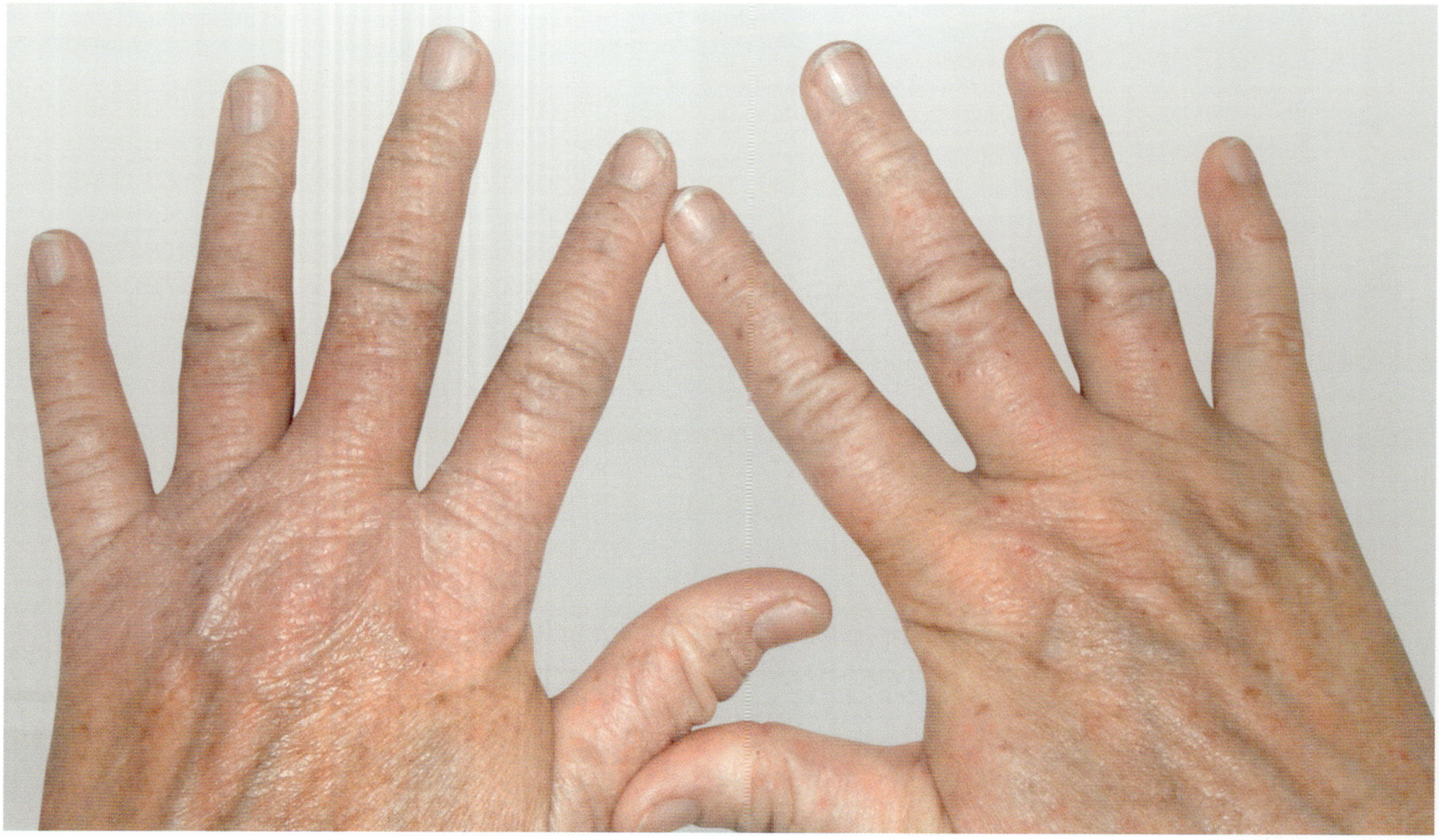

Case 9: Photodamage and advanced skin aging in a 54-year-old woman. Additional finding: hand eczema.

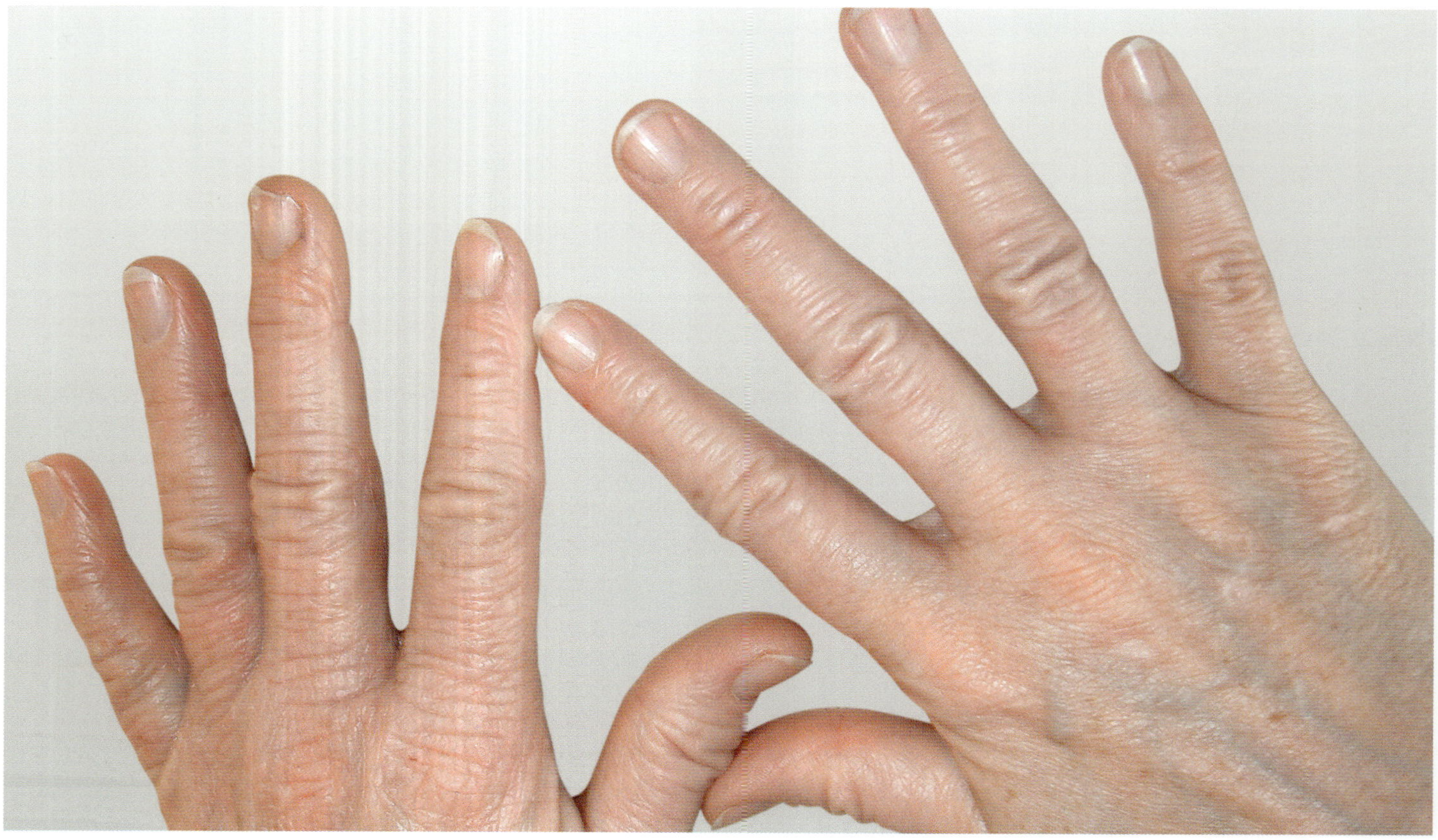

Case 9: Rejuvenation of the skin on the backs of the hands and fingers after three Mesolift treatments.

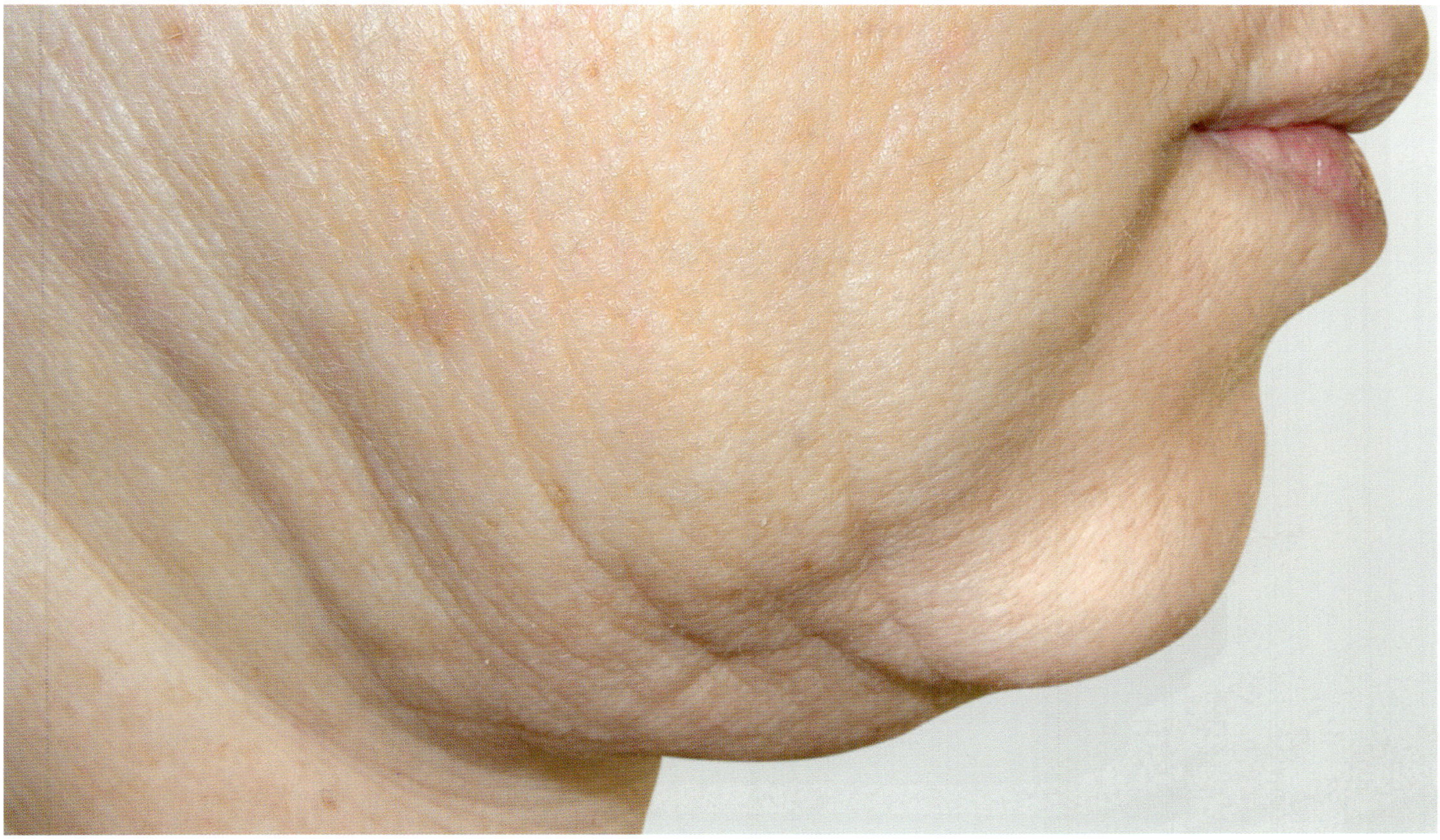

Case 10: Sagging skin, photodamage and double chin in the same patient as case 9.

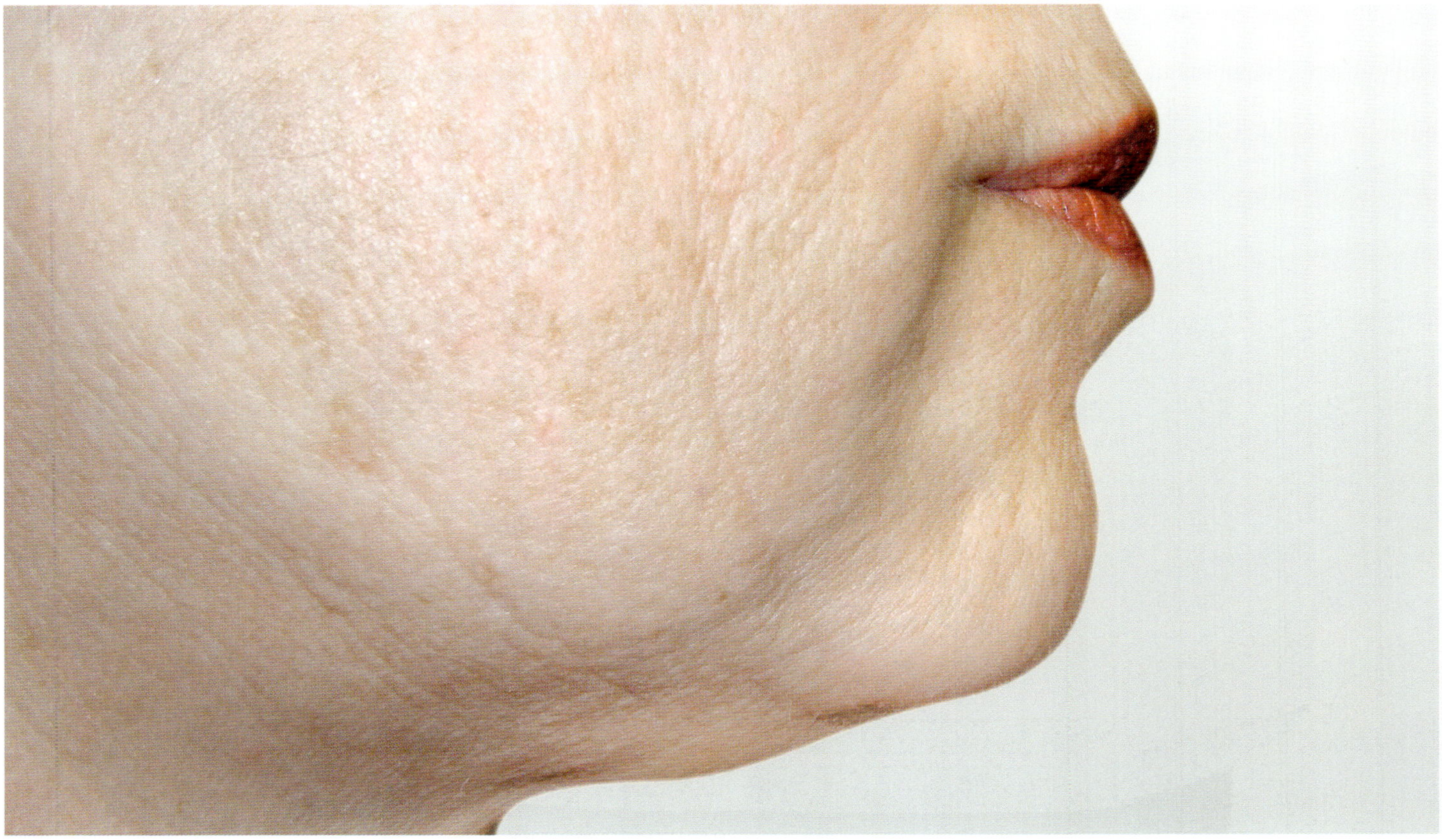

Case 10: Result after three Mesolift sessions and a single initial lipolysis treatment.

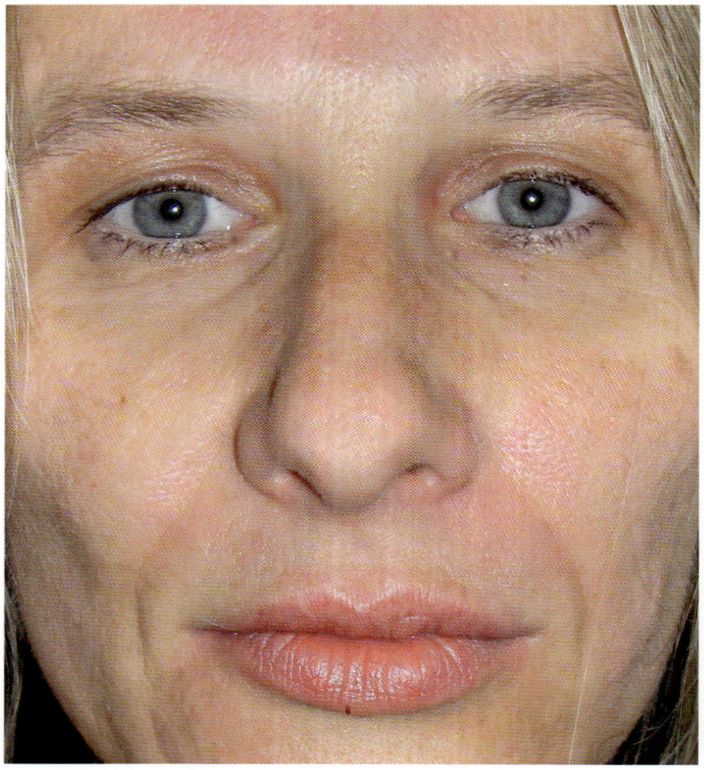

Case 11: Baseline status immediately after one Mesolift session.

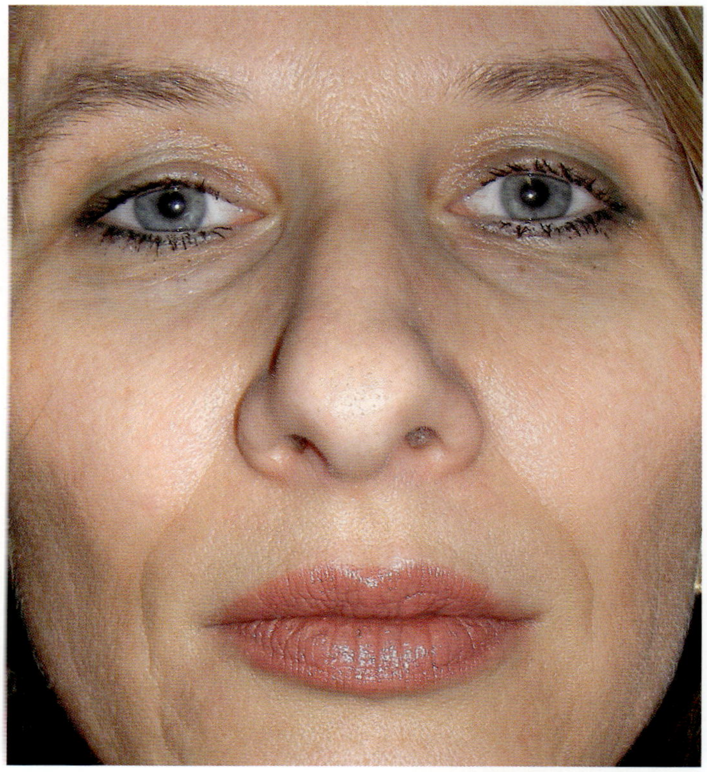

Case 11: Result after three Mesolift sessions and the supplementary administration of 1 ml Teosyal deep lines into the nasolabial region during the first session. There has been a marked improvement in skin texture with a youthful radiance.

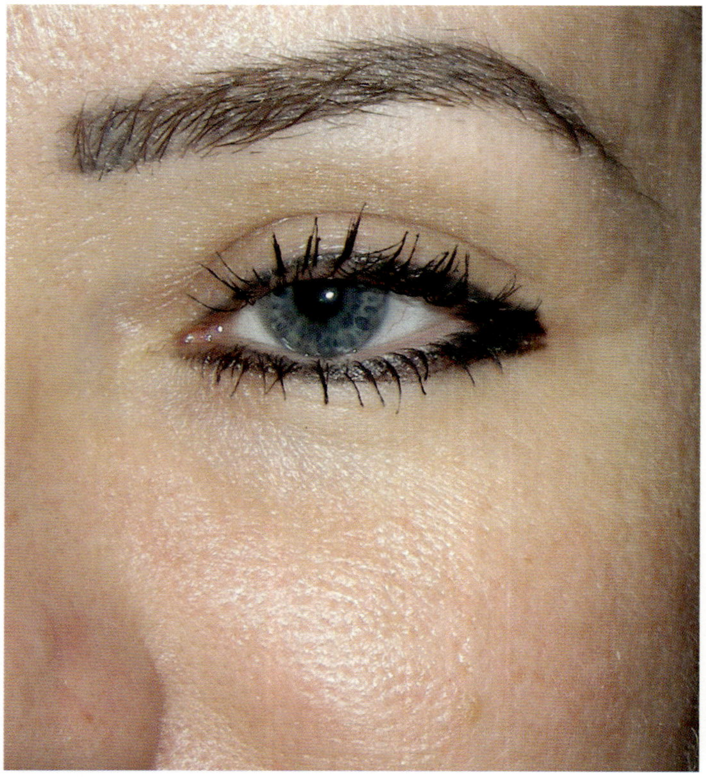

Case 12: Baseline status before preventative treatment in a 40-year-old woman.

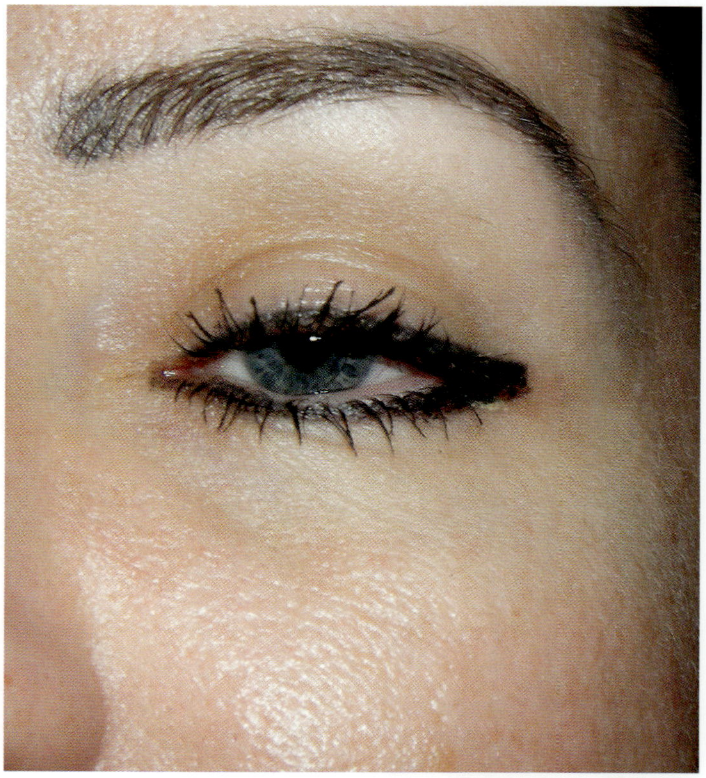

Case 12: The younger and smoother the skin, the less impressive are the visual results. The skin has been plumped up slightly and shows the typical glow effect.

9.2 MesoHair

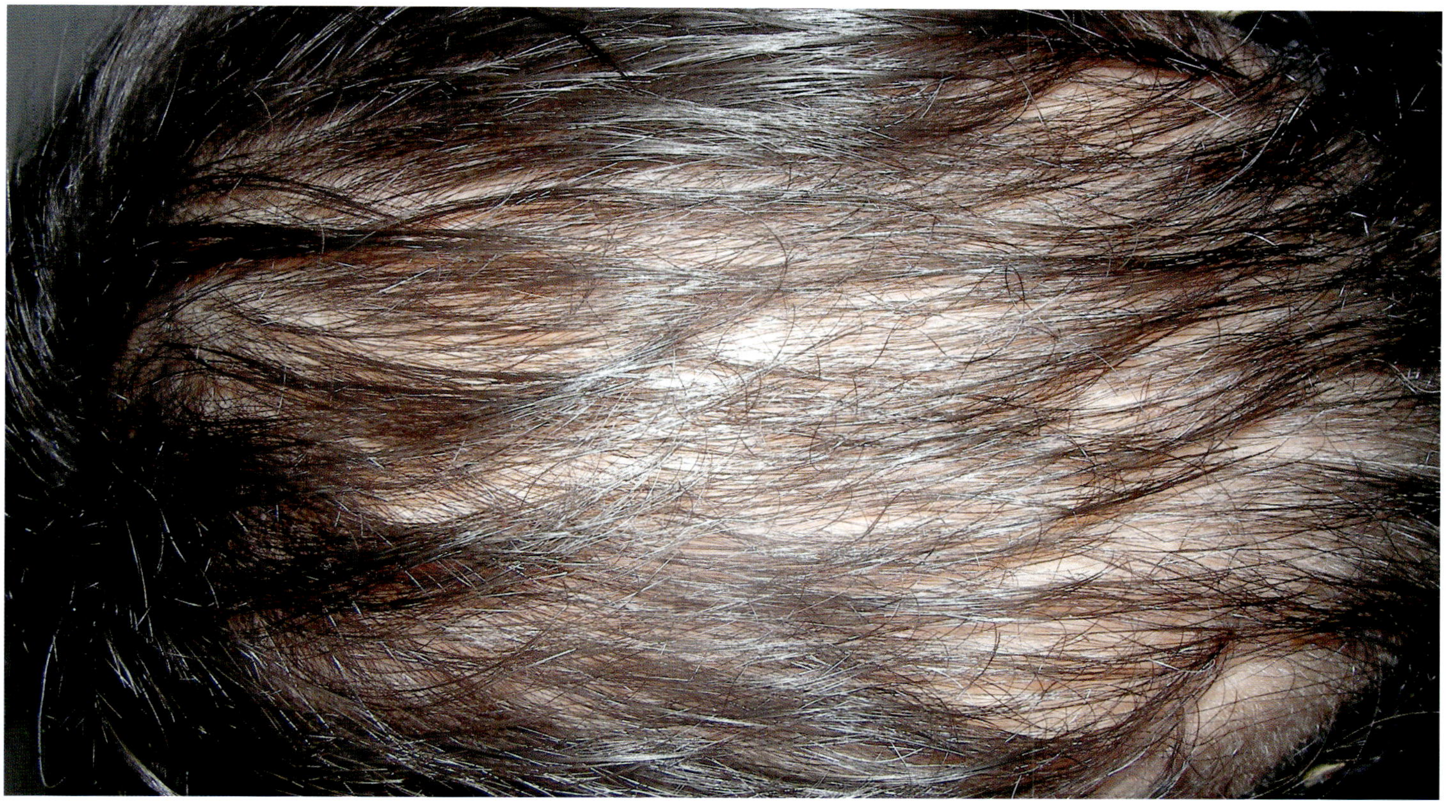

Case 13: Florid androgenetic hair loss in a 30-year-old man.

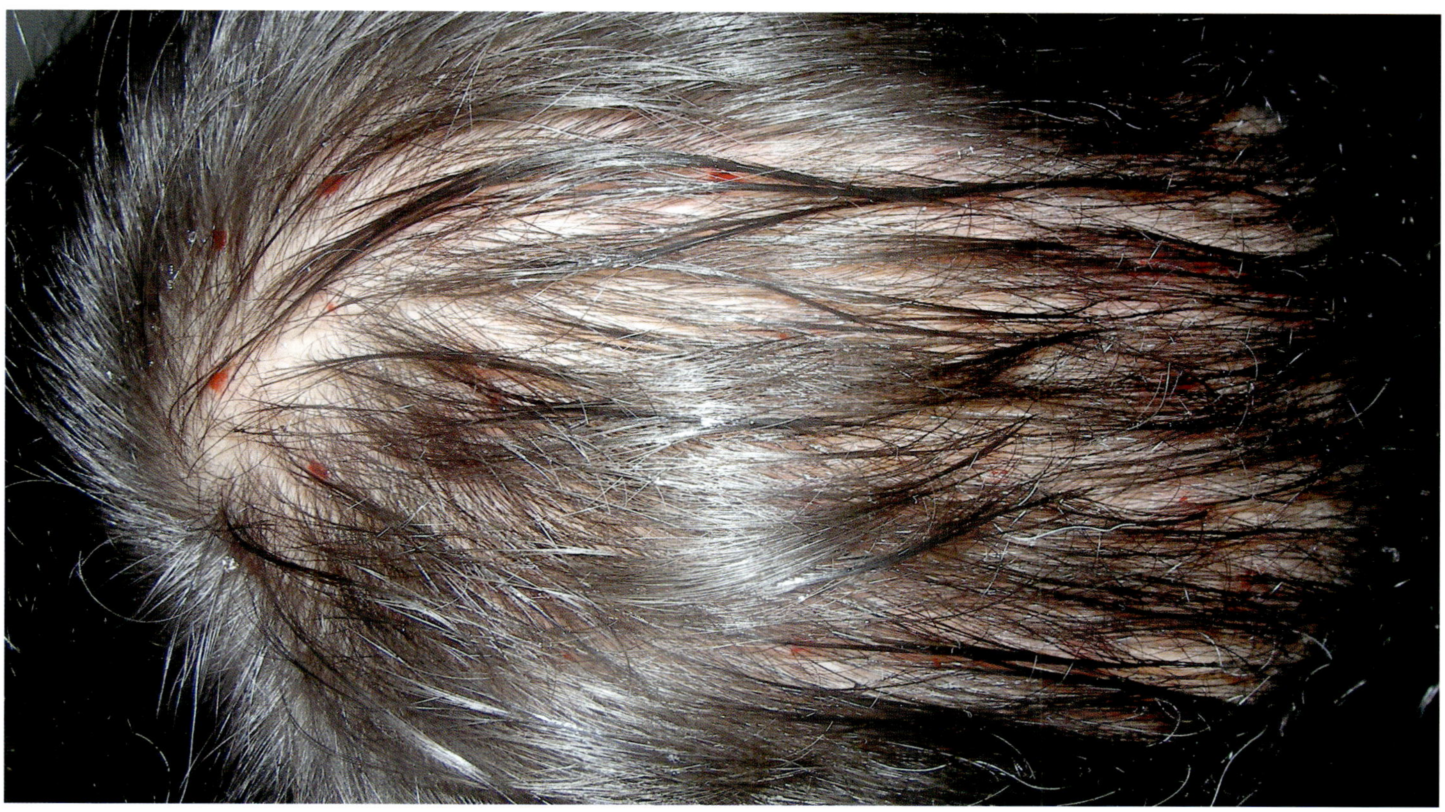

Case 13: Result after 2 months: less hair loss, considerably denser hair growth, better hair quality. Long-term, monthly maintenance therapy is needed in this case.

9.3 Cellulite treatment

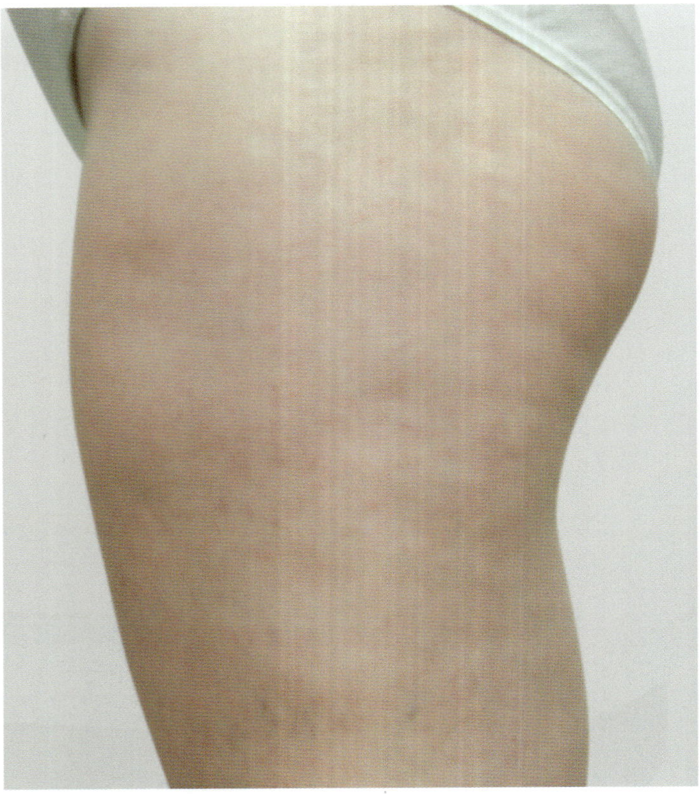

Case 14: Discrete cellulite on the thigh of a slim female patient.

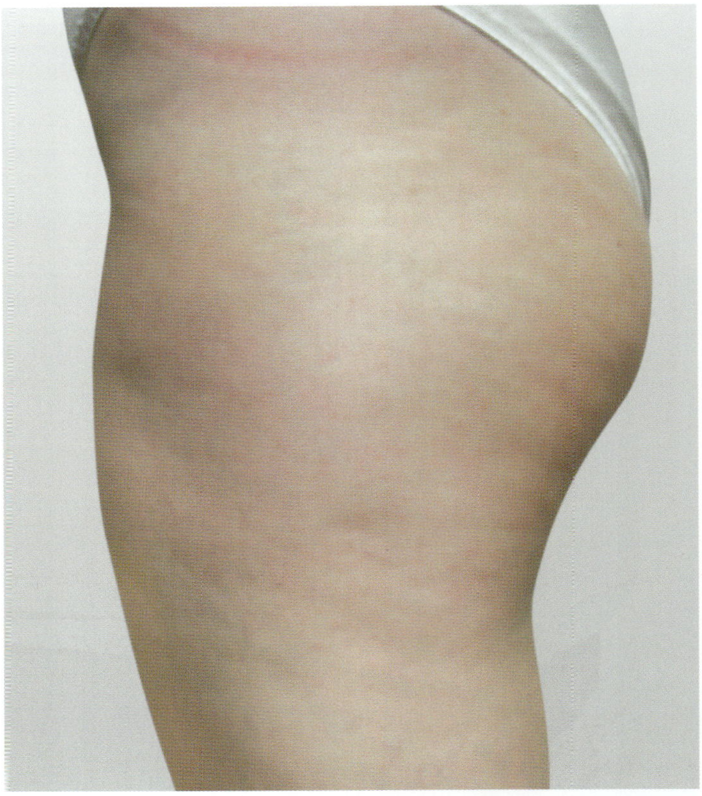

Case 14: Marked slimming and improvement in connective tissue structure following a combined MesoCellulite and lipolysis session.

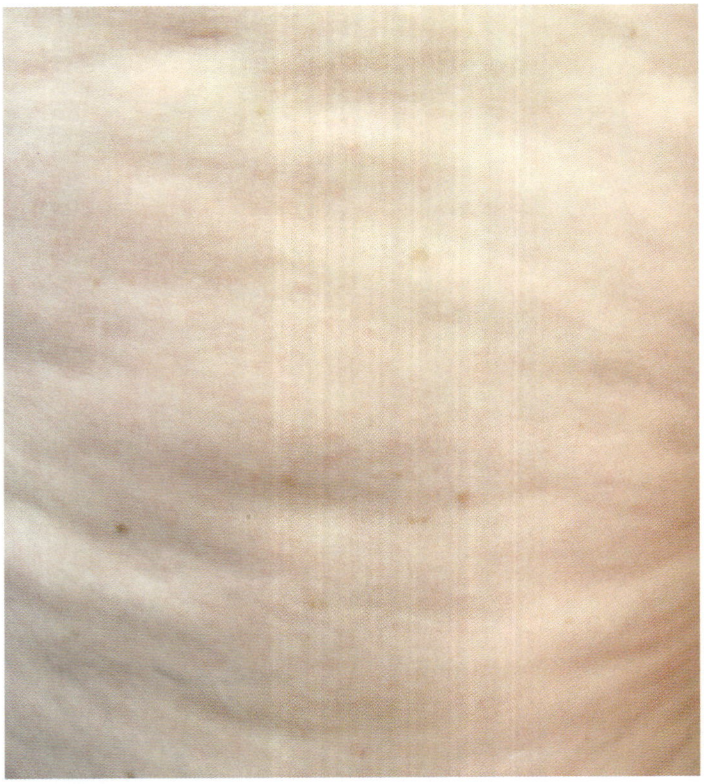

Case 15: Severe cellulite in an overweight female patient.

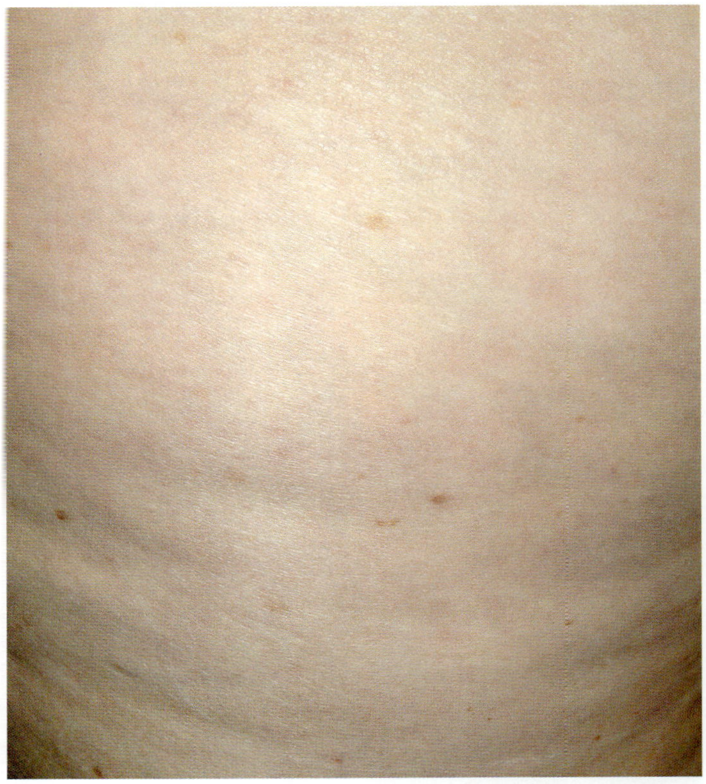

Case 15: Improvement in connective tissue structure and a 1 cm reduction in the thickness of the adipose tissue layer 6 weeks after the combination treatment.

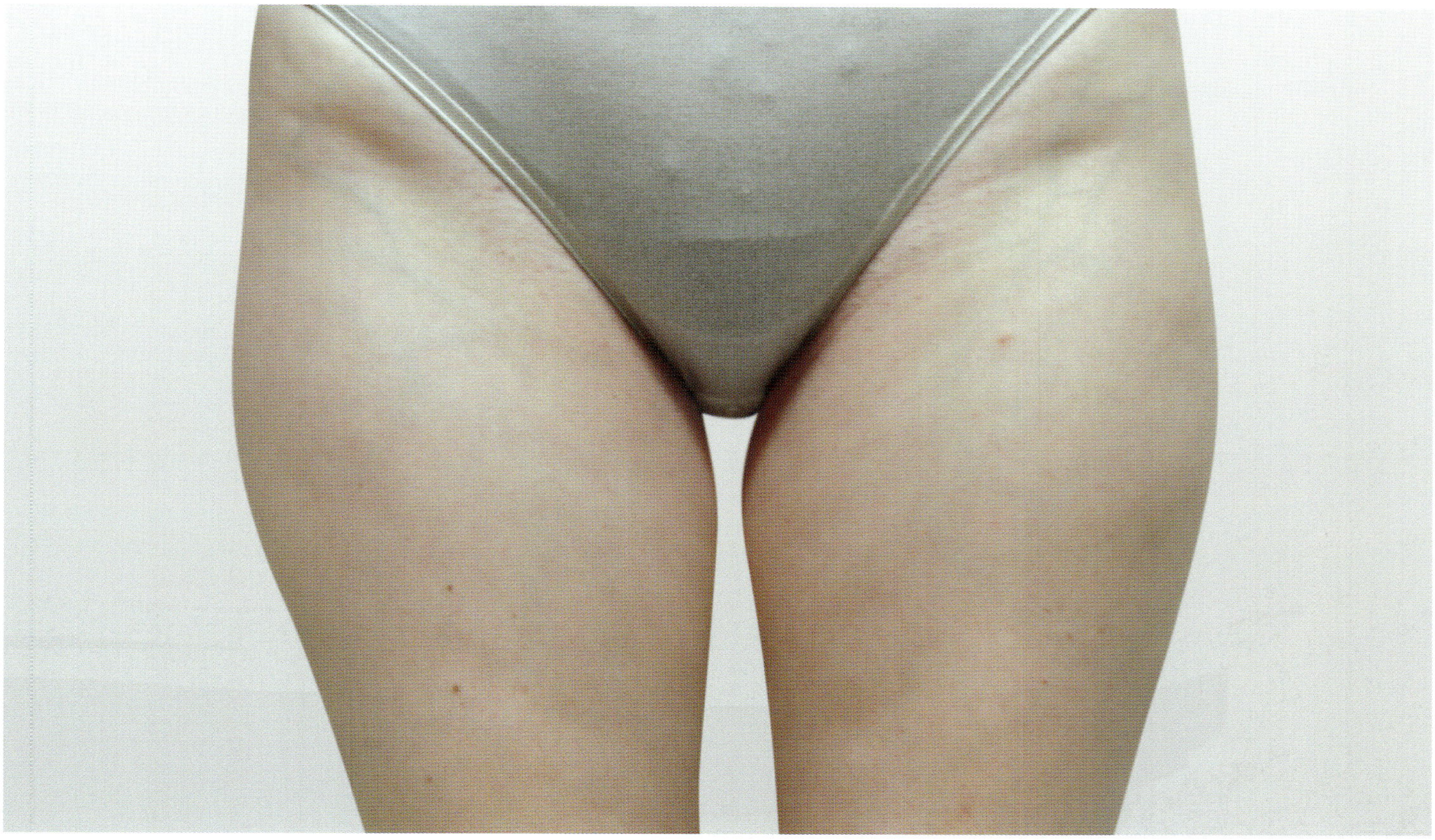

Case 16: Discrete cellulite on the thighs (female patient case 14).

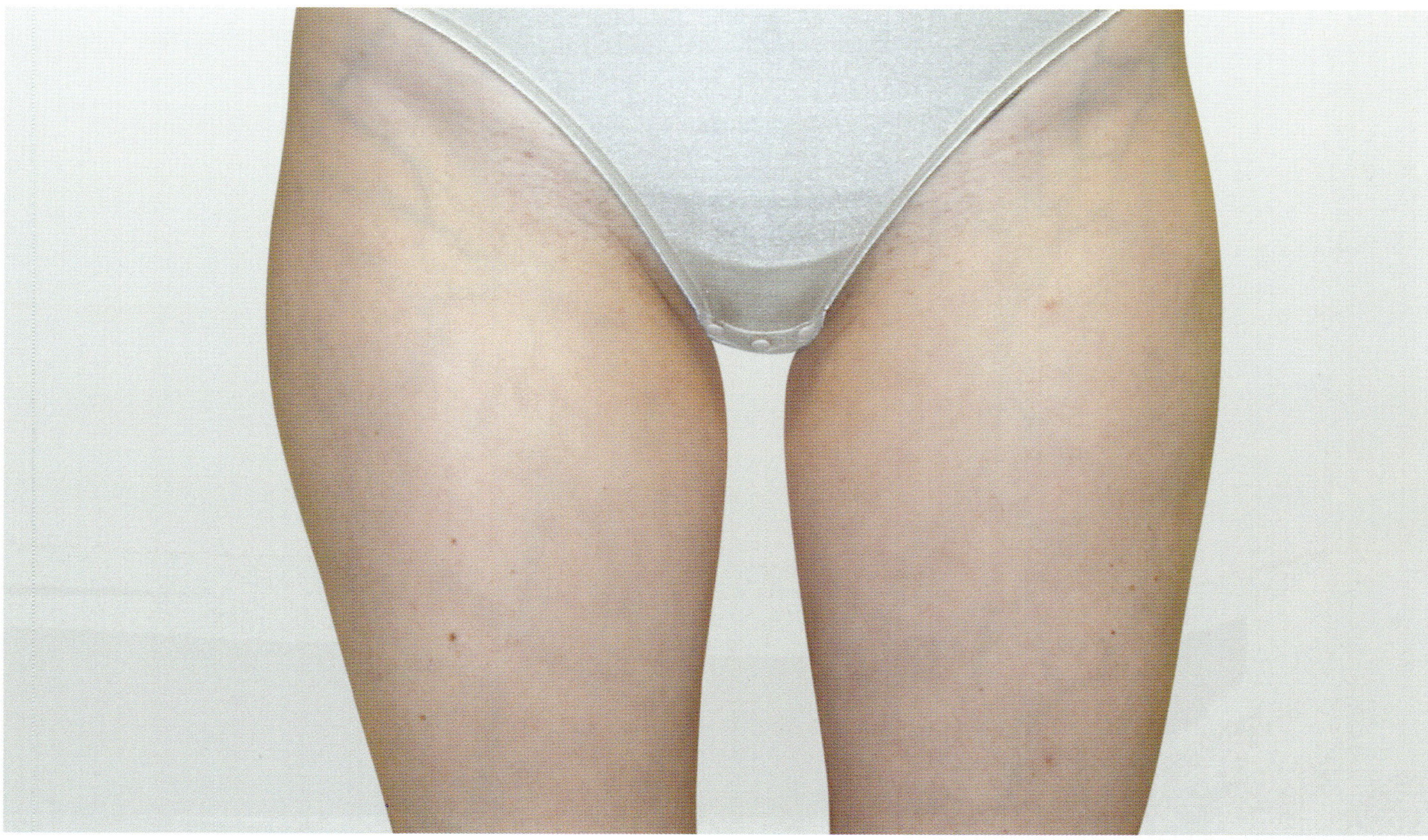

Case 16: Marked slimming and improvement in connective tissue structure 6 weeks after the combination treatment.

9

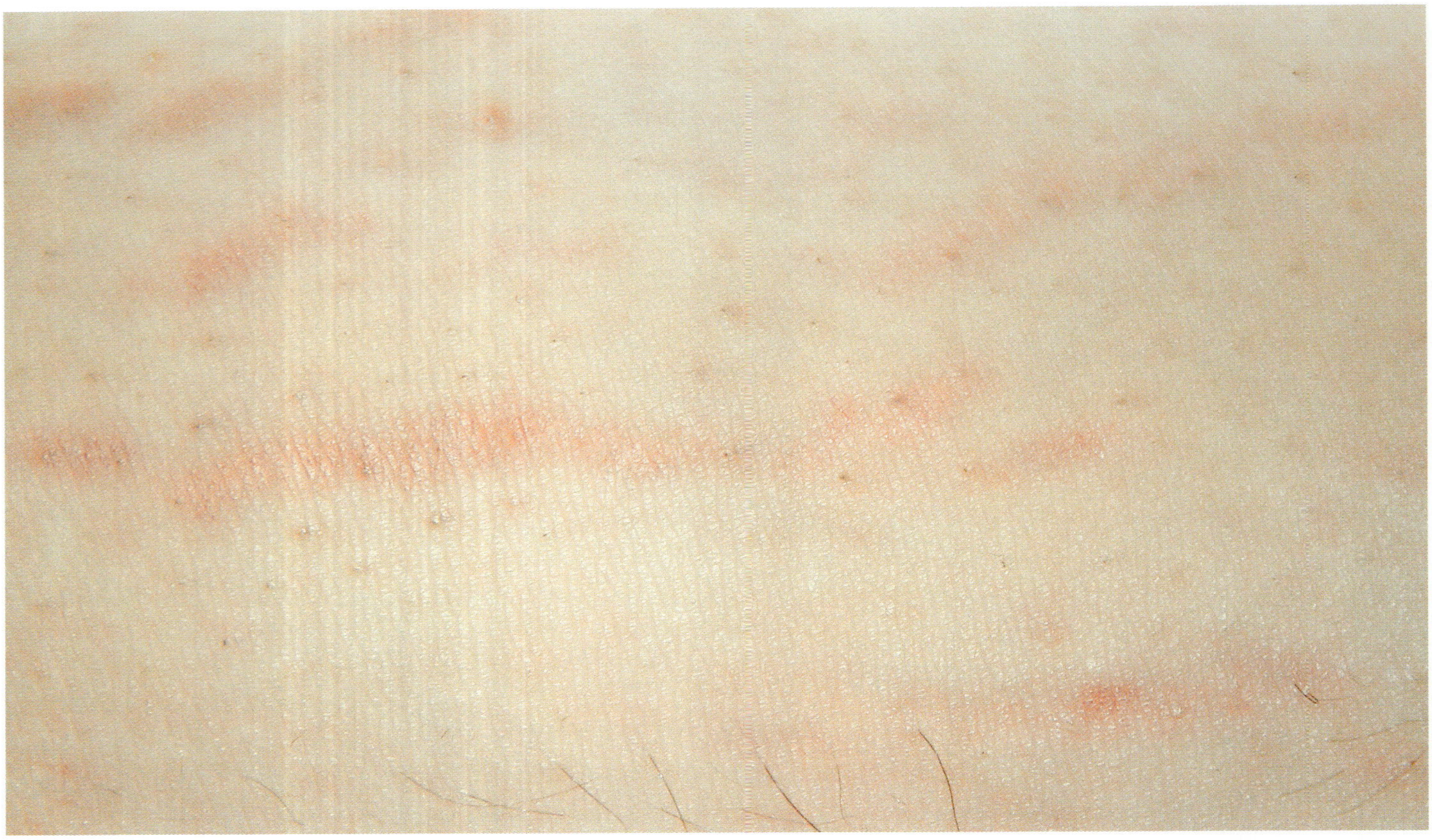

Case 17: Fresh stretch marks in a young woman.

Case 17: Treatment result after 2 weeks (a single mesotherapy session).

10 Aids for the therapist

Information sheet and consent form for injection lipolysis treatment

Injection lipolysis, also known as the "fat-away" injection, is intended for the reduction of localized fat pads or small lipomas (fat nodules or lumps), if a surgical procedure is not desired. The prescription-only active substance Lipostabil® is injected directly into the area being treated. Lipostabil® consists of the natural active substances soy lecithin (PPC) and a bile acid (DC) and is licensed for the intravenous treatment of fat embolisms. The injections into the fatty connective tissue cause little pain, but they are immediately followed by itching, reddening, tenderness, and possibly hematomas (bruises) or nodules (lumps) at the treatment site, which persist for 3–4 days. These local side-effects are normal and attributable to the effects of the substances used. No signs and symptoms of overdose or intoxication have been reported to date. Approximately 1 cm of the fat layer is lost per treatment, accompanied by firming of the skin at the treatment site. There has to be an interval of 4–6 weeks between the individual treatment sessions. The fat breakdown effect also persists for this length of time. You may need to have 2–6 sessions per body region, depending on severity. As with any medical treatment, there is no guarantee of success.

Your statutory medical insurance does not cover the costs of lipolysis. By signing this document, you confirm that you are aware that you will need to meet the treatment costs yourself. You have been given detailed information about alternative treatment options, such as diet, fitness training or a surgical procedure (e.g. liposuction).

The following absolute contraindications (conditions that rule out having this treatment) and relative contraindications (conditions which increase the treatment risk) apply to injection lipolysis:

Absolute contraindications: Age less than 16 years, pregnancy, nursing mother, diabetes with blood vessel complications (microangiopathy)

Relative contraindications:
- Active autoimmune disorders, e.g. of the thyroid, multiple sclerosis, Crohn's disease, rheumatic disease
- Severe liver or kidney disorders
- Acute infection or chronic immune deficiency
- Obesity with a BMI of over 30
- Known hypersensitivity or intolerance to one of the ingredients, e.g. soy allergy
- Coagulation disorders, menstrual problems and irregularities

All deeper injections carry the following rare risks:
- Nerve damage, which may be permanent in certain circumstances
- Infection with subsequent scarring, e.g. injection abscess

Frequent side-effects which you must expect to get:
- Swellings and overheating at the injection site
- Reddening of the skin, which may persist for longer periods
- Itching, pain and tenderness at the injection site
- Hematomas (bruises)
- Nodules (lumps) at the treatment site, which may persist for longer periods
- Dents/hollows caused by irregular fat breakdown

Possible general bodily reactions:

- Symptoms such as nausea, vomiting, increased salivary flow, circulatory reaction
- Diarrhea (also with mucus), breakthrough bleeds
- Allergic reactions such as nettle rash, asthma, symptoms of shock (very rare!)

Off-label use

The use of medicines in conditions other than those for which they have been licensed is known as off-label use. This term refers not only to the range of uses of a medicine, but also to the method of its administration. When medicines like Lipostabil are administered locally into the connective/fatty tissue, in pure or diluted form, this constitutes off-label use, and we are required to inform you about this.

In many cases, however, certain medicines have also become established for indications outside their licensed range of uses. This is the case with lipolysis, even though it is not generally recognized in medicine and not licensed as a medicine for local fat reduction.

I have read the Information Sheet through carefully and have understood it.

I was given the opportunity to discuss all the contents of this Information Sheet with

.... and to ask any questions that I had.
(name of doctor)

I was given sufficient time to consider my decision to undergo the treatment.

Name of patient: . . . .

Body region to be treated: . . . .

Body region to be treated: : . . . .

Costs per session . . . .

. . . .	. . . .	. . . .
Place, date	Signature of patient	Doctor

☐ Copy to patient

Patient information sheet for mesotherapy

In skilled hands, mesotherapy is not dangerous and only rarely causes side-effects which require the treatment to be discontinued.

Undesirable effects include pain during the injection, local reddening, itching or allergic reactions, circulatory collapse in anxious/sensitive patients, skin granulomas, skin necrosis (very rare) or pigment disruptions on the skin, infections (very rare), damage to nerves (extremely rare). The following are relatively common: hematomas (= bruising; a treatment break is necessary until they disappear completely), surface scratches.

To avoid pain during the injection, the therapist may work with a mesotherapy injector gun and/or apply an anesthetic cream beforehand. Some active substances are used on an off-label basis, i.e. they are not licensed to be used for that indication.

Rules for the patient

Before the treatment

- Do not take any aspirin or enzyme products two days before the mesotherapy.
- Inform the therapist about any regular medication (e.g. oral anticoagulants) and previous illnesses.
- Inform the therapist about all allergies or intolerances (e.g. predisposition to keloids).
- Only cleanse the skin with water and soap, without applying any skincare products or make-up to the area being treated.
- Do not have any immunizations (particularly BCG) before the mesotherapy.

After the treatment

- No full baths, saunas, massages, mudpacks or lymphatic drainage for 24 hours.
- Do not sunbathe for 48 hours.
- Do not wear any colored, new or very tight clothing (e.g. pre-worn jeans) over the treated area.
- Do not use any ointments, creams or powders, unless prescribed by the physician.
- No X-rays/radiotherapy or electrotherapy for the next three days.
- Your usual skincare may be resumed after 24 hours.

I have read this Information Sheet and give my agreement to it. I would like to have mesotherapy treatment.

. . . .
Place, date

. . . .
Signature of Patient

Advantages of mesotherapy

- Evidence-based medical treatment method (minimally invasive injection procedure)
- Use of medicinal products licensed in curative medicine, in low-dose mode, administered via the skin directly to the site of the disorder, taking into account the anatomy and physiology of the skin
- Immediate and long-term effect at the desired location
- Pharmacological effect on the local microcirculation, immunoregulation, the neurovegetative system, cell function and the extracellular matrix
- Physical stimulus (acupuncture effects) through multiple microinjections
- Avoids compliance problems
- Strong bond with the patient
- Avoids problems of bioavailability, absorption and the first-pass effect, as encountered when medicinal products are administered systemically
- Avoids side-effects and complications caused by high-dose systemic treatment
- Particularly suitable in chronic disorders and multiple morbidity
- Savings on prescription costs (confirmed savings potential, particularly with antibiotics, analgesics and anti-inflammatory agents)
- Quick and efficient to administer
- Established interdisciplinary uses
- Little or no investment cost
- Easy to learn and may be implemented at the practice straight away
- Internationally standardized training with examination option
- Regular annual update courses for continuing professional development
- International contacts and inclusion by the SIM (Société Internationale de Mésothérapie, the International Mesotherapy Society)

Indication spectrum outside medical esthetics

- Treatment of pain
- Degenerative arthritic conditions
- Headache and back pain
- Tendinopathies
- Musculoskeletal disorders
- Sports medicine
- Immune disorders
- Recurrent infections, allergies, hay fever
- Psychosomatic symptoms
- Exhaustion, sleep problems
- Menopausal syndrome
- Quitting smoking
- Perfusion and wound healing disorders
- To repel mosquitoes, etc.

Merz Scales® (TM) Documentation form

Name of patient | Date of birth | Medical Insurance

Lines on forehead – static

A

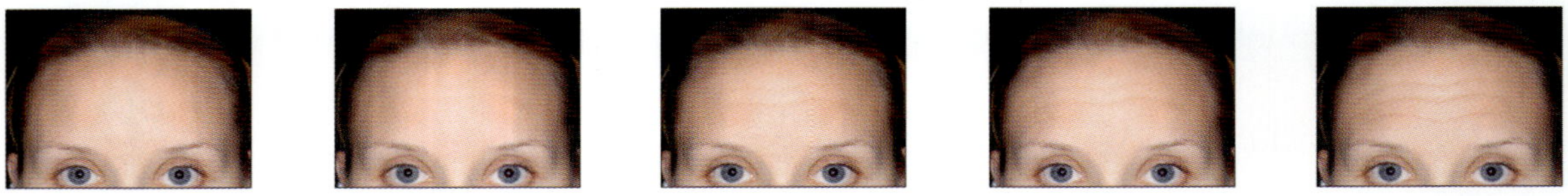

0 1 2 3 4

Lines on forehead – dynamic

B

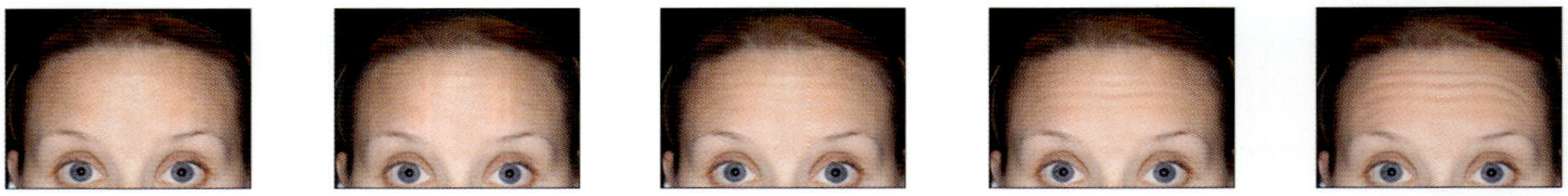

0 1 2 3 4

Position of eyebrows

C

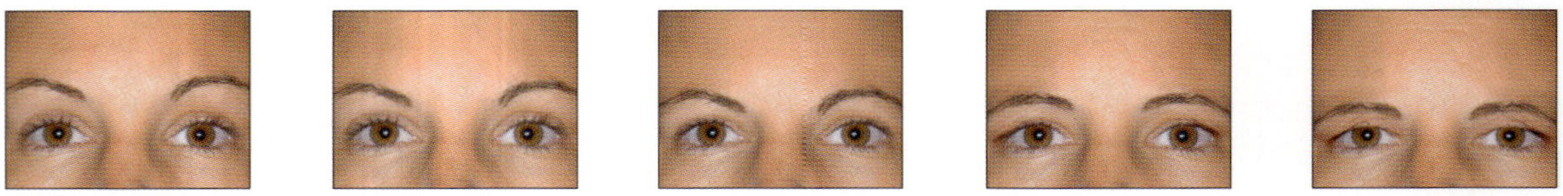

0 1 2 3 4

Crow's feet – static

D

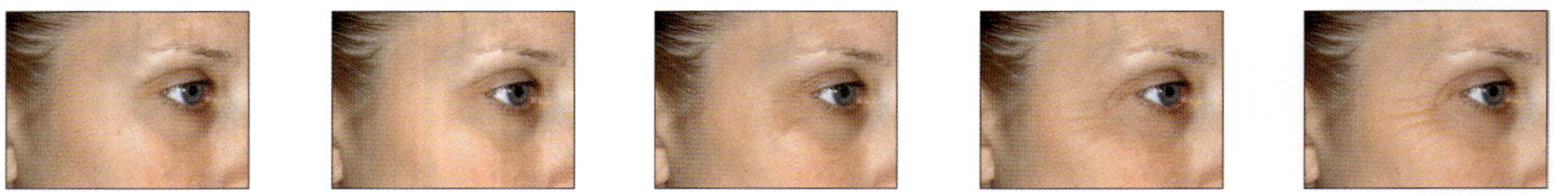

0 1 2 3 4

Crow's feet – dynamic

E

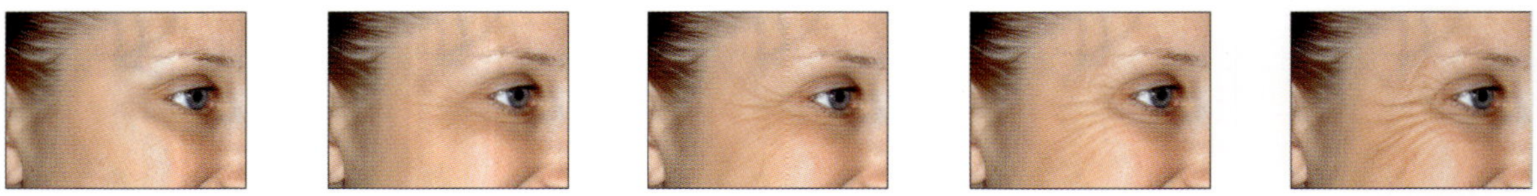

0 1 2 3 4

Marionette lines

F

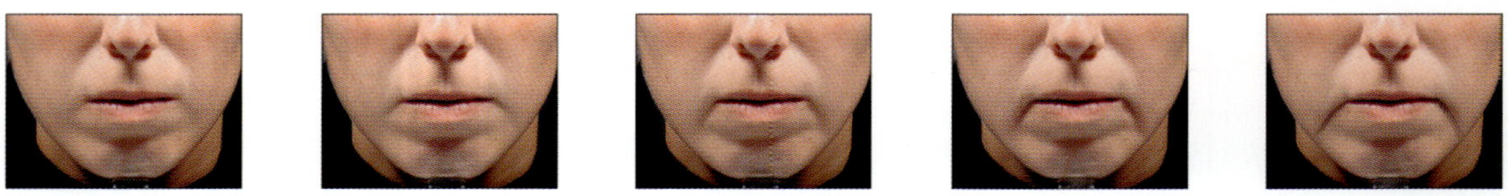

0 1 2 3 4

Neck

G

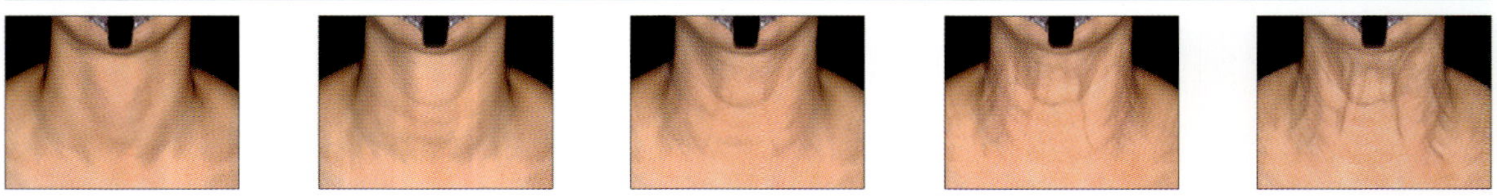

0 1 2 3 4

PHOTOCOPYING TEMPLATE

Documentation form for esthetic treatments

Name of patient | Date of birth | Medical Insurance

Treatment with: ☐ *Botulinum toxin* ☐ *Filler*

Products:

Batch numbers:

Units (ml):

Merz Scale:	A	B	C	D	E	F	G
Value:							

Date:

Photo today: ☐ *Yes* ☐ *No*

Treatment with: ☐ *Botulinum toxin* ☐ *Filler*

Products:

Batch numbers:

Units (ml):

Merz Scale:	A	B	C	D	E	F	G
Value:							

Date:

Photo today: ☐ *Yes* ☐ *No*

Treatment with: ☐ *Botulinum toxin* ☐ *Filler*

Products:

Batch numbers:

Units (ml):

Merz Scale:	A	B	C	D	E	F	G
Value:							

Date:

Photo today: ☐ *Yes* ☐ *No*

Treatment with: ☐ *Botulinum toxin* ☐ *Filler*

Products:

Batch numbers:

Units (ml):

Merz Scale:	A	B	C	D	E	F	G
Value:							

Date:

Photo today: ☐ *Yes* ☐ *No*

Treatment with: ☐ *Botulinum toxin* ☐ *Filler*

Products:

Batch numbers:

Units (ml):

Merz Scale:	A	B	C	D	E	F	G
Value:							

Date:

Photo today: ☐ *Yes* ☐ *No*

Treatment with: ☐ *Botulinum toxin* ☐ *Filler*

Products:

Batch numbers:

Units (ml):

Merz Scale:	A	B	C	D	E	F	G
Value:							

Date:

Photo today: ☐ *Yes* ☐ *No*

Case documentation for mesotherapy: I

Patient's name (abbrev.) .... Date of birth: ....

Nature of problems/symptoms: ....

Diagnosis(es): ....

Diagnosis(es) confirmed by means of: ....

Additional diagnosis(es): ....

Particulars from the history

Previous treatment, since when? ....

Nature of previous treatment with rating (on a scale of 1–6, where 1 = very good, 2 = good, 3 = satisfactory, 4 = adequate, 5 = poor and 6 = inadequate): ....

....

....

....

Side-effects? ....

....

Accompanying treatments? ....

....

Mesotherapy

Findings of relevance to mesotherapy (clinical and pathophysiological):

....

....

Mesotherapy mixture (active substances, dose/quantity):

....

Mesotherapy (location and injection technique): ....

Mesotherapy interval: .... Number of sessions: ....

Accompanying therapy? ....

Progress assessment

Treatment period: from .... to ....

Global success rating: ....

Global efficacy of the mesotherapy (on a scale of 1–6, where 1 = very good, 2 = good, 3 = satisfactory, 4 = adequate, 5 = poor and 6 = inadequate): ....

Evaluation of efficacy:

- Physician: ....
- Patient: ....

Satisfaction:

- Physician: ....
- Patient: ....

Observed or reported side-effects:

....

Final comments:

....

....

....

....	....	....
Date	Signature	Practice stamp

Case documentation for mesotherapy: II

....

Name of patient (abbrev.)

....

Date of birth

....

Nature of problems/symptoms

....

Diagnosis(es)

....

Diagnosis (es) confirmed by means of

....

Additional diagnosis (es)

....

Particulars from the history

....

Previous treatment since when?

....

Nature of previous treatments with rating (on a scale of 1–6, where 1 = very good, 2 = good, 3 = satisfactory, 4 = adequate, 5 = poor and 6 = inadequate)

....

Side-effects

....

Accompanying treatments

11 Appendix

Supplier information

Aesthetic Dermal S.L.C (Reparistim®)
Spain, www.aestheticdermal.com

Filorga (NCTF 135®)
Paris, France

FOREVERMED
Ina Bergner,
Practice telephone number: 08178-868861, cell phone (mobile): 0177-6130400, www.meso-forever.com

FotoFinder Systems GmbH
Aichner-Schmied-Straße 3, 84364 Bad Birnbach, Germany
Tel. +49 (0) 8563 977200, Fax +49 (0) 8563 9772010, www.fotofinder.de, info@fotofinder.de

Handelsagentur Bourgett (provides a wide range of mesotherapy services, distributor for Toskani Cosmeceuticals), Lanzinger Str. 2, 83250 Marquartstein, Germany, Tel. 08641-696178, Fax 08641-696187, www.mesotherapie-shop.de

Living Nature® (Rescue Gel)
New Zealand, www.livingnature.com

Magnet aktiv GmbH (elha injectables, Fuculacca)
Postfach 1380, 69154 Wiesloch, Germany, www.elha-web.de

Merz Pharmaceuticals GmbH (cross-linked and non-cross-linked HA, Botulinum toxin)
60048 Frankfurt, Germany, Tel. 069-1503-1

Receptura Apotheke
Altenhöferallee 3, D-60438 Frankfurt am Main, Germany,
Tel. +49 (0) 69 92 880-300, Fax +49 (0) 69 92 880-333, www.receptura.de

Revitacare®
95310 Saint Ouen l'Aumône, France, www.revitacare.net

St. Johanser-Naturmittelvertrieb GmbH (Matricell® Königinnen Trank)
Postfach 1462, 82119 Gauting, Germany

Teoxane GmbH (cross-linked and non-cross-linked HA, pre-/post-treatment products)
Am Lohmühlbach 17, 85356 Freising, Germany, Tel. 08161-14805-0, Fax 08161-14805-15, www.teoxane.de

Wiedemann Pharma GmbH (Wiedemann Homöokomplex BH)
82541 Münsing-Ambach, Germany, www.wiedemann-pharma.de

Manufacturers' details

Mesoject® needles: Thiebaud Biomedical Devices, Margencel, France
Mesoram® needles: Rimos srl., Mirandola, Italy
Mesorelle® needles: Biotekne srl., Bologna, Italy
Pistor 4 and Pistor 5: MI-MEDICAL-Innovation Parc d'activités, F-48230 Chanac, France, Tel. 0033-4-66482279, Fax 0033-4-66482699, www.mi-medicalinnovation.com
Syringes and Microlance® needles: BD, Franklin Lakes, USA
Sterican® needles: Terumo, Leuven, Belgium
Toskani cosmetics, Barcelona, Spain, Tel. 0034-938418289 www.toskanicosmetics.com

Web links

www.mesotherapie.org
Deutsche Gesellschaft für Mesotherapie e.V. (German Mesotherapy Association), Munich
www.mesotherapie-shop.de
Mesotherapy service, events organization
www.simeso.org
International Mesotherapy Society, Paris

Sources

Figures
10, 48, 50 (bottom): with the kind permission St. Johanser GmbH, Gauting, Germany
27, 29, 33 FotoFinder Systems GmbH, Bad Birnbach, Germany
38: Bernd Kardorff (Archive)
58: David Kühn, Marburg, Germany
63 (top, left): fotolia.de
68: Teoxane GmbH, Freising, Germany
89, 109, 110, 111, 112, 113, 114, 115: Britta Knoll (Archive)
108 (bottom), 109 (bottom), 122: Merz Pharmaceuticals GmbH, Frankfurt am Main, Germany

Text
Chapter 3: Documentation and organization (extracts): FotoFinder Systems GmbH, Bad Birnbach, Germany

British Library Cataloguing in Publication Data

ISBN-13: 978-1-85097-232-7

QUINTESSENCE PUBLISHING

Quintessence Publishing Co, Ltd
Quintessence House, Grafton Road, New Malden, Surrey KT3 3AB
United Kingdom
www.quintpub.co.uk

Translation: Rosana Jelaska, London
Editing: Quintessence Publishing Co, Ltd, London
Layout and Production: Quintessenz Verlags-GmbH, Berlin, Germany
Printed and bound by AZ Druck- und Datentechnik, Berlin, Germany

Important note:

Like every other science, medicine is subject to constant development. Research and clinical experience widen our knowledge base, particularly with regard to medicines and other forms of treatment. If any dosages or methods of administration are mentioned in this book, the reader may have confidence that the authors, editors and publishers have taken great care to ensure that this information is in line with the latest knowledge available at the time of publication.

However, the publisher cannot give guarantees for any information regarding dosing instructions and methods of administration. All users are requested to take great care to check the package insert leaflets of the products used to establish whether the dosage recommendations or details of contraindications given therein differ in any way from the information given in this book. This sort of check is particularly important with rarely used or recently launched products. The use of any medication dose or method of administration takes place at the user's own risk. The author and publisher appeal to all users to inform them if they spot any obvious inaccuracies. The author and publisher are grateful for feedback of any kind.

References

Arch Dermatol 2009 (145), S. 1375-1379

Atlas of Mesotherapy in Skin Rejuvenation. Informa Health Care. 2007

Beilin, Ghislaine: The mesolift, in: Mesotherapy Journal, USA

Bonnet, Laurens, Perrin, Masson: Guide Pratique de Mesotherapie. 2008

Coz, le, J.: Mesotherapy and Lipolysis. EstheticMedic. 2008

DGM: Ästhetik-Skript

DGM: Jahresupdates. Band 3-10

DGM: Mesotherapie Kurskompendium

DGM: Praxis der Mesotherapie nach M. Pistor

Fahr, Alfred: Studie zur Wirksamkeit eines neuartigen Gerätes zur verbesserten Einschleusung von Wirkstoffen in die Haut. Der Dermaroller®.Philipps-Universität Marburg. Institut für Pharmazeutische Technologie und Biopharmazie 2001

Greco, Joseph F.: Micro Needling and Injecting Platelet Rich Plasma to Enhance Collagen Synthesis and Skin Tightening, in: Mesotherapy Journal, USA

Heine, Hartmut: Lehrbuch der biologischen Medizin. Grundregulation und Extrazelluläre Matrix. Hyppokrates Verlag. 2007, 3. Auflage

Informa Health Care: Atlas of Mesotherapy in Skin Rejuvenation. 2007

Informa Healthcare: Aesthetic Mesotherapy and Injection Lipolysis in Clinical Practice. Madhère 2007

Klein, Schreml et al.: In Vitro Studies Investigating the Effect of Subcutaneous Phosphatidylcholine Injections in the 3T3-L1 Adipocyte Model: Lipolysis or Lipid Dissolution? Plastic and Reconstructive Surgery. 2009 (124) 2, S. 419–427

Mang, Werner L. V. (Hrsg.) et.al.: Das Medizinproduktegesetz und dessen Auswirkungen, in: Ästhetische Chirurgie. Einhorn-Presse-Verlag 1998 (II), S. 138

Philipps-Universität Marburg. Institut für Pharmazeutische Technologie und Biopharmazie

Pitié-Salpêtrière Hospital: Impact of Injection mode on the anti-aging effect of mixture composed of hyaluronic acid and multivitamins injected using the U 225 biophymed mesotherapy gun into human skin maintainded in survival. Paris 2006

Plastic Surgery. April 2009 (36) 2, S. 181–192

Rittes, Patricia: Mesolift treatment the micro-injections facial mesotherapy, in: Mesotherapy Journal, USA

Sattler, G.: Bildatlas der ästhetischen Boulinumtoxin-Therapie. KVM – Der Medizinverlag. Marburg 2010

Tordjman, M.: Hautverjüngung des Dekolletés durch Mesotherapie. Zeitschrift für Schönheitsmedizin und dermatologische Chirurgie. Paris 2003 18, S. 111–118

Matarasso, A., Pfeifer, T. M.: Mesotherapy and injection lipolysis.
The first part of this article familiarizes the reader with the evolution of mesotherapy, injection lipolysis, and the use of phosphatidylcholine and deoxycholate for subcutaneous fat reduction. There is an emphasis on the underlying basic science of fat metabolism and the biochemistry of phosphatidylcholine, so that practitioners will be able to understand future published research on these topics. The second half details some personal experience with injection lipolysis.
a Department of Plastic and Reconstructive Surgery, Albert Einstein College of Medicine, New York, NY, USA
b Department of Plastic Surgery, Manhattan Eye, Ear and Throat Hospital, New York, NY, USA
c Division of Plastic Surgery, Lenox Hill Hospital, New York, NY, USA
d Private Practice, 1009 Park Avenue, New York, NY 10028, USA
e Private Practice, 565 Park Avenue, New York, NY 10028, USA
PII:S0094-1298(08)00121-1, doi:10.1016/j.cps.2008.11.002, © 2009 Published by Elsevier Inc.

Growth factor studies

Skin

Fitzpatrick, R. E.; Rostan, E. F.: Reversal of photodamage with topical growth factors: A pilot study. J Cosmet Laser Ther. 2003 Bd. 4, S. 25–34

Gerstein, A. D.; Phillips, T.J.; Rogers, G.S.; Gilchrest, B.A.: Wound healing and aging. Dermatol Clin. 1993, (11), S. 749–757

Pilcher, B. K.; Gaither-Ganim, J.; Parks, W. C.; Welgus, H. G.: Cell type-specific inhibition of keratinocyte collagenase-1 expression by basic fibroblast growth factor and keratinocyte growth factor. A common receptor pathway. The journal of biological chemistry. 18. Juli 1997 (272) 29, S. 18147–18154

Rao, J.; Ehrlich, M.; Goldman, M.P.: Facial skin rejuvenation with a novel topical compound containing transforming growth factor beta-1 and vitamin C.Cosmet Dermatol. 2004, Bd. 17, S. 705–713

Shen, S.; Alt, A.; Wertheimer, E.; Gartsbein, M.; Kuroki, T.; Ohba, M.; Braiman, L.; Sampson, S. L.; Tennenbaum, M.: A Divergence point in the signaling of insulin and IGF-1–induced Proliferation of skin keratinocytes. Diabetes. Februar 2001 (50)

Hair

DANILENKO, D.M.; RING, B. D.; YANAGIHARA, W.;BENSON, B.; WIEMANN, C.; STARNES, O; PIERCE, G. F: Keratinocyte growth factor is an important endogenous mediator of hair follicle growth, development, and differentiation. Normalization of the nu/nu follicular differentiation defect and amelioration of chemotherapy-induced alopecia". Am J Pathol. Juli 1995, (147) 1, S. 145–154

ITAMI, S.; KURATA, S.; TAKAYASU, S.: Androgen induction of follicular epithelial cell growth is mediated via insulin-like growth factor-I from dermal papilla cells. Biochemical and biophysical research communications. 26. Juli 1995, (212) 6, S. 988–994

KIICHIRO, Y.; LAWRENCE, F.; BROWN, D. M.: Control of hair growth and follicle size by VEGF-mediated angiogenesis. The Journal of Clinical Investigation. Februar 2001 (107), 4

SU HY; HICKFORD, J.G.; BICKERSTAFFE, R.; PALMER, B.R.: Insulin-like growth factor 1 and hair growth. Dermatol Online J. November 1999, (5) 2, S. 1

DMAE studies

GROSSMAN, R.: The role of dimethylaminoethanol in cosmetic dermatology. Am J Clin Dermatol. 2005; 6 (1), S. 39–47

UHODA, I. ET AL.: Split face study on the cutaneous tensile effect of 2-dimethylaminoethanol (deanol) gel skin. Research and technology. August 2002, (8), S. 164

Silicon studies

CALOMME, M. R.; VANDEN BERGHE, D. A.: Supplementation of calves with stabilized orthosilicic acid. Effect on the Si, Ca, Mg, and P concentrations in serum and the collagen concentration in skin and cartilage. Biol Trace Elem Res 1997 (56), S. 153–65

LASSUS, A,: Colloidal silicic acid for oral and topical treatment of aged skin, fragile hair and brittle nails in females. J Int Med Res. Juli/August 1993, (21) 4, S. 209–215

MANCINELLA, A.: Silicon, a trace element essential for living organisms. Recent knowledge on its preventive role in atherosclerotic process, aging and neoplasms. Clin Ter. Juni 1991, (15); 137 (5), S. 343– 0

PAILLET C.: Application of silicium for cosmetics. Skin and silicium". Fragr J. 2000, (28) 11, S. 23–26

Q10 and ferulic acid studies

CRANE, F.: Biochemical functions of coenzyme Q10, In: Journal of the American College of Nutrition. 2001, (20), 6, S. 591–598

HOPPE, U.; BERGMANN, J.; DIEMBECK, W.; ENNEN, J.; GOHLA, S.; HARRIS I.; JACOB, J.; KIELHOLZ, J.; MEI, W.; POLLET, D.; SCHACHTSCHABEL, D.; SAUERMAAN, G.; SCHREINER, V.; STAB, F.; STECKEL, F.: Coenzyme Q10. A cutaneous antioxidant and energizer. BioFactors. 1999, (9), 2–4, S. 371–378

LIN, F. H. ET AL.: Ferulic acid stabilizes a solution of vitamins C and E and doubles its photoprotection of skin. J Invest Dermatol. Oktober 2005, 125 (4), S. 826–832

MATHEW, S.; ABRAHAM, T. E.: Ferulic acid. An antioxidant found naturally in plant cell walls and feruloyl esterases involved in its release and their applications. Crit Rev Biotechnol. 2004, (2–3), 24, S. 59–83

Phosphatidylcholine studies

HEXSEL, D.; SERRA, M.; MARUZZO, R.; DAL FORNO, T.; ZECHMEISTER, D.: Phosphatidylcholine in the treatment of localized fat. J Drugs Dermat. Oktober 2003, (5), 2, S. 511–518

MOY, L. S.: Phosphatidylcholine injections. A study measuring decreased subcutaneous fat thickness. American Society for Dermatologic Surgery and the American Society of Mohs mocrographic surgery and cutaneous oncology combined annual meeting. San Diego. 30. September – 3. Oktober 2004

RITTES, P. G.: The use of phosphatidylcholine for correction of localized fat deposits. Aesthetic Plastic Surg. Juli/August 2003, (4), 27, S. 315–318

RITTES, P. G.: The use of phosphatidylcholine for correction of localized fat deposits. Aesthetic Plastic Surg. November 2003, S. 12

ROTUNDA, A. M.; SUZUKI, H.; MOY, R.L.; KOLODNEY, M.S.: Detergent effects of sodium deoxycholate are a major feature of an injectable phosphatidylcholine formulation used for localized fat dissolution. Dermatol Surg. 2004 (30), S. 1001–1008

SERRA, M.; PEREIRA, F.: Subcutaneous infiltration with phosphatidylcholine solution for treatment of „buffalo hump" and „fatty pads". 3rd International workshop on the adverse drug reactions and lipodystrophy in HIV. Athen. October 2001

YOUNG, V.L.: Lipostabil. The effect of PPC on subcutaneous fat. Aesthet Surg J. 2003 (23), S. 413–417

Copper peptide studies

PHILIPOTT, M. P.; GREEN, M. R.; KEALEY, T.: Human growth in vitro. Journal of Cell Science. (97) 3, S. 463–471

PICKART, L.: Improving hair growth with skin remodeling copper peptides. Cosmetics & Medicine Journal. Russland 2004

SAWAYA, M.: Alopecia. Unapproved treatments or indications. Clinics in Dermatology. (18) 2, S. 177–186

SAWAYA, M.: Novel agents for the treatment of alopecia. Seminars in Cutaneous Medicine and Surgery. Clinics in Dermatology. Dezember 1998, (17) 4, S. 276–283

Index